MW00514276

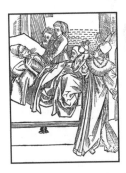

Mark A. Marinella, MD, FACP, CNSP

Department of Internal Medicine
Wright State University School of Medicine
and
Hematology and Oncology
Dayton Physicians, LLC
Dayton, OH

JONES & BARTLETT
LEARNING

World Headquarters

Jones & Bartlett Learning
40 Tall Pine Drive
Sudbury, MA 01776
978-443-5000
info@jblearning.com
www.jblearning.com

Jones & Bartlett
  Learning Canada
6339 Ormindale Way
Mississauga, Ontario L5V 1J2
Canada

Jones & Bartlett Learning
  International
Barb House, Barb Mews
London W6 7PA
United Kingdom

Jones & Bartlett Learning books and products are available through most bookstores and online booksellers. To contact Jones & Bartlett Learning directly, call 800-832-0034, fax 978-443-8000, or visit our website, www.jblearning.com.

Substantial discounts on bulk quantities of Jones & Bartlett Learning publications are available to corporations, professional associations, and other qualified organizations. For details and specific discount information, contact the special sales department at Jones & Bartlett Learning via the above contact information or send an email to specialsales@jblearning.com.

Production Credits

Sr. Acquisition Editor: Nancy Anastasi Duffy
Editorial Assistant: Sara Cameron
Production Editor: Dan Stone
Medicine Marketing Manager: Rebecca Rockel
V.P., Manufacturing and Inventory Control: Therese Connell
Composition: Newgen Imaging Systems Pvt. Ltd.
Cover Design: Kate Ternullo
Cover Image: Courtesy of National Library of Medicine
Printing and Binding: Cenveo
Cover Printing: Cenveo

ISBN 13: 978-0-7637-9315-9

6048

Printed in the United States of America
14 13 12 11 10   10 9 8 7 6 5 4 3 2 1

Tarascon Pocket Oncologica

Table of Contents

Tarascon Pocket Oncologica

Table of Contents

BACKGROUND

- Glioblastoma multiforme (GBM) is the most common malignant brain tumor of adults and one of the most aggressive cancers in oncology, with median survival of less than 1 year in most series.
- Mean age at diagnosis is 55 years; more common in males and whites.
- Risk factors include familial syndromes (e.g., familial polyposis/Turcot syndrome, Li-Fraumeni syndrome, neurofibromatosis; <5% of cases) and radiation; questionable evidence that cell phone use may increase risk.

PATHOBIOLOGY

- Most adult GBMs arise *de novo*, resulting from sequential accumulation of gene aberrations and dysregulation of cell growth/proliferation pathways—usually in older patients with rapid presentation.
  - Epidermal growth factor receptor (EGFR) amplification in 60%, loss of heterozygosity (LOH) of chromosome 10q in 70%, deletion/mutation of phosphatase and tensin homologue on chromosome 10 (PTEN) in 40%.
- Secondary GBM arises from low-grade astrocytoma, typically in younger patients; transformation may take years.
  - p53 mutation characteristic in over 60%; retinoblastoma (Rb) gene mutation in 25%; LOH 10 q in 70%; PTEN less common than in *de novo* GBM.
- GBM contains malignant neural and stromal tissues; neural, stromal, and inflammatory cells produce vascular endothelial growth factor (VEGF), which induces angiogenesis—the hallmark of GBM; high VEGF content confers aggression and poor prognosis.
- Histology of GBM: nuclear and cellular pleomorphism, high cellularity, numerous mitoses, necrosis, and endothelial proliferation; neoplastic cells invade adjacent tissue and spread via white-matter pathways—infiltrative nature renders R0 resection impossible.
- Overexpression of the enzyme O^6-methylguanine DNA methyltransferase (MGMT) confers resistance to alkylator chemotherapy.

CLINICAL PRESENTATION

- Symptoms of GBM are often acute and related to mass effect, parenchymal infiltration, tumoral hemorrhage, tissue destruction, and /or hydrocephalus.
- New-onset headache is most common (35% to 50% of patients) symptom; often occurs in morning or worse with Valsalva or bending over.
- Seizures, focal weakness, aphasia, personality changes, nausea, and vomiting are not uncommon; intracranial bleed in 3% may cause headache, vomiting, or syncope.
- Lethargy and coma may occur with hydrocephalus.

PHYSICAL FINDINGS

- Examination may be normal if GBM involves frontal lobe; subtle mental status changes may be detected.
- Focal signs include cranial nerve palsy, aphasia, papilledema, focal limb weakness.

DIAGNOSTIC TESTS AND STAGING

- Cerebral magnetic resonance imaging (MRI) is the diagnostic test of choice; gadolinium reveals characteristic ring enhancement; edema and necrosis common; multifocal lesions may occur.
  - Postoperative MRI at 24–72 hours to determine resection extent.
- Cerebral contrast-enhanced computed tomography (CT) is an alternative if contraindication for MRI.
  - Typically reveals contrast-enhancement and vasogenic edema.

TREATMENT

- Surgery: maximal resection should be attempted unless the tumor is in an eloquent area; complete (R0) resection is not possible due to infiltrative nature of GBM.
  - Craniotomy with resection improves survival compared to biopsy alone.
- Chemoradiation: postoperative radiation improves survival and quality of life; addition of the oral alkylator, temozolamide, improves overall survival (OS) and progression-free survival (PFS).
  - 60 Gy of radiation in fractions of 1.8–2.0 Gy daily 5 days weekly.
  - Daily oral temozolomide (75 mg/m^2) during radiation improved survival by 2.5 months (14.6 vs. 12.1 months, $p<.001$) and 2-year survival (26.5% vs. 10.4%) compared to radiation alone in EORTC trial.

- Chemotherapy.
  - Following chemoradiation, oral temozolomide 150–200 mg/m^2 daily for 5 days every 28 days for 6 months is current standard of care for resected GBM and results in increased survival (see chemoradiation).
  - Biodegradable carmustine wafers placed into resection bed increased survival by 2.3 months in one study (11.6 vs. 13.9 months, p=.03).
  - GBM typically progresses within several months; recent data suggests benefit from VEGF inhibitor, bevacizumab, with or without irinotecan.
  - Other single-agent agents with minimal benefit at relapse include carboplatin, procarbazine, etoposide, and nitrosoureas; numerous targeted agents in clinical trials.
- Ancillary drugs.
  - Dexamethasone: decrease tumoral edema/intracranial pressure; slow taper usually necessary.
  - Antiepileptic drugs (e.g., phenytoin, carbamazepine, levtiracetam): indicated if seizures occur; no data to support prophylactic use; levtiracetam may be agent of choice due to lack of drug interactions.
  - Trimethoprim-sulfamethoxazole: 1 double-strength (DS) tab orally twice daily three times per week during chemoradiation for prophylaxis against *Pneumocystis jirovecii* pneumonia.
  - Low-molecular-weight heparins: thromboembolism prophylaxis; safe if no cerebral hemorrhage evident.

Table 1–1 Regimens for GBM

First-line chemoradiation
Temozolomide 75 mg/m^2 by mouth daily during radiation with 60 Gy (two Gy fractions 5 days per week for 6 weeks)
Temozolomide 150–200 mg/m^2 by mouth days 1–5 every 28 days for 6 months following chemoradiation
Salvage treatment
Bevacizumab 10 mg/kg IV every 2 weeks
Bevacizumab 10 mg/kg IV and irinotecan 340 mg/m^2 IV (if on antiepileptic drugs) or 125 mg/m^2 IV (if not on antiepileptic drugs) every 2 weeks for 6-week cycles

COMPLICATIONS OF TREATMENT

- Chemoradiation: fatigue, headache, cerebral edema, nausea/vomiting, *P. jirovecii* pneumonia, cytopenia.
- Radiation: radiation necrosis (may mimic recurrent tumor), leukoencephalopathy (dementia, ataxia, urine incontinence; months to years later), second tumors (sarcoma, skin cancers).
- Chemotherapy: nausea, vomiting, cytopenia, fatigue, photosensitivity, hepatitis, infection.

- Bevacizumab: headache, bleeding, venous/arterial thrombosis, proteinuria, hypertension, perforated viscus.
- Corticosteroids: infection, hyperglycemia, myopathy, delirium, skin breakdown, ecchymoses, thrush, cataracts, osteopenia, avascular necrosis.

FOLLOW-UP CARE

- Because postsurgical treatment is not truly adjuvant due to infiltrative nature and inability to achieve R0 resection, history and neurologic examination should be performed every 4 to 6 weeks; MRI should be performed if clinical evidence of progression occurs or every few months.
  - Initial postradiation MRI may reveal phenomena of "pseudoprogression" due to radiation-induced vascular permeability changes; important to repeat MRI several weeks later, because misdiagnosis of pseudoprogression as tumor progression may lead to premature administration of second-line therapy.

PROGNOSIS

- Advanced age (>70 years) and poor performance status associated with very poor prognosis (<6 month survival).
- Improved survival associated with age <40 years, Eastern Oncology Cooperative Group (ECOG) 0–1, frontal tumor, and gross total resection.
- Prognosis directly correlated with extent of resection:
  - Mean survival times: gross total resection, 11.3 months; partial resection, 10.4 months; and biopsy, 6.6 months.
- Temozolomide with radiation therapy median OS of 14.6 months; patients with methylated MGMT gene have superior survival compared to unmethylated tumors.

REFERENCES

N Engl J Med 2005;352:987.
N Engl J Med 2008;359:492.
J Natl Cancer Inst 1993;85:704.
J Neurooncol 2009;93:1.
J Clin Oncol 2007;25:4722.
Clin Cancer Res 2007;13:1253.
Semin Radiat Oncol 2009;19:150.

2 ■ PRIMARY CENTRAL NERVOUS SYSTEM LYMPHOMA

- Primary central nervous system lymphoma (PCNSL) is an uncommon subtype of non-Hodgkin's lymphoma (NHL) that, by definition, is confined to the CNS; although the cerebral parenchyma is the most commonly affected site, the vitreous body of the eyes, the meninges, or spinal cord may be involved.
  - PCNSL must be distinguished from nodal/extranodal NHL that secondarily involves the CNS.
- PCNSL accounts for approximately 2% of all brain tumors but has significantly increased in incidence over the last two decades in both immunocompetent and immunocompromised patients (mainly those infected with the human immunodeficiency virus [HIV]); this discussion is limited to immunocompetent patients.
- The mean age at diagnosis in immunocompetent patients with PCNSL is 55 years, with a slight male predilection.
- Risk factors include HIV infection (confers over 3000-fold higher risk than general population), organ transplantation, primary immunodeficiency syndromes, and autoimmune diseases.

PATHOBIOLOGY

- Approximately 90% of cases of PCNSL are of the diffuse large B-cell lymphoma (DLBCL) subtype, to which this discussion will be limited.
  - Malignant cells are approximately three times larger than normal lymphocytes and immunohistochemically express CD45, CD20, and, often, BCL6.
  - Deletion of the tumor suppressor gene p16 is present in approximately one-half of patients.
- The malignant cell may originate from lymphocytes normally trafficking through the CNS or from malignant cells originating in an extraneural site that possess tropism for the CNS; the latter theory is favored, because many immunocompetent cases of PCNSL express the BCL6 protein, which arises from the germinal center, a structure not present in the brain/CNS.

- Malignant lymphocytes of PCNSL are thought to arise from centroblasts derived from the germinal center or immunoblasts that arise from outside germinal center.
  - PCNSL that stains positive for the BCL6 protein, a marker for cells that have been exposed to the germinal center, have a superior survival to BCL6-negative tumors.
- PCNSL is a diffusely infiltrative neoplasm, which makes surgical extirpation impossible in most patients; malignant cells characteristically spread along perivascular Virchow-Robin spaces to reach beyond the primary tumor mass; involvement of the eyes, leptomeninges, and spinal cord may occur.

CLINICAL PRESENTATION

- Subacute cognitive dysfunction (confusion, memory loss, personality change) and headache are the most common symptoms of PCNSL.
- Neurologic deficits such as paresis, dysarthria, dysphagia, or paresthesia may occur, but seizures are uncommon because the cortex is typically uninvolved.
- Ocular involvement typically presents with "floaters" or visual loss.
- Gait problems and ataxia are common in late PCNSL.

PHYSICAL FINDINGS

- Patients with cognitive dysfunction may fare poorly on a mini-mental status examination (MMSE); they may manifest delirium, somnolence, or become psychotic.
- Cranial nerve paresis, limb hemiparesis, or decreased sensation may be noted.
- Slit-lamp examination may reveal a cell-fluid level in the anterior chamber or vitreal changes.

DIAGNOSTIC TESTS AND STAGING

- Brain CT typically reveals isodense to hyperdense lesions in a periventricular distribution that ring-enhance with intravenous contrast; involvement of the corpus collosum and contralateral brain may occur; edema is typically less than that of a similar-sized glial tumor.
- MRI is the imaging study of choice for suspected PCNSL and exhibits the following characteristics:
  - Isointense-to-hypointense lesions on T2-weighted imaging that enhance with gadolinium; have a predilection for the corpus collosum; and manifest edema, often with ring-enhancement.
  - PCNSL most often involves the cerebral hemispheres, frequently in deeper structures or in a periventricular location.

- Enhancement of the Virchow-Robin spaces, which appear as wispy, linear-enhancing structures that radiate from the lesion margin, is highly specific for PCNSL (neurosarcoid is the only other disease in which this MRI finding occurs).
- Stereotactic needle biopsy is the diagnostic procedure of choice for most patients and is relatively safe when performed by an experienced neurosurgeon.
- Slit-lamp examination of the eyes is recommended because vitreous involvement may occur in 15% to 20% of patients and, when present, is bilateral in approximately 80% of patients; anterior-chamber paracentesis with cytologic analysis or vitreal aspiration with cytopathology may be considered for diagnosis, especially if no brain lesions are evident or brain biopsy is contraindicated.
- Lumbar puncture with cerebrospinal fluid (CSF) cytology and flow cytometry is suggested, unless severe mass effect is present, because 15% to 50% of patients will exhibit malignant cells at some point of their disease.
  - Patients with positive cytology, lymphocytosis, or elevated protein should undergo MRI to exclude spinal cord involvement.
- CT scans of the chest, abdomen, and pelvis as well as scrotal ultrasound and bone marrow biopsy are required to exclude extraneural sites of involvement.
  - Some physicians do not routinely perform marrow biopsy unless spinal cord involvement is present.
- Blood tests should include a complete blood count (CBC), lactate dehydrogenase (LDH), serum chemistries, and serologic testing for hepatitis B/C viruses and HIV.
- PCNSL, by definition, is stage IE (one localized involved area, extranodal disease) but has a much worse prognosis than non-CNS NHL of identical stage.

TREATMENT

- Surgical resection, unlike in glial tumors, plays no therapeutic role in the management of PCNSL due to the diffuse nature of the neoplasm, which renders complete (R0) resection impossible; patients with life-threatening edema/mass effect may benefit from urgent decompression.
  - Median survival is 3 months for patients treated with resection alone.
- Corticosteroids may cause rapid tumoral lympholysis and vascular stabilization with edema resolution, which may significantly alter appearance on MRI; furthermore, malignant cytolysis from steroids may render histologic diagnosis impossible; steroids should not be administered prior to biopsy if PCNSL is suspected, unless life-threatening cerebral edema is present.

- Radiation therapy is more efficacious than surgical resection as mono-therapy but is not curative, with a median survival of approximately 12 months and 5-year survival <5%.
  - Due to the diffuse nature of PCNSL, radiation must encompass the whole brain (WBRT) and is typically administered in 1.8–2.0 Gy fractions without boost, but there does not appear to be a dose response over 40 Gy; radiation is associated with late-term neurotoxicity, especially in patients >60 years of age, and is often fatal.
  - Patients with intraocular involvement without brain disease are treated with orbital radiation; chemotherapy should be considered because over 90% of patients will relapse or develop PCNSL; patients with PCNSL and simultaneous intraocular disease can receive high-dose methotrexate (MTX, 8 g/m^2 IV for four cycles) as long as vision and examination improve; consolidation orbital radiation is suggested for patients with persistent disease following MTX.
- High-dose MTX is currently the therapy of choice for PCNSL; MTX may be combined sequentially with WBRT in patients <60 years of age but should NOT be administered concurrently or sequentially to patients >60 years due to the very high risk of late neurotoxicity.
  - Most agents utilized in the management of NHL (e.g., cyclophosphamide, doxorubicin, vincristine) are not effective for PCNSL due to poor penetration of the blood–brain barrier (BBB).
  - The BBB excludes the cerebral capillary from the systemic capillary circulation, preventing exogenous xenobiotics from reaching the CNS.
  - The vessels of the BBB are characterized by the presence of tight junctions, thick basal membranes, absence of capillary fenestrations, and expression of the P-glycoprotein system, which serves as an efflux mechanism for most chemotherapy drugs.
  - The blood–tumor barrier (BTB) capillaries, in contrast to the BBB vessels, display fenestrations, disrupted tight junctions, and an abundance of pinocytotic vessels—all of which allow for drug penetration into tumor tissue.
- MTX, an antimetabolite folate antagonist, penetrates the BBB when intravenously administered in high doses (>1 g/m^2 every 14 days; most practicing oncologists utilize 3.5 g/m^2, whereas some use 8 g/m^2) and has been shown in several trials to increase PFS when used as mono-therapy or combined with WBRT compared to WBRT alone.
  - High-dose MTX followed by WBRT is the current regimen of choice for most patients <50–60 years of age with PCNSL; the median survival is 30–51 months with a 5-year survival of 20% to 35%; patients >60 years should not receive chemotherapy and radiation due neurotoxicity risk.
    - MTX should be administered prior to radiation due to decreased neurotoxicity and improved drug delivery, because XRT may lead to repair of the BBB, thereby impeding MTX penetration.

- Single-agent MTX is associated with radiographic response in 52% to 100% of patients and may result in long-term survival, with a median survival of 55 months reported in some studies; unfortunately, the majority of patients relapse at variable time intervals following first-line MTX; patients with intraocular lymphoma may achieve response from high-dose MTX alone.
- Supportive care includes intravenous hydration with 2.5–3.5 liters/m^2/day; urinary alkalinization with one to two ampules of sodium bicarbonate per liter of fluid to attain urine pH >7; and rescue with intravenous leucovorin calcium 10 mg IV every 6 hours starting 24 hours after MTX until the serum MTX level is <0.10 μmol/L.

Table 2–1 Regimens for PCNSL

First-line regimen[*][†]
High-dose MTX[‡]: MTX 3.5 g/m^2 IV day 1 every 21 days for four cycles followed approximately 4 weeks later by WBRT with 36 Gy to those with CR after MTX; an additional 9 Gy administered to bed in those with partial response following MTX; patients >60 years generally should not receive WBRT due to neurotoxic effects
High-dose MTX and cytarbine[‡]: MTX 3.5 g/m^2 IV day 1 and cytarabine 2 g/m^2 IV days 2,3 every 21 days for four cycles followed approximately 4 weeks later by WBRT with 36 Gy to those with CR after MTX; an additional 9 Gy administered to bed in those with partial response following MTX; patients >60 years generally should not receive WBRT due to neurotoxic effects
High-dose MTX (Batchelor et al., J Clin Oncol 2003;21:1044): MTX 8 g/m^2 IV day 1 every 2 weeks for up to eight cycles; may be repeated monthly

Relapse regimen
High-dose MTX may be repeated if prolonged relapse-free period after initial treatment
Temozolamide 150–200 mg/m^2 by mouth days 1–5 every 28 days
Temozolamide 150 mg/m^2 by mouth days 1–5 and rituximab 375 mg/m^2 IV day 1 every 28 days for four cycles followed by temozolamide 150 mg/m^2 by mouth days 1–5 every 28 days for up to eight cycles (premedication with acetaminophen 650–1000 mg by mouth and diphenhydramine 50 mg by mouth/IV prior to rituximab)
Topotecan 1.5 mg/m^2 IV days 1–5 every 21 days

[*]High-dose MTX supportive care: alkalinization of urine with bicarbonate-containing fluids, leucovorin calcium rescue (10-mg IV every 6 hours beginning 24 hours after IV MTX until serum MTX level <0.10 μmol/L), and filgrastim or pegfilgrastim

[†]Various regimens of MTX ranging from 1–8 g/m^2 IV have been published; optimal schedule not defined, but 3.5 g/m^2 used by many oncologists; patients should have adequate performance status, renal, hepatic, and hematologic function.

[‡]Lancet 2009;374:1512

- A recent large multicenter randomized phase II trial (*Lancet* 2009;374:1512) utilized four cycles of high-dose MTX (3.5 g/m^2 IV day 1) and high-dose cytarabine (2 g/m^2 IV twice daily on days 2 and 3) every 3 weeks followed by WBRT for patients <75 years (36 Gy for those in complete remission following chemotherapy and at the physician's discretion in those >60 years) versus MTX (at same dose) alone every 3 weeks for four cycles; the complete response (CR) rate following chemotherapy was 46% vs. 18%, with an overall response rate of 69% vs. 40%, for MTX/cytarabine and MTX, respectively; the 3-year survival was 46% vs. 32% (*p*=0.07, HR 0.65); administration of pegfilgrastim and prophylactic antibiotics are recommended due to infection risk; although there were three deaths in the cytarabine arm (compared to one in the MTX arm), this regimen may be a reasonable option in younger patients with preserved organ function; whether it will become a new treatment standard remains to be seen.
- Relapsed PCNSL has no standard treatment, but high-dose MTX may be readministered if there has been a long disease-free interval (>1 year), with up to two-thirds of patients achieving complete remission, some of whom may experience long-term survival; patients who have been treated initially with MTX alone may be treated with WBRT with a median survival of 7 months; small, uncontrolled series have reported some response from topotecan, carboplatin/etoposide/cyclophosphamide, procarbazine/CCNU/vincristine, temozolamide, and temozolamide/rituximab.
  - Oral temozolamide with or without rituximab may be an option in heavily pretreated or elderly patients with relapsed PCNSL; a few patients have experienced significant responses with tolerable toxicity.

COMPLICATIONS OF TREATMENT

- High-dose MTX has the following complications: nausea, vomiting, oral mucositis, diarrhea, seizures, aphasia, headaches/nuchal rigidity/fever-syndrome due to arachnoidits, pneumonitis, rash, myelosuppression, acute renal failure (intratubular MTX precipitation; prevented with urinary alkalinization), urate nephropathy, hepatitis.
- Delayed neurotoxicity from combined MTX and WBRT is universal in patients >60 years and may occur in approximately 20% to 30% of younger patients by 96 months; results from pathologic small vessel sclerosis, white matter gliosis, and widespread loss of myelin and axons; radiation generates free radicals that may damage endothelial cells and oligodendroglia production of myelin; the incidence of neurotoxicity increases markedly if MTX is administered following WBRT.
  - Most cases occur a year or more following treatment (with an increased incidence over time) and present with a characteristic constellation of symptoms, including cognitive impairment/memory

loss, ataxia, and urinary incontinence; somnulence, abnormal MMSE, and a wide-based shuffling gait with postural instability; dementia eventually ensues.

- Autonomic neuropathy may manifest as dysphagia, pseudobulbar palsy, and urinary/fecal incontinence.
- MRI of the brain typically reveals hydrocephalus due to cortical/subcortical atrophy and diffuse white matter changes.

- Cytarabine has the following complications: nausea, vomiting, diarrhea, oral mucositis, cerebellar toxicity (ataxia, dysmetria), delirium, seizures, pneumonitis, noncardiogenic pulmonary edema, rash/hidradenitis, conjunctivitis (prevented with corticosteroid eye drops), and sepsis.

FOLLOW-UP CARE

- No standard follow-up regimen is defined for patients with PCNSL, but patients with complete response should be followed at frequent intervals (every 3 months) with careful history, neurologic, and ocular examination; relapse may occur as long as 5 years following initial therapy, although most occur within 2 years.
- Cerebral imaging with MRI should be performed in patients with any neurologic symptoms or signs; routine imaging can also be considered to detect early relapse.
- Neurotoxicity may develop years later, especially in elderly patients treated with MTX and WBRT; patients who develop memory loss, ataxia, and/or urinary incontinence should undergo MRI evaluation.

PROGNOSIS

- Generally, age and performance status are among the most consistent prognostic factors for patients with PCNSL.
- A useful prognostic scoring system devised by the International Extranodal Lymphoma Study Group (IELSG) includes five factors determined by multivariate analysis to be predictive of a poor prognosis:
  - Age >60 years, ECOG performance status >1, elevated lactate dehydrogenase (LDH), elevated CSF protein level, and tumor involving deep brain region(s).
  - Two-year survival based on number of adverse features: 0–1, 80%; 2–3, 48%; or 4–5, 15%.
- Patients with BCL6-positive (germinal center B-cell-like) tumors had a 100-month OS of approximately 70% compared to <20% for BCL6-negative (activated B-cell-like) tumors.
- Lymphoma-free patients who develop delayed neurotoxicity following combined modality treatment have a median survival of 1.8 years following symptom onset.

REFERENCES

Ann Oncol 2006;17:1141.
Arch Neurol 2005;62:1595.
Cancer 2004;101:139.
Clin Cancer Res 2003;9:1063.
Clin Cancer Res 2004;10:5643.
Int J Radiat Oncol Biol Phys 2001;51:419.
J Clin Oncol 1998;16:864.
J Clin Oncol 2003;21:266.
Lancet 2009;374:1512.
Lancet Oncol 2001;2:354.
N Engl J Med 2005;352:185.
Neurology 2004;62:532.
Neurology 2006;66:1435.

3 ■ TESTICULAR CANCER

- Germ cell tumor (GCT) of the testis is the most common solid tumor among men aged 15 to 35 years.
- There are approximately 8100 cases annually in the United States, with 370 deaths.
  - Seminoma and nonseminomatous GCT (NSGCT) each account for approximately 50% of cases.
- Worldwide incidence of GCT is increasing for unknown reasons.
- Most curable of all solid tumors, with an overall cure rate of 80%.
  - The introduction of cisplatin revolutionized treatment of testicular GCT.
- Risk factors: white race, cryptorchid testis, family history of GCT, infection with human immunodeficiency virus (HIV).
  - Increased risk of mediastinal GCT in men with Klinefelter syndrome.

PATHOBIOLOGY

- GCT are cancers of primordial germ cells—cells destined to become spermatozoa.
- GCT hallmark is extra chromosome 12 material, most commonly isochromosome 12p (i12p).
  - Various genes residing on chromosome 12 lead to malignant transformation and cell proliferation.
  - Hyperploidy is common in GCT.
- Primary area of testicular lymphatic drainage ("landing zone") is the retroperitoneal lymph nodes; supraclavicular nodes can be involved in some cases.
- Seminoma.
  - 50% of testicular cancers; retain totipotentiality; exquisite sensitivity to radiation.
  - 20% produce β-human chorionic gonadotropin (β-HCG), but NOT oncofetal protein α-alpha fetoprotein (AFP).
  - Spermatocytic variant occurs in elderly men and is indolent.
- NSGCT.
  - 50% of testicular cancers; less sensitive to radiation.
  - Embryonal carcinoma: most aggressive and undifferentiated subtype.
  - Yolk sac tumor (endodermal sinus tumor).
  - Choriocarcinoma (uncommon).

- Teratoma: composed of somatic germ cell layers (e.g., ectoderm, mesoderm, endoderm).
  - Lack metastatic capability, but can evolve into somatic malignancies (e.g., carcinoma, sarcoma).
- Most are composed of more than one cell type.
- Tumor cells may produce AFP and/or β-HCG.

CLINICAL PRESENTATION

- Most testicular cancers present as a painless, firm, unilateral testicular lump, which is pathognomonic for GCT of testis.
- Other symptoms include diffuse testicular pain, swelling, and firmness.
  - May be mistaken for epididymoorchitis.
- Metastasis to retroperitoneal nodes may result in back pain.
- Pulmonary metastasis may cause dyspnea, cough, or hemoptysis, but this is rare at presentation.
- Tumor production of large amounts of β-HCG may result in bilateral gynecomastia.

PHYSICAL FINDINGS

- Isolated testicular mass most common; rare patients may have palpable synchronous contralateral tumor.
- Signs of metastatic disease include palpable supraclavicular nodes, pulmonary rales/dullness, abdominal mass, or neurologic signs if brain metastases are present.

DIAGNOSTIC TESTS AND STAGING

- A solid testicular mass in any male should prompt an ultrasound of the testes.
  - Scrotal ultrasound typically reveals a discrete solid mass lesion.
- Transscrotal biopsy is CONTRAINDICATED due to risk of seeding of scrotal tissue.
- Radical inguinal orchiectomy with ligation of the spermatic cord at the internal inguinal ring is diagnostic and therapeutic.
- Staging evaluation.
  - Chest radiograph, CT of the abdomen and pelvis, and tumor markers (AFP, β-HCG, and LDH).
    - Tumor-marker elevation more prevalent with advanced disease.
    - Levels should decrease to normal after orchiectomy based on serum half-lives: β-HCG, 5 to 7 days, and AFP, 30 hours.
    - Serum level of tumor markers is part of TNM staging system and form a part of the International Germ Cell Cancer Collaborative Group (IGCCCG) risk stratification based on degree of elevation.

Table 3–1 TNM Staging Criteria

Primary tumor (T)
Tis: *in situ* neoplasia; **T1:** limited to testis/epididymis without vascular/lymphatic invasion; may invade tunica albuginea but not vaginalis; **T2:** limited to testis/epididymis with vascular/lymphatic invasion or involvement of tunica vaginalis; **T3:** invades spermatic cord with or without vascular/lymphatic invasion; **T4:** invades scrotum with or without vascular/lymphatic invasion

Regional lymph nodes (N)
N0: no lymph node metastases; **N1:** lymph node <2 cm or ≤5 nodes all <2 cm; **N2:** lymph node >2 cm but <5 cm or >5 nodes all <5 cm; extranodal extension; **N3:** any node(s) >5 cm

Distant metastases (M)
M0: no distant metastases; **M1A:** nonregional nodes or lung metastases. **M1B:** nonlung visceral metastases (e.g., liver, brain)

Serum tumor markers (S)
S0: LDH, HCG, and AFP levels normal; **S1 (good risk):** LDH <1.5× normal; HCG <5000; AFP <1000; **S2 (intermediate risk):** LDH 1.5–10× normal; HCG 5000–50,000; AFP 1000–10,000; **S3 (poor risk):** LDH >10x normal; HCG >50,000; AFP >10,000

Stage groupings
Stage I: limited to testis, epididymis, spermatic cord **Stage II:** limited to retroperitoneal nodes (IIA: nodes <2 cm; IIB: nodes 2–5 cm; IIC: nodes >5 cm **Stage III:** metastasis above diaphragm and all visceral sites

IGCCCG risk Stratification
NSGCT **Good risk:** Testis/retroperitoneal primary and good markers and no nonlung visceral metastases **Intermediate risk:** Testis/retroperitoneal primary and intermediate markers and no nonlung visceral metastases **Poor risk:** Mediastinal primary or testis/retroperitoneal primary with either nonlung visceral metastases or poor markers **Seminoma*** **Good risk:** Any primary and any markers and no nonlung visceral metastases. **Intermediate risk:** Any primary and any markers and presence of nonlung visceral metastases.

*There is no high-risk seminoma group.

TREATMENT

- Radical inguinal orchiectomy with ligation of the spermatic cord at the internal inguinal ring is the standard of care.
- Adjuvant treatment of testicular cancer is stage and histology dependent.

- Embryonal-predominant NSGCT and any testis cancer with lymphovascular invasion, rete testis invasion, or a tumor >4 cm are especially high-risk for relapse and may not be optimal for surveillance.
- NSGCT adjuvant therapy.
  - Stage I [40% to 50% have clinical stage I at diagnosis; may be upstaged at retroperitoneal lymph node dissection (RPLND)].
    - Patients may be risk-stratified based on poor tumor histologic features of lymphovascular invasion, absence of yolk sac component, and/or presence of embryonal component; 50% of stage I patients with lymphovascular invasion have positive nodes at RPLND and will relapse during surveillance.
    - Surveillance: requires follow-up every 1 to 2 months with tumor markers and chest radiographs and abdominal CT every 3 to 6 months during the first 2 years, because 92% of relapses occur during this time; positron emission tomography (PET) scanning not sensitive to detect relapse and is not recommended.
      - Relapse following surveillance treated with three cycles of bleomyycin/etoposide/cisplatin (BEP) or four cycles of etoposide/cisplatin (EP).
    - RPLND: most accurate method to differentiate between pathologic stage I and II disease (may upstage up to 50% of patients).
      - Cure rates of 50% to 90% with surgery alone in patients with low-volume stage II disease.
      - Post-RPLND BEP or EP for two cycles recommended if more than six positive nodes, nodes >2 cm, or extranodal spread.
      - pN3 disease should receive four cycles of EP or three cycles of BEP.
      - Post-RPLND relapse almost never occurs in retroperitoneum.
    - Chemotherapy: should be considered with high-risk histologic features noted above and typically consists of one or two cycles of BEP with some studies showing 4-year relapse rates of 1% with one cycle.
      - Stage 1S disease with persistent marker elevation but normal imaging should receive four cycles of EP or three cycles of BEP.
      - Carboplatin is inferior to cisplatin and should not be substituted.
  - Stage IIA.
    - Normal markers: EP for four cycles, BEP for three cycles, or RPLND.
    - Elevated markers: EP for four cycles or BEP for three cycles.
  - Stage IIB/III.
    - EP for four cycles or BEP for three cycles.
    - Brain metastasis: chemotherapy and radiation, with or without surgery:

- Patients with intermediate or poor-risk NSGCT should receive BEP for four cycles as standard of care (based on IGCCC).
- Management of residual CT masses after chemotherapy.
  - RPLND and excision of all residual masses: 45% contain necrosis/fibrosis; 40% contain teratoma (unresponsive to chemotherapy); 15% contain viable GCT.
  - If viable GCT found in specimen, two cycles of post-RPLND chemotherapy with EP, vinblastine/ifosfamide/cisplatin (VeIP), or paclitaxel/ifosfamide/cisplatin (TIP).
- Relapsed/refractory disease.
  - 20% to 30% of patients do not achieve CR after first-line treatment and should receive some type of salvage treatment.
    - Four cycles of VeIP, up to 25% CR rate; four cycles of TIP up, to 70% CR rate.
    - High-dose therapy with autologous stem cell rescue should be considered for patients failing to achieve CR with initial salvage chemotherapy or poor risk disease with lack of CR with initial chemotherapy.
      - Carboplatin and etoposide (high dose).
      - Can result in CR in 15% to 20% of patients.

Table 3–2 Regimens for GCT of Testis

First-line regimen
BEP: bleomycin 30 U IV days 1,8, 15; etoposide 100 mg/m² IV days 1–5; cisplatin 20 mg/m² IV days 1–5 every 21 days.
EP: etoposide 100 mg/m² IV days 1–5; cisplatin 20 mg/m² IV days 1–5 every 21 days.

Second-line/salvage regimen
VeIP: vinblastine 0.11 mg/kg IV days 1–2; ifosfamide 1200 mg/m² IV days 1–5; cisplatin 20 mg/m² IV days 1–5; MESNA 400 mg/m² IV days 1–5 every 21 days.
TIP: paclitaxel 250 mg/m² IV day 1; ifosfamide 1500 mg/m² IV days 2–5; cisplatin 25 mg/m² IV days 1–5; MESNA 500 mg/m² IV before and 4 and 8 hours after ifosfamide (can use oral route for 4- and 8-hour doses) every 21 days.
VIP: etoposide 75 mg/m² IV days 1–5; ifosfamide 1200 mg/m² IV days 1–5; cisplatin 20 mg/m² IV days 1–5; MESNA 120 mg/m² IV slow push day 1 then 1200 mg/m² /day by continuous infusion days 1–5 every 21 days.
High-dose: carboplatin 700 mg/m² IV and etoposide 750 mg/m² IV administered 5, 4, and 3 days before stem cell infusion for two cycles.

Palliative
GemOx: gemcitabine 1000–1250 mg/m² days 1 and 8; oxaliplatin 130 mg/m² day 1 every 21 days.

- Patients without CR to high-dose therapy are incurable and can be considered for palliative chemotherapy with gemcitabine and oxaliplatin (GemOx).
- Consideration of surgical resection of a solitary site of relapse (e.g., brain, lung, retroperitoneum) should always be considered.

- **Seminoma adjuvant therapy.**
  - Stage IA and IB (70% of patients):
    - Infradiaphragmatic radiation (20–30 Gy), including paraaortic nodes with or without ipsilateral inguinal nodes.
    - Single dose of carboplatin (AUC 7, by Calvert formula): no difference in 5-year relapse-free rates compared to radiation (95% vs. 96%) and lower incidence of new testicular cancers.
    - Surveillance: requires meticulous follow-up with regular tumor markers, chest radiographs, and abdominal CT scans and dedicated, compliant patient, because 15% to 20% of stage I patients relapse in <2 years if they do not undergo adjuvant radiation or chemotherapy.
  - Stage IS:
    - Infradiaphragmatic radiation as for IA/IB.
  - Stage IIA and IIB:
    - 35–40 Gy radiation, including paraaortic and ipsilateral inguinal nodes.
    - If contraindication for radiation (e.g., prior radiation, horseshoe kidney, bowel disease) then four cycles of EP.
  - Stage IIC and III:
    - All IIC and III is good risk except for nonlung visceral metastases, which indicates intermediate risk.
    - Four cycles of EP or three cycles of BEP for good risk and four cycles of BEP for intermediate risk.
    - After chemotherapy, CT scan of abdomen and tumor markers obtained.
      - No mass, normal markers: no further treatment; surveillance.
      - Residual mass, normal markers: PET scan at 6–8 weeks to assess for viable tumor or necrotic mass; PET-negative, no treatment but observe for recurrence; PET-positive, biopsy followed by excision or salvage chemotherapy or radiotherapy.
  - Relapse:
    - Recurrence treated with chemotherapy according to stage at recurrence and recommended with increasing tumor markers or new mass on surveillance CT (regimens similar to NSGCT, see above).
    - 90% of patients with advanced/relapsed seminoma cured with cisplatin-based chemotherapy.

COMPLICATIONS OF TREATMENT

- Orchiectomy: Bleeding and infection.
- RPLND: Bleeding, wound infection, lymphocele, retrograde ejaculation (uncommon in experienced centers with nerve-sparing surgery), chylous ascites, bowel obstruction, deep vein thrombosis/pulmonary embolism.
  - Overall, RPLND morbidity of 10% to 23% and mortality of 0.3%.
- Radiation: pulmonary fibrosis/pneumonitis, cardiovascular disease, solid visceral tumors (e.g., stomach, pleura, pancreas, bladder).
- Chemotherapy: Divided into immediate and long-term complications.
  - Immediate: All agents: myelosuppression, febrile neutropenia, sepsis, bleeding, anemia; cisplatin: nephrotoxicity, ototoxicity, electrolyte loss, neuropathy, venous thrombosis, stroke, arterial ischemia; bleomycin: Raynaud phenomenon, pneumonitis/pulmonary fibrosis; etoposide: hypersensitivity.
  - Long-term: cardiovascular disease, mesenteric ischemia, infection, pulmonary fibrosis, metabolic syndrome, hypertension, obesity, Raynaud phenomenon, second malignancies (e.g., solid tumors, leukemia/myelodysplasia from etoposide), infertility, anxiety/depression.

FOLLOW-UP CARE

- Because metachronous testicular cancers can occur in up to 2% of patients, regular testicular examination is recommended.
- Physical examination and history, measurement of tumor markers, and chest radiography should be performed every 1 to 2 months and abdominal CT every 3 months during the first 2 years of follow-up because the majority of recurrences occur during this time.
- The interval of follow-up can be lengthened after 2 years, realizing that late relapses can occur.
- Close observation for development of hypertension, hyperglycemia, hyperlipidemia, anxiety, and second malignancies should be performed at least annually.

PROGNOSIS

- Long-term prognosis of testicular patients with good-risk and/or low-stage disease is excellent, with overall cure rates of 95% and 80%, respectively, for metastatic disease.
- Patients with poor response to initial standard chemotherapy and first-line salvage therapy have a very poor prognosis and are generally incurable.
- Deaths from causes other than testicular cancer are more common in this population.

REFERENCES

Ann Intern Med 1988;109:540.
Crit Rev Hematol Oncol 2009;70:114.
Crit Rev Hematol Oncol 2009;71:22.
Eur Urol 2008;53:260.
J Clin Oncol 1988;6:1231.
J Clin Oncol 2005;23:6549.
JAMA 2008;299:672.
Lancet 2005;366:293.
N Engl J Med 1987;316:1435.

4 ■ RENAL CELL CARCINOMA

- Renal cell carcinoma (RCC) accounts for >90% of kidney cancers, with the clear-cell variant accounting for 85% of all cases—this chapter will pertain to this subtype.
- Approximately 58,000 annual cases in United States, with 13,000 deaths.
- Median age of 65 years, more common in men.
- Third most common genitourinary malignancy next to prostate and bladder cancer.
- Risk factors: smoking, obesity, asbestos and petroleum exposure, hypertension, acquired cystic disease from hemodialysis, familial syndromes (Birt-Hogg-Dube syndrome, von-Hippel Lindau (VHL) disease; rare).

PATHOBIOLOGY

- RCC is an immunologically reactive tumor, which may explain rare spontaneous regressions and response to immunotherapy.
- VHL syndrome is an autosomal-dominant disease characterized by loss of chromosome 3p material that predisposes affected patients to RCC, retinal angiomas, cerebellar hemangioblastoma, and pheochromocytoma.
  - The VHL gene is a tumor-suppressor gene located on chromosome 3p that encodes a protein that normally destroys hypoxia-inducible factor (HIF), a protein that stimulates production of tumor-stimulating factors such as vascular endothelial growth factor (VEGF) and platelet-derived growth factor-β (PDGF-β).
- Mutation or methylation-induced silencing of the VHL-suppressor gene is very common in sporadic RCC and results in increased VEGF levels, which play a role in the characteristic vascular nature of these tumors.
- The mammalian target of rapamycin (mTOR) is another growth factor frequently active in sporadic RCC and has recently become a target of drug treatment.

- RCC exhibits a propensity to grow into the renal vein and inferior vena cava; occasional tumor embolism to the pulmonary arteries or serpiginous tumor growth into the right atrium may occur.
- RCC may produce a variety of cytokines that result in various paraneoplastic and immune-mediated phenomena.

CLINICAL PRESENTATION

- RCC is known for protean systemic manifestations such as fever, anorexia, and weight loss ("the internist's tumor") that result from cytokine release and effects on the immune system.
- Gross hematuria and flank/back pain are the most common symptoms.
- Approximately 30% of patients may present with metastatic disease resulting in a variety of symptoms, including bone pain, headache, paralysis, seizures, dyspnea, hemoptysis, and abdominal pain.

PHYSICAL FINDINGS

- Patients with localized RCC may have no clinical manifestations if the tumor is detected incidentally during abdominal imaging for another problem.
- Palpable flank mass or tenderness.
- Varicocele from compression of the testicular vein.
- Plethora may indicate paraneoplastic erythrocytosis.
- RCC has a predilection for CNS spread, which may result in cranial nerve deficits, limb weakness, or paralysis due to spinal cord compression.

DIAGNOSTIC TESTS AND STAGING

- Abdominal-pelvic CT and ultrasound to assess size and for local invasion/metastases.
- Chest radiography to exclude pulmonary metastases.
- Abdominal MRI to exclude renal vein/vena cava involvement before surgery.
- Bone scan if bone pain or suspicion of bone metastasis.
- MRI of the brain if neurologic symptoms present.
- PET scan not routinely indicated during initial evaluation.
- Transesophageal echocardiogram if extension to inferior vena cava/heart suspected.
- Lab studies: CBC (anemia, erythrocytosis, thrombocytosis), serum calcium (paraneoplastic hypercalemia or bone metastases), liver function tests (paraneoplastic hepatitis is Stauffer syndrome), LDH (prognostic factor), creatinine.

Table 4–1 TNM Staging Criteria

Primary tumor (T)
T1: <7 cm, limited to kidney; **T2:** >7 cm, limited to kidney; **T3:** extends into major veins, adrenal gland, or perinephric tissues but not beyond Gerota's fascia; **T4:** extends beyond Gerota's fascia.

Regional lymph nodes (N)
N0: no lymph node metastases; **N1:** metastasis involving 1 node; **N2:** metastasis involving >1 node.

Distant metastasis (M)
M0: none; **M1:** present

Stage grouping
Stage I: T1 N0 M0
Stage II: T2 N0 M0
Stage III: T3 N0 M0; T1–3 N1 M0
Stage IV: T4 N0–1, M0; Tany N2 M0; Tany Nany M1

TREATMENT

- Treatment for RCC continues to evolve and depends upon stage, prognostic factors, tumor-related symptoms (e.g., hematuria, pain), and patient performance status.
- For localized RCC, radical nephrectomy is the historic gold-standard therapy, although nephron-sparing surgery is acceptable for smaller tumors located at the pole.
  - Cryoablation of small peripheral tumors may be utilized in poor surgical candidates, although long-term survival data are not available.
  - Adjuvant drug or radiation therapy has not shown survival benefit to-date after resection of localized (stage I-III) RCC and is not indicated at present.
  - Enrollment in clinical adjuvant trials is advised if available.
- Treatment of metastatic RCC.
  - Cytoreductive nephrectomy should be considered in good-performance-status patients or in those with ongoing hematuria or pain.
    - Nephrectomy followed by interferon-α (IFN) showed survival benefit in randomized trials; relevance of this data with newer drugs is unclear.
  - Resection of solitary metastases (e.g., lung, brain) if systemic disease controlled.
  - RCC is resistant to cytotoxic chemotherapy, but gemcitabine and fluorouracil (5-FU) or capecitabine have shown modest salvage activity.
  - High-dose interleukin (IL)-2: 600–720,000 Units/kg IV every 8 hours, up to 14 doses, is the only drug that has resulted in durable (curative) responses in a minority of patients (10% to 15% experience major response and 5% to 7% long-term survival).

- Should be administered in ICU setting due to severe systemic symptoms and capillary-leak syndrome; mortality rate 1% to 4%.
  - Consider restricting to patients with good performance status, minimal metastatic sites, and >85% tumor expression of carbonic anhydrase IX.
- Interferon-α: may result in partial responses in 15% of patients, but are not typically durable; significant toxicity.
- Sunitinib: a multitargeted tyrosine kinase inhibitor (TKI) indicated for first-line therapy in clear-cell RCC; increased PFS, response rate, and survival time with 50 mg daily for 28 days, 14 days off, repeated every 6 weeks.
- Sorafenib: multitargeted kinase inhibitor indicated in pretreated/cytokine-refractory patients; can also be used first-line.
- Temsirolimus: an mTOR inhibitor indicated as first-line treatment in patients with three or more poor prognostic factors from Memorial Sloan-Kettering Cancer Center (MSKCC) criteria (with addition of sixth factor of more than one site of metastasis); increased PFS and OS with weekly temsirolimus.
- Everolimus (RAD001): oral mTOR inhibitor for patients who progress on sunitinib or sorafenib showed increased PFS compared to placebo.
- Bevacizumab and IFN: increased VEGF production by RCC is targeted by the monoclonal antibody, bevacizumab; increased response rates and PFS when bevacizumab combined with IFN.

Table 4–2   Regimens for Metastatic RCC

High-dose IL-2: 600–720,000 Units/kg IV every 8 hours up to 14 doses repeated 2–3 weeks later constitutes one cycle; may be repeated if no progression
Interferon-α 9 million units SQ three times weekly with bevacizumab 10 mg/kg IV every 2 weeks
Sunitinib 50 mg daily by mouth day 1–28 every 42 days
Sorafenib 400 mg by mouth twice daily
Temsirolimus 25 mg IV weekly
Everolimus 10 mg by mouth daily

COMPLICATIONS OF TREATMENT

- Nephrectomy: wound infection, venous thromboembolism, bleeding, renal failure.
- IL-2: fever, hypotension, arrhythmia, edema, infection, cytopenia, hepatitis, electrolyte loss, respiratory failure, acute renal failure, rash, myocardial infarction, stroke.
- IFN: headache, fever, anorexia, myalgia, rash, depression, fatigue, hypothyroidism, cytopenia, hepatitis.

- Sunitinib/sorafenib: fatigue, stomatitis, hypertension, diarrhea, hand-foot syndrome, cytopenia.
- Temsirolimus/everolimus: fatigue, cough, dyspnea, nausea, stomatitis, hyperglycemia, hyperlipidemia, cytopenia, renal failure, edema, pneumonitis.
- Bevacizumab: fatigue, hypertension, epistaxis, headache, proteinuria, hemorrhage, bowel perforation, poor wound healing.

FOLLOW-UP CARE

- Localized disease: clinical examination, LDH, CBC, and chest radiography should be considered every 3 to 6 months; abdominal and chest CT for baseline, then as clinically indicated.
- Metastatic disease: CT of sites of measurable disease, PET scan, LDH; studies are often individualized but frequently performed at 3 to 6 month intervals.

PROGNOSIS

- The average 5-year OS for RCC is approximately 65% for all stages and 15% for metastatic RCC.
  - Poor prognostic determinants affecting 5-year survival include grade, local extent, nodal involvement, and metastases.
- The MSKCC survival criteria are applicable to stage IV RCC and are based on five clinical variables (although these were compiled in the pre-TKI era): no nephrectomy, Karnofsky score <80, anemia, hypercalcemia, and elevated LDH.
  - 0 risk factors (good risk): median survival 24 months.
  - 1–2 risk factors (intermediate risk): median survival 12 months.
  - ≥3 risk factors (poor risk): median survival 5 months.

REFERENCES

Crit Rev Hematol Oncol 2009;69:56.
J Clin Oncol 1999;17:2530.
J Clin Oncol 2006;24:2505.
JAMA 2006;295:2516.
Lancet 2008;372:449.
N Engl J Med 2007;356:115.
N Engl J Med 2007;356:2271.

BACKGROUND

- Bladder cancer (BC) is the second most common genitourinary malignancy and the fourth most common cancer in men, with a male predominance of 3:1 and median age at diagnosis of 65 years.
- 69,000 cases in the United States in 2008, with 14,000 deaths.
- Risk factors: smoking, occupational toxins (e.g., dyes, hydrocarbons), drugs (e.g., cyclophosphamide).

PATHOBIOLOGY

- Over 90% of BC are transitional cell carcinoma (TCC) histology, and are the only type discussed here.
- A variety of oncogenes (e.g., RAS), chromosomal deletions (e.g., 9p/q, 11p,13q), and altered tumor-suppressor genes (e.g., p53) are involved in the development and progression of invasive BC.
- Pathologically, BC can range from recurrent, superficial disease (noninvasive papillary tumors, carcinoma *in situ* [CIS]) to a deeply invasive, metastatic phenotype.
  - Virtually all invasive BC is poorly differentiated (grade 3).

CLINICAL PRESENTATION

- Hematuria most common symptom; dysuria, frequency, and urgency may occur.
- Flank/back pain may indicate locally invasive disease, and metastatic symptoms may include bone pain or dyspnea.

PHYSICAL FINDINGS

- With metastatic disease, palpable groin nodes or bone tenderness may be present.
- Mass at bladder outlet may present with large, palpable bladder.

DIAGNOSTIC TESTS AND STAGING

- An adult with persistent hematuria should undergo cystoscopy.
  - Papillary lesions are readily identified; CIS appears as red, abnormal mucosa; invasive tumors are typically large, irregular, and friable.

- Abdominal-pelvic CT indicated if a large or invasive tumor suspected; evaluation of the upper tract with intravenous pyelogram (IVP) or retrograde pyelogram suggested.
- Transurethral resection of bladder tumor (TURBT) and exam under anesthesia (EUA) indicated if cystoscopy abnormal.
  - Papillary tumors may be removed *in toto*.
  - Adequate, deep biopsy of muscle tissue to determine degree of invasion; large invasive tumors should be considered for neoadjuvant chemotherapy followed by cystectomy or combined-modality bladder-sparing treatment—in both cases the entire tumor is not removed at TURBT.
  - CIS requires biopsies of adjacent and random sites.
- Urine cytology: insensitive; negative result does not exclude BC.
- Metastatic evaluation: chest radiograph and bone scan if metastases suspected (e.g., respiratory symptoms, bone pain, elevated alkaline phosphatase), PET scan, MRI/CT of brain if neurologic symptoms.

Table 5–1 TNM Staging Criteria

Primary tumor (T)
Ta: noninvasive papillary tumor; **Tis:** carcinoma *in situ*; **T1:** invades subepithelium; **T2:** invades superficial (2a) or deep muscle (2b); **T3:** invades perivesical tissue (microscopic 3a, macroscopic 3b); **T4:** invades prostate, uterus, vagina (4a) or pelvic/abdominal wall (4b)

Regional lymph nodes (N)
N0: no node metastases; **N1:** <2 cm metastasis in one node; **N2:** 2–5 cm metastasis in single node; multiple node metastases <5 cm; **N3:** node metastasis >5 cm

Distant metastasis (M)
M0: none; **M1:** present

Stage grouping
Stage 0a: Ta N0 M0
Stage 0is: Tis N0 M0
Stage I: T1 N0 M0
Stage II: T2a/b N0 M0
Stage III: T3a–T4a N0 M0
Stage IV: T4b N0 M0; Tany N1–3 M0; Tany Nany M1

TREATMENT

- TURBT with or without intravesical bacillus-calmette Guerin (BCG) or mitomycin-C for high-grade Ta or CIS—under purview of urologist.
  - CIS requires intensive surveillance cystoscopy and cytology due to high-grade nature and precursor to invasive BC.

- Radical cystectomy: removal of bladder, prostate (males), uterus (females), and urinary diversion/neobladder procedure in patients with muscle invasion (T2a/b, T3); neoadjuvant chemotherapy should be strongly considered.
  - Pelvic lymph node dissection (PLND) is diagnostic and therapeutic; extended dissection associated with lower local recurrences and improved survival.
  - Node metastasis and/or perivesical tumor are indications for adjuvant chemotherapy or radiation; no proven survival benefit from adjuvant chemotherapy alone.
- Partial cystectomy: limited to lesions in dome of bladder.
- Neoadjuvant chemotherapy: administration of three cycles of cisplatin-containing regimen preoperatively for T2–T4a tumors.
  - Better tolerated than postoperative treatment and provides a survival benefit.
  - Neoadjuvant methotrexate, vinblastine, doxorubicin, cisplatin (MVAC) improved median survival from 46 to 77 months compared to surgery alone in a recent trial; 5-year survival was 43% vs. 57% ($p=0.06$) for the surgery and MVAC arm, respectively; this survival advantage has been subject of much debate.
  - Gemcitabine and cisplatin (GC) has emerged as a widely utilized neoadjuvant regimen due to similar efficacy and lower toxicity than MVAC in a phase III trial in patients with metastatic BC.
  - Meta-analysis demonstrated 5% absolute survival benefit at 5 years.
  - Pathologic CR predicts long-term survival (85% 5-year OS).
- Bladder preservation: applicable in 20% of patients (T2/T3a) if entire tumor can be resected with minimal bladder dysfunction and low recurrence risk.
  - Combination of chemotherapy, radiation, and transurethral resection results in pathologic CR rates of 20% to 40% and 5-year survival of 49% to 62%.
  - Less than an early CR via cystoscopy/biopsy requires cystectomy.
- Radiation therapy: not standard curative treatment for muscle-invasive BC unless combined with chemotherapy; radiation alone may be palliative for infirm patients.
  - Cisplatin, alone or in combination with 5-FU.
  - Low-dose carboplatin (AUC 2) and paclitaxel (45 mg/m^2) administered weekly during radiation an option in nonsurgical candidates.
- Unresectable disease (T4a/b): if significant perivesical tumor or large adenopathy (>2 cm) is noted at staging or surgery, chemotherapy with or without radiation may render the patient operable.
- Metastatic disease: metastatic BC is incurable, but chemosensitive and palliative chemotherapy extends survival and improves quality of life.
  - Patients with significant visceral metastases and/or poor performance status derive little, if any, benefit from combination chemotherapy.

- GC is better tolerated than MVAC with similar survival and less toxicity.
- Other active agents: paclitaxel, docetaxel, carboplatin, pemetrexed.

Table 5–2 Regimens for BC

Neoadjuvant/adjuvant
MVAC: methotrexate 30 mg/m^2 IV days 1, 15, 22; vinblastine 3 mg/m^2 IV days 2, 15, 22; doxorubicin 30 mg/m^2 IV day 2; cisplatin 70 mg/m^2 IV day 2 every 28 days × 3 cycles
GC: 1000 mg/m^2 IV days 1,8,15; cisplatin 75 mg/m^2 IV day 1 every 28 days × 3 cycles

First-line metastatic
GC: gemcitabine 1000 mg/m^2 IV days 1,8,15; cisplatin 75 mg/m^2 IV day 1 every 28 days (may substitute carboplatin AUC 5–6 for cisplatin)

COMPLICATIONS OF TREATMENT

- Cystectomy: wound infection, venous thromboembolism, myocardial infarction, electrolyte/acid-base disorders (if ileal conduit created).
- Radiation: hematuria, urgency, frequency, tenesmus, pelvic pain, skin irritation, late malignancies (sarcoma, rectal cancer).
- Chemotherapy: fatigue, alopecia, neuropathy, anemia, thrombocytopenia, neutropenia, fever, septic death (4% with MVAC), heart failure.

FOLLOW-UP CARE

- Cystoscopy and urine cytology following intravesical therapy, because Ta and T1 tumors have a 50% to 70% rate of recurrence by 5 years.
- Postcystectomy: Urine cytology and CT of abdomen/pelvis/chest every 3 to 6 months for 2 years.
- If diversion performed, monitor electrolytes and B12 status periodically.

PROGNOSIS

- 5-year survival for localized BC with combined modality therapy may exceed 60% in select patients; patients in the neoadjuvant MVAC trial had a median survival of 77 months.
- Patients with untreated metastatic BC rarely survive >6 months; median survival of patients treated with GC is 15 months, and 5-year OS is 13%.
- Patients with a poor performance status and/or visceral metastases have a very poor prognosis.

REFERENCES

Cancer 2002;95:1022.
J Clin Oncol 2000;17:3068.
J Clin Oncol 2000;18:1921.
J Clin Oncol 2005;23:4602.
Lancet 2003;361:1927.
N Engl J Med 2003;349:859.
Urology 2004;64:479.

6 ■ PROSTATE CANCER

- Prostate cancer is the most common male cancer (235,000 cases in 2008 with 27,000 deaths), affecting one in six men.
- Many men will die with, but not of, prostate cancer (8.5:1 incidence/mortality ratio) due to variability in tumor aggressiveness.
- 70% of men >80 years have autopsy evidence of prostate cancer.
- Risk factors: age, black race, family history, familial syndromes (e.g., BRCA2 mutation), dietary fat.

PATHOBIOLOGY

- Most cases do not result in death; others are aggressive and fatal.
- 99% of prostate cancers are adenocarinomas; rare variants include small cell, lymphoma, and sarcoma.
  - Aggressive neuroendocrine component may supervene late in course; histologically small, dense cells with neuroendocrine markers on immunohistochemical staining (e.g., neuron-specific enolase, chromogranin, synaptophysin).
- Tumor phenotype develops in stepwise fashion with acquired mutations of various genes controlling cell proliferation/differentiation.
- Androgens are the primary regulator of neoplastic cell growth; castration/blockade slows tumor growth.
- Tumor morphology dictates Gleason score (discussed under Treatment, p. 33).

CLINICAL PRESENTATION

- Most cases of prostate cancer are discovered through prostate specific antigen (PSA) screening during asymptomatic stage.
- Advanced-stage disease may present with urgency, frequency, dysuria, hematuria, impotence, or urine retention.
- Metastatic disease often presents with back pain—the most common site of initial symptomatic metastases—or dyspnea due to lung metastases (via Batson's plexus).

PHYSICAL FINDINGS

- Rectal exam: palpable nodule or area of induration most common; bilateral lobe or extracapsular involvement or seminal vesical mass indicates locally advanced disease.
- Inguinal nodes, spine tenderness, supraclavicular nodes, leg edema, or neurologic findings if advanced/metastatic.
- Rarely, cranial nerve palsies may result from base-of-skull metastasis.

DIAGNOSTIC TESTING AND STAGING

- PSA screening is widely utilized in the United States and, although there is no evidence that screening improves outcome, is the most common reason for prompting prostate biopsy and diagnosis.
  - 15% of patients with normal PSA (<4 ng/mL) have cancer and 2% have high-grade cancer.
  - Risk of recurrence PSA categories: low, PSA <10 ng/dL; intermediate, PSA 10–20 ng/dL; high, PSA >20 ng/dL.
- Rectal examination is the primary clinical staging tool for primary tumor.
  - Nonpalpable or palpable (one or both lobes and/or extracapsular/ seminal vesical invasion).

Table 6–1 TNM Staging Criteria

Primary tumor (T)
T1: clinically unapparent tumor not palpable or visible on imaging; incidentally found at TURP histology: <5% of tissue (T1a) or >5% of tissue (T2b); diagnosed based on PSA-driven biopsy (T1c); **T2:** tumor confined to prostate; <one-half of 1 lobe (T2a); >one-half of 1 lobe (T2b); both lobes (T2c); **T3:** tumor beyond capsule; extracapsular (T3a); seminal vesicle(s) (T3b); **T4:** tumor fixed to or invades bladder, rectum, pelvic wall

Regional lymph nodes (N)
N0: metastases absent; **N1:** metastases present

Distant metastases (M)
M0: none; **M1:** present

Stage grouping
Stage I: T1a (GS 2–4) N0 M0
Stage II: T1a (GS 5–10) N0 M0; T1b/c N0 M0; T2 N0 M0
Stage III: T3 N0 M0
Stage IV: T4 N0 M0; Tany N1 M0; Tany Nany M1

- Transrectal ultrasound-guided prostate biopsy with 10 to 12 cores.
  - Gleason score (GS): sum of dominant and secondary malignant gland patterns scored from 1 (well-differentiated) to 5 (poorly-differentiated).
    - GS risk categories: low (2–6), intermediate (7), high (8–10).
- CT or MRI may reveal extent of prostatic, seminal vesical, and/or local tissue involvement, but sensitivity imperfect.
- Imaging studies (e.g., bone scan, CT) to detect metastases are based on symptoms (e.g., bone pain, dyspnea), high-risk GS (≥8), and PSA >20 ng/dL.
- Blood studies: high alkaline phosphatase may indicate bone metastasis; anemia/thrombocytopenia may indicate bone marrow involvement; elevated creatinine may indicate urinary tract obstruction.

TREATMENT

- Localized disease.
  - Radical prostatectomy (RP) should be considered if life expectancy >10 years and patient is acceptable surgical risk: open, laparoscopically, or robotically (faster recovery, less blood loss with latter two methods) with similar oncologic results/survival.
    - PLND if risk of positive nodes >7% (many nomograms).
    - RP reduces cancer-specific mortality, but not overall mortality.
  - External beam radiotherapy (EBRT).
    - Three-dimensional or intensity-modulated radiation therapy (IMRT) with 70–79 Gy to prostate with or without seminal vesicles for low-risk tumors; 75–80 Gy for intermediate- and high-risk tumors.
    - High-risk and some intermediate-risk tumors derive survival benefit from neoadjuvant, concurrent, and 3 years of adjuvant androgen deprivation therapy (ADT) (e.g., leuprolide 7.5 mg IM monthly, goserelin 3.6 mg IM monthly).
  - Brachytherapy.
    - Placement of radioactive seeds (iodine^{125} or palladium^{103}) under anesthesia for low-risk cancers yields results similar to surgery and EBRT.
- Pelvic lymph node involvement.
  - High-risk cancers may benefit from pelvic node radiation and 2 to 3 years of ADT; intermediate-risk cancers may benefit from radiation and 4 to 6 months of ADT; low-risk tumors should not receive either treatment.
  - Patients with pathologically involved pelvic nodes have improved survival and metastasis-free periods from adjuvant radiation and immediate ADT with goserelin 3.6 mg IM monthly.

- Metastatic disease.
  - Initial treatment in patients with symptoms or radiographic metastases is surgical (bilateral orchiectomy) or medical castration via ADT with a luteinizing hormone-releasing hormone (LHRH) agonist (e.g., monthly or trimonthly goserelin or leuprolide).
    - Patients with PSA-only recurrence may not require immediate ADT unless the doubling time is rapid, the initial disease was high risk, or the PSA is >50 ng/dL.
  - Addition of an antiandrogen such as bicalutamide 50 mg orally daily or flutamide 250 mg orally twice a day to LHRH analogue (complete androgen blockade, CAB) improves survival modestly at expense of more adverse effects.
  - Patients with epidural or retroperitoneal tumor bulk should receive 7 to 10 days of an antiandrogen (e.g., bicalutamide 100–150 mg orally daily) to avoid acute spinal cord compression or urinary obstruction, respectively, due to LHRH agonist "flare" from initial testosterone surge.
  - Progression during ADT (castrate refractory prostate cancer, CRPC) may briefly respond to administration or withdrawal of antiandrogen, ketoconazole, or estrogens.
  - Chemotherapy with docetaxel every 3 weeks for CRPC is the only regimen demonstrated in phase III trials to prolong survival of patients with adequate performance status (19.2 vs. 16.3 months compared to mitoxantrone).
  - Monthly zoledronic acid (2–4 mg IV every 4 weeks) decreases skeletal complications in patient with bone metastases.
  - Bone-seeking radiopharmaceuticals, strontium-89 and samarium-153, may benefit patients with refractory skeletal pain but do not improve survival.

Table 6–2 Regimens for CRPC

Docetaxel 75 mg/m^2 IV day 1 and prednisone 5 mg by mouth twice daily every 21 days
Mitoxantrone 12 mg/m^2 IV day 1 and prednisone 5 mg by mouth twice daily every 21 days

COMPLICATIONS OF TREATMENT

- Radical prostatectomy: bleeding, impotence, incontinence, wound infection, venous thromboembolism, myocardial infarction, urethral stricture.
- Radiation therapy: impotence, incontinence, dysuria, diarrhea, hematochezia, radiation proctitis, rectal stricture, second malignancy (e.g., rectal cancer, sarcoma).
- ADT: fatigue, gynecomastia, hot flashes, anemia, osteoporosis, fractures, sarcopenia, obesity, insulin resistance/diabetes, cardiovascular disease, hyperlipidemia.

- Antiandrogen therapy: hot-flashes, impotence, painful gynecomastia, galactorrhea, constipation, hepatitis, diarrhea, nausea.
- Chemotherapy: fatigue, mucositis, neutropenia, infection, anemia, thrombocytopenia.
- Bisphosphonates: flulike symptoms, hypocalcemia, renal dysfunction, osteonecrosis of the jaw (ONJ).

FOLLOW-UP CARE

- Localized disease treated with radiation/surgery: annual rectal examination and PSA every 6 months for 5 years, then yearly; imaging for detection of metastasis based on symptoms and PSA elevation.
- Metastatic disease: history, physical examination, and PSA every 3 to 6 months; imaging based on symptoms and/or PSA rise; oral examination to detect ONJ; monitoring renal function if on bisphosphonate; patients on ADT: screening and treatment for osteoporosis (e.g., zoledronic acid 4 mg IV annually or alendronate 70 mg orally weekly if high fracture risk; vitamin D 400 IU and calcium 500 mg daily), monitoring glucose and lipids, treatment of hot flashes (e.g., clonidine 0.1 mg orally daily), treatment of gynecomastia (e.g., breast radiation).

PROGNOSIS

- Patients with low- risk tumors (PSA <10 ng/dL, GS 2–6, T1–T2a) have <10% chance of cancer-death at 20 years.
- Patients with high-risk tumors (PSA >20 ng/dL, GS 8–10, ≥T3a) have a high-risk of relapse after treatment, with some patients having progression-free survival of only 28–36% after surgery.
- Median survival of CRPC is 18–24 months from initiation of hormonal therapy.

REFERENCES

J Clin Oncol 2003;21:3972.
J Clin Oncol 2005;23:800.
J Clin Oncol 2007;25:1038.
J Clin Oncol 2007;25:1596.
JAMA 1999;281:1598.
N Engl J Med 2002;347:781.
N Engl J Med 2004;351:1502.
N Engl J Med 2009;360:2516.

7 ■ BREAST CANCER

- Breast cancer (BC) results from malignant transformation and proliferation of the epithelium lining the ducts (ductal carcinoma) or lobules (lobular carcinoma) of the breast; less common variants, such as lymphoma, sarcoma, tubular, medullary, or adenoid cystic carcinomas will not be discussed.
- BC is the most common malignancy in women, accounting for 31% of cancers, and the second most common cause of cancer death; the lifetime risk of the average woman surviving to age 80 is 1 in 9.
- There are approximately 184,000 cases of invasive BC and 41,000 deaths annually in the United States; male breast cancer is relatively rare, with 1700 cases and 400 deaths annually.
  - Ductal carcinoma in situ (DCIS), malignant cells within a duct limited by basement membrane without metastatic potential, has increased in incidence (approximately 68,000 annual cases), primarily from screening mammography; lobular carcinoma in situ (LCIS) does not require therapy (although tamoxifen can be considered), but indicates an increased future risk (1–2% per year) of developing invasive BC, warranting close follow-up and screening.
  - Invasive BC refers to cancer cells that spread beyond the basement membrane of the duct (invasive ductal carcinoma, IDC) or the lobule (invasive lobular carcinoma, ILC).
- Mortality from BC has been declining in recent years due to early diagnosis and improved treatments; although incidence of BC is higher in whites, mortality is higher in black women, often due to a more aggressive phenotype (often hormone-receptor negative) and later stage at diagnosis.
- Risk factors: age and family history are the predominant risk factors; having a first-degree relative with BC increases risk modestly; however, only 5–10% of cases are due to a genetic defect, most commonly mutations in the BRCA 1 or 2 genes, which confer a lifetime risk of 60–80%; mutations of BRCA genes are more common in women of Ashkenazi Jewish heritage.
  - Other risk factors: early menarche, late menopause, atypical hyperplasia, estrogen replacement therapy, mammographically dense breasts, nulliparity, late first childbirth, obesity, high-fat diet,

thoracic radiation (especially mantle radiation prior to age 30 for Hodgkin's disease), alcohol intake.

- Predictive risk models, such as the Gail model, are available to calculate an individual patient's risk.
- BC complicates 1 in 3000–4000 pregnancies and is often diagnosed in advanced stages, because breast abnormalities are often attributed to pregnancy changes; ANY abnormal, persistent lump/mass during pregnancy should be pursued as possible BC.

- The importance of BC being an estrogen-driven neoplasm is demonstrated by a decreased risk of BC in women taking selective estrogen receptor modulators (SERMs, tamoxifen or raloxifene) or whom have undergone bilateral oophorectomy either prophylactically or for other reasons.
  - Meta-analysis of SERM prevention trials in high-risk women demonstrated a 38% reduction in BC incidence.
- Screening for BC via mammography has been shown in multiple trials to conclusively decrease risk of breast cancer death by 25–39% in women >50 years, with 26% reduction in meta analysis; women 40 to 50 years still enjoy a reduction, although to a lesser degree.
  - Patients carrying BRCA 1 or 2 mutations may develop cancer at young age and should begin screening by age 25; these patients may develop interval cancers, so mammography every 6 months should be considered; breast MRI should be strongly considered in BRCA carriers due to improve sensitivity over mammography.
  - False-positive rate of screening mammography of 10–15%, especially in young women with dense breasts; this reinforces importance of monthly self-exams and at least annual physician exam.

PATHOBIOLOGY

- BC represents a heterogeneous group of malignancies characterized by differences in histology, surface receptor status, and gene expression.
- BC is primarily an estrogen-driven neoplasm; after estrogen binds to estrogen receptor (ER), it is internalized and transported to nucleus where genes controlling cell proliferation are up-regulated, leading to neoplastic growth.
- The majority of BC is due to IDC, which will be the focus of this discussion.
  - DCIS, by definition, is limited by basement membrane and possesses nil metastatic potential if properly treated; tumor cell biology similar to IDC, although acquisition of additional lesions conferring invasive phenotype likely leads to IDC.
    - Histologic subtypes of DCIS include solid, cribiform, comedonecrotic, and micropapillary; necrosis and high-grade forms portend increased recurrence risk; axillary metastasis in <1% of cases.
  - A subtype (1–5% of cases) of invasive BC is inflammatory BC (IBC), which is vital to recognize due to its very aggressive nature and need for timely, multimodality therapy.

- Pathologic hallmark is invasion of dermal lymphatic vessels by tumor cells resulting in characteristic clinical presentation (erythema, warmth, swelling); most are ER-negative; expression of E-cadherin increased and mutation of p53 common.
- Most cases of sporadic breast cancer result from stepwise acquisition of acquired damage to DNA.
  - After cell transformation, tumor growth usually progresses in stepwise fashion: benign hyperplasia leads to atypical hyperplasia, which leads to *in situ* cancer, which leads to invasive cancer; this process may occur over years (as in estrogen-receptor [ER] positive cancers) or rather rapidly (as in tumors not expressing ER, progesterone receptor [PR], or HER-2/*neu*—"so called triple-negative" tumors [approximately 10–15% of BC] or HER-2/*neu* expressing tumors [approximately 20% of BC]).
    - HER2/*neu* is a receptor-tryosine kinase of the EGFR family; overexpression results in increased proliferation, invasiveness, and angiogenesis and decreased tumor cell apoptosis.
    - Mutation of tumor-suppressor gene p53 common in sporadic BC; mutated PTEN gene in 10%; increased expression of HER-2/*neu* in 20% of BC cases and confers more aggressive phenotype.
- BRCA 1/2 mutation carriers develop aggressive tumors that may elude mammographic detection, occurring between screening intervals ("interval" cancers).
  - BRCA-1 is a tumor-suppressor gene located on chromosome 17q that is integral to DNA repair; mutated ductal cells are unable to properly repair DNA damage, leading to malignant phenotype; patients carrying BRCA-1 mutation have lifetime BC risk of 70–80% and ovarian cancer risk of 30–40%; more common in Ashkenazi Jewish women.
  - BRCA-2 has similar role to BRCA-1 and is found on chromosome 13q; lifetime risk of BC similar to BRCA-1 mutation, but less risk for ovarian cancer; increased risk of prostate cancer, male breast cancer, and melanoma with BRCA-2 mutation.
- Histopathologic features of aggressive tumors include high cytologic or nuclear grade, increased mitotic activity, lymphovascular invasion, neural invasion, tumor necrosis, dermal lymphatic invasion, or extracapsular lymph node extension.
- Circulating VEGF binds to receptors on tumor vessels stimulating neovascularization and increased tumor growth; the resulting disordered vasculature confers a chemotherapy-resistant phenotype.
- The importance of tumor genomic profiles in determining tumor aggressiveness and potential benefit from adjuvant treatment is being demonstrated.
  - Gene expression array analyses have been shown to correlate with different tumor phenotypes:
    - ER-positive BC classified "luminal" A and B, with the luminal A variant typically of lower grade and less likely to express HER-2/*neu*

than luminal B; overall, luminal tumors have a favorable prognosis when treated with antiestrogen therapy; luminal tumors expressing HER-2/*neu* behave clinically/biologically between ER-positive/HER-2 negative and "triple-negative" tumors (see below).

- ER/PR-negative tumors are characterized by presence of (ER-, PR-, HER2/*neu*+) HER-2/*neu* receptor, which confers more aggressive phenotype than luminal cancers (but treatable with trastuzumab) or absence of (ER-, PR-, HER2/*neu*-) HER2/*neu* receptor, the so-called "triple-negative" BC or basal-like phenotype, which is associated with early relapse and a predilection for cerebral metastasis.
- A clinically available 21-gene assay (Oncotype-DX©) to assess various genes conferring tumor invasiveness, proliferative capacity, and metastatic potential is available for predicting recurrence risk on paraffin-embedded samples of BC tissue in postmenopausal women with ER-positive tumors <3 cm with more than three positive nodes.

CLINICAL PRESENTATION

- Most cases of localized BC are asymptomatic and diagnosed during screening mammography.
- Breast symptoms include a palpable lump, nipple changes (e.g., inversion, discharge), or skin changes (e.g., redness, warmth, tenderness) in the case of IBC.
- General symptoms of metastatic breast cancer (MBC) may include weight loss, anorexia, or fatigue.
- Specific symptoms of MBC include headache, diplopia, limb weakness/paresthesia, seizures (brain metastasis); abdominal pain (liver metastasis); dyspnea, cough, hemoptysis (lung metastasis); back pain, leg weakness, or bowel/bladder incontinence or retention (spine metastasis with spinal cord compression).

PHYSICAL FINDINGS

- Localized disease: palpable breast lesion (typically <3–5 cm), moveable axillary nodes; eczema-like nipple lesion in Paget disease.
- Locally advanced breast cancer (LABC): large mass (>5 cm) or mass fixation to chest wall; large axillary nodes—may be matted or fixed; palpable supraclavicular (N3) nodes.
- Inflammatory breast cancer (IBC): erythema, warmth, skin thickening/induration, and *peau-de-orange* changes; mass may or may not be palpable; enlarged axillary nodes common; often misdiagnosed as cellulitis/mastitis, which leads to diagnostic delay.

DIAGNOSTIC TESTS AND STAGING

- Most cases of BC are diagnosed after screening mammography, although many women present to their physician after finding a breast lump on self-exam—these women should undergo diagnostic mammogram.
- Diagnostic mammogram: includes magnification, spot compression, and oblique views to assess for characteristic radiographic changes of malignancy.
  - DCIS: typically appears as clustered microcalcifications, segmentally or linearly, often with a branching pattern; soft-tissue abnormality may be noted.
  - LCIS: intralobular proliferation of atypical cells; by definition, a pathologic diagnosis and nonpalpable.
- Ultrasound: useful to confirm nature of mass on mammogram; cystic lesions are readily identified and may be immediately aspirated—if cyst collapses and nonbloody fluid that is cytologically negative is obtained, routine follow-up is all that is required; solid or complex lesions should be referred to a surgeon and/or interventional radiologist for tissue diagnosis.
- MRI: very sensitive, often detects benign lesions or very small cancers; rapid inflow and washout of gadolinium into mass consistent with hypervascular nature of malignancy; although may be useful to assess equivocal lesions, MRI not indicated for screening average-risk women, but is recommended in patients with BRCA mutations or very strong family history of BC.
- Tissue diagnosis: any lesion suspicious on imaging or examination should be biopsied to exclude cancer; some common approaches include:
  - Fine-needle aspiration (FNA): can be performed on palpable mass in surgeon's office with minimal pain; requires expert cytopathologist; false-positive rate <5%; although excellent way to diagnose BC, drawback is lack of tissue core to determine invasive or *in situ* BC or receptor analysis.
  - Core needle biopsy (via stereotactic or needle-localization approach) best way to assess tissue/cellular architecture, presence of invasion, and obtain ample tissue for immunohistochemical (IHC) stains for ER, PR, and HER-2/*neu* (3+ on IHC indicative of pathologic overexpression and indication for HER-2 directed therapy with trastuzumab; 2+ IHC should be confirmed with fluorescence *in situ* hybridization [FISH]; 0–1+ IHC is negative assay for HER-2).
  - Incisional biopsy not indicated in most cases; useful if core biopsy inconclusive, yielded insufficient material, or IBC is suspected.
- Evaluation for metastatic disease not warranted at presentation unless history or physical examination suggest concern (e.g., headache, weight loss, bone pain); diagnostic modalities for MBC include:

- CT of chest (lung metastasis, malignant pericardial/pleural effusion) and abdomen/pelvis (liver metastasis, ascites, ovarian metastasis, malignant bowel obstruction).
- Brain imaging to detect metastasis or leptomeningeal involvement; gadolinium-enhanced MRI test of choice; CT with intravenous contrast alternative.
- PET scanning may be useful to diagnose metastasis if CT equivocal or if detecting distant disease would change management; some clinicians monitor response to treatment of MBC by measuring size and standard uptake value (SUV) of tumor deposits.
- Radionuclide bone scan should be considered if bone pain or increase in serum alkaline phosphatase; often unnecessary if good quality PET obtained.

Table 7-1 TNM Staging Criteria

Primary tumor (T)
T1: tumor <2 cm; T1mic: ≤0.1 cm; T1a: >0.1–≤0.5 cm; T1b: >0.5–≤1.0 cm; T1c: >1 cm–≤2.0 cm; **T2:** tumor >2 cm–≤5 cm; **T3:** tumor >5 cm; **T4:** T4a: extension to chest wall (not including pectoralis); T4b: edema (including IBC) or ulceration of breast skin or ipsilateral satellite skin nodules

Regional lymph nodes (N)
Clinical: N0: node metastasis absent; **N1:** metastasis involving mobile ipsilateral axillary node(s); **N2:** metastasis involving fixed/matted ipsilateral axillary nodes, or clinically apparent (by imaging) ipsilateral internal mammary nodes in absence of clinically evident axillary node metastasis; **N3:** metastasis involving infraclavicular node(s), or metastasis involving ipsilateral internal mammary node(s) and axillary node(s), or metastasis involving ipsilateral supraclavicular node(s)
Pathologic: pN0: histologic node metastasis absent; **pN1:** pN1mic: micrometastasis (>0.2–<2.0 mm); **pN1:** metastasis involving 1–3 axillary nodes; **pN2:** metastasis involving 4–9 axillary nodes (with at least one tumor deposit >2.0 mm), or clinically apparent internal mammary node(s) in absence of axillary node metastasis; **pN3:** metastasis involving ≥10 axillary nodes or metastasis to infraclavicular node(s), or clinically apparent ipsilateral internal mammary node(s) in the presence of ≥1 positive axillary nodes, or metastasis involving supraclavicular node(s)

Distant metastasis (M)
M0: present; **M1:** absent

Stage grouping
Stage I: T1 * N0 M0
Stage II: IIA: T0–1 N1 M0; T2 N0 M0; **IIB:** T2 N1 M0; T3 N0 M0
Stage III: IIIA: T0–T3 N2 M0; T3 N1 M0; **IIIB:** T4 N0–2 M0; **IIIC:** Tany N3 M0
Stage IV: Tany Nany M1

*All T1 include T1mic.

- Cytologic analysis of body fluids: CSF via lumbar puncture (carcinomatous meningitis), pleural fluid via thoracentesis or tube thoracostomy (malignant pleural effusion), pericardial fluid via pericardiocentesis (malignant pericardial effusion), ascitic fluid via paracentesis (malignant ascites/peritoneal carcinomatosis).
  - Serum tumor markers such as CA 27–29 and CA 15–3 may be useful if significantly and persistently elevated if radiographic evidence of MBC is equivocal; decreasing levels during treatment of MBC may be assumed to be indicative of favorable response, whereas significant elevation may indicate progression; however, because markers are not 100% sensitive or specific, instituting or discontinuing therapy based solely on levels is discouraged.
- Assessment of axillary nodes: presence of axillary nodal metastasis is a powerful predictor of recurrence; presence of abnormally palpable nodes (especially if fixed or matted) is indication for full axillary lymph node dissection (ALND) at initial breast surgery (either lumpectomy or mastectomy).
  - Sentinel lymph node biopsy (SLNB) based on premise that lymphatics predictably drain into one to four nodes (sentinel nodes) before spreading to higher-echelon nodes; if sentinel nodes are pathologically negative, there is very small risk of metastasis in other nodes, sparing patient morbidity of ALND; SLNB indicated in patients with ≥T1 tumors (DCIS rarely associated with axillary metastasis) and absence of pathologically palpable axillary nodes, which mandates ALND; peritumoral or periareloar injection of blue dye and radioactive tracer are taken up by local lymphatics and empty into sentinel node, which is identified by visual observation and radioactivity with handheld gamma probe.

TREATMENT

- DCIS (stage 0): because DCIS has nil metastatic potential (<1%), SLNB is not indicated unless there is a large mass (>5 cm) and/or extensive high-grade DCIS; the two most common surgical treatment modalities are mastectomy or breast-conservation surgery (BCS) with lumpectomy followed by radiation; both options should be followed by 5 years of tamoxifen.
  - Mastectomy for DCIS: the local failure rate for total mastectomy is <2%, with an approximate 98% disease-free survival; radiation unnecessary following mastectomy.
  - BCS: randomized trials (such as NSABP B-17) have conclusively shown that lumpectomy and radiation (1.8–2.0 Gy daily to 45–50 Gy over 5 to 6 weeks) produce long-term outcomes identical to mastectomy; as such, BCS is popular for women who wish to preserve their breast without compromising disease control; there is essentially no patient group undergoing lumpectomy that does not benefit from

radiation (except perhaps for >70 year old women with a small, low-grade, ER-positive DCIS focus and >1 cm surgical margin).

○ Adjuvant tamoxifen: the randomized NSABP B-24 trial demonstrated a 31% reduction in local recurrence and a 53% decrease in contralateral BC in women treated with 5 years of tamoxifen following BCS.

- Localized BC: patients with localized BC typically have stage I/II or disease with nonbulky axillary nodes and freely mobile, resectable primary tumors; standard treatment typically involves BCS and, if indicated, adjuvant chemotherapy, trastuzumab in HER-2/*neu* positive patients, and hormone therapy in ER/PR-positive patients.
  ○ BCS provides identical disease control and survival benefit compared to mastectomy; indications for postmastectomy radiation generally include tumor >5 cm and/or four or more positive nodes; contraindications to BCS include pregnancy, prior chest wall radiation, connective tissue disease (especially lupus and scleroderma), or positive margins (patients with positive margins should undergo reexcision to ensure a negative margin; mastectomy is indicated for persistently positive margins despite reexcision); radiation should commence after completion of adjuvant chemotherapy.
  ○ Adjuvant chemotherapy has been shown in numerous randomized trials and meta-analyses to reduce risk of recurrence (23%) and death (17%) from invasive breast cancer; the magnitude of benefit is greatest in women <50 years (approximate 30% reduction in death) and least in women >70 years (approximate 13% reduction in death); chemotherapy is more effective for hormone-receptor-negative tumors.
  ○ Selection of localized BC patients for chemotherapy is dependent on several factors, but generally is indicated for tumors >1 cm (T1c), especially if triple-negative or HER2/*neu*-positive.
    ◦ Postmenopausal patients with an ER-positive BC <3 cm and one to three positive nodes (N1) are candidates for a 21-gene array (Oncotype-DX®) to determine risk of recurrence within 10 years (recurrence score) and predict degree of benefit from adjuvant chemotherapy; tumors with score >31 have recurrence risk of 30.5% and an absolute decrease in recurrence of 27.6% at 10 years (HR 0.26) compared to patients with score of <18 who have a recurrence risk of 6.8% and an absolute decrease in recurrence of –1.1% at 10 years.
    ◦ Patients who are candidates for chemotherapy (e.g., >0.5–1 cm [≥T1b] triple negative, or HER-2/*neu*-positive with or without positive nodes), are best treated with combination chemotherapy as soon as surgical incisions are healed; radiation should commence shortly after completion of chemotherapy and followed by endocrine therapy.

- The classic CMF regimen (cyclophosphamide, methotrexate, 5-FU) may be considered for elderly patients or those with low-risk tumors; however, trials have demonstrated superiority of anthracycline-containing regimens such as AC (doxorubicin and cyclophosphamide) over CMF; addition of taxanes also provide disease-free and survival benefit; recent trials show superiority of the TC regimen (docetaxel and cyclophosphamide) compared to the AC regimen in terms of recurrence and survival at 7 years and allows avoidance of potentially cardiotoxic anthracyclines.
  - Dose-dense AC and paclitaxel administered every 14 days with growth-factor support are more efficacious than every-21-day regimens; weekly paclitaxel also shown to provide improved outcome compared to every-21-days in node-positive and node-negative patients with T2–3 tumors.
  - Nonanthracycline regimens increasing in popularity; the TCH regimen (docetaxel, carboplatin, trastuzumab) appears as efficacious as anthracycline-containing regimens for HER-2/*neu*-positive BC, with lack of cardiotoxicity.
  - Trastuzumab, a humanized monoclonal antibody directed at HER2/*neu* receptor, in combination with chemotherapy demonstrated unequivocally in several phase III trials to decrease recurrence risk by 50% and improve survival in node-positive and high-risk node-negative patients with HER2-*neu*-positive disease; typically administered for total of 52 weeks; regular monitoring of ventricular function is necessary due to 3–4% risk of cardiac dysfunction.
- Radiation: whole breast radiation therapy (WBRT) following chemotherapy was shown in several randomized trials to decrease local recurrence in all subgroups of invasive BC; Early Breast Cancer Trialists' Collaborative Group (EBCTCG) data from 42,000 patients demonstrated improved local control and overall survival at 15 years; 45–50 Gy delivered in 1.8–2.0 Gy doses over 6 weeks followed by local 16 Gy "boost" to tumor bed further decreases recurrence risk by approximately 3%.
  - Partial breast irradiation (PBI) with interstitial balloon-based catheters placed into surgical cavity can deliver therapeutic doses of brachytherapy over 5 days in patients <45 years with T1, node-negative tumors with negative margins; data are still accumulating and WBRT remains standard of care.
- Adjuvant endocrine therapy with tamoxifen for 5 years (with or without ovarian ablation with gonadotropin-releasing hormone [GnRH] analogues or oophorectomy) in premenopausal women or an aromatase inhibitor (AI) for postmenopausal women.
  - Tamoxifen (20 mg orally daily) for 5 years was shown to decrease risk of recurrence by 40–50% and death by 33% in pre- and postmenopausal women in Oxford meta-analysis; inhibitors of CYP2D6, such as paroxetine and fluoxetine, should be avoided, because

these inhibit transformation of tamoxifen into the active metabolite, endoxifen, thereby decreasing efficacy and increasing risk of recurrence.

- Als (letrozole 2.5 mg orally daily, anastrozole 1 mg orally daily, and exemestane 25 mg orally daily) decrease circulating estrogen by >95% and are adjuvant endocrine agents of choice in postmenopausal women with BC; several large randomized trials (BIG-98, ATAC, ASBCG, IES) have demonstrated superiority of all three agents compared to tamoxifen in regard to disease-free survival (approximately 20%) without increased survival; some data have shown slight survival benefit for exemestane and extended 5 years of letrozole following 5 years of tamoxifen in node-positive patients (MA-17).

- **LABC**—neoadjuvant therapy: patients with large (T3) tumors, tumors fixed to chest wall (T4), or those with bulky axillary nodes may initially present with unresectable disease; neoadjuvant therapy, most commonly with combination chemotherapy, may render unresectable BC operable—either BCS or mastectomy without compromised survival; patients with a clinically negative axilla should optimally undergo prechemotherapy SLNB: if positive, then ALND at breast surgery is indicated; if negative, ALND is omitted at breast surgery; patients not undergoing prechemotherapy SLNB should undergo ALND or, at least, a SLNB at surgery.

  - Multiagent chemotherapy, similar to regimens utilized in the adjuvant setting, are administered for several cycles before surgery; 20–30% pathologic complete response expected with modern taxane-containing regimens; the NSABP B-27 regimen consisting of four cycles of AC followed by four cycles of docetaxel prior to breast surgery is popular amongst U.S. oncologists; radiation and endocrine therapy as indicated postoperatively; patients who experience a complete pathologic response have superior outcomes to those with a partial pathologic response; patients with hormone-negative BC have superior response to neoadjuvant chemotherapy compared to hormone-positive BC, but have a lower overall survival due to early systemic relapse.

  - Postmenopausal patients with strongly ER-positive tumors may be treated with neoadjuvant endocrine therapy, preferably anastrozole or letrozole, based on published data.

  - Patients with HER2/*neu*-positive LABC should receive neoadjuvant trastuzumab-containing regimens; Buzdar *et al.* reported a very high pathologic complete response (pCR) rate (65%) with a concurrent trastuzumab and epirubicin-containing regimen with minimal cardiotoxicity—caution needs to be exercised if anthracyclines are administered with trastuzumab, although epirubicin is less cardiotoxic than doxorubicin.

  - Patients with minimal or no response to neoadjuvant chemotherapy can be administered preoperative radiation to improve resectability; patients at high risk of relapse can be considered for radiation with concomitant capecitabine as a radiation sensitizer.

- Indications for postmastectomy radiation to the chest wall and regional nodes generally include four or more positive axillary nodes (and consideration for one to three positive nodes); tumor >5 cm with or without one to three positive nodes; positive postmastectomy margins.

- Inflammatory BC: a subset of stage III BC and the most aggressive type of BC; multimodality therapy consisting of neoadjuvant multiagent chemotherapy, mastectomy, and radiation produce 5-year survival rates approaching 40%; most cases are hormone negative, but should receive endocrine therapy as indicated and trastuzumab if HER2/neu-positive.

- MBC: with rare exception, MBC is an incurable illness; however, with improving drug therapies, some patients are managed as a chronic disease, especially those with ER-positive BC with predominantly bone/soft-tissue metastasis.

  - The principles of therapy for MBC include preservation of quality of life, limiting treatment-induced toxicity, and prolonging survival.

  - Generally, single-agent chemotherapy regimens are preferred due to improved tolerability and less toxicity compared to doublet regimens; with the exception of gemcitabine–paclitaxel and capecitabine–docetaxel, multiagent regimens do not provide significant survival benefit compared to single-drug regimens and add significant toxicity.

  - Because treatment is palliative, patients typically should be offered treatment holidays to limit toxicity; many oncologists will treat with a few cycles past optimal response, until undue toxicity develops or until progression occurs.

  - There is no standard-of-care chemotherapy regimen, although the most active single-agents include anthracyclines, taxanes, vinorelbine, and capecitabine; patients with HER2/neu-positive BC should receive trastuzumab, alone or with chemotherapy, until progression occurs, at which time the combination of lapatanib (dual inhibitor of EGFR and HER2/neu) and capecitabine should be considered (produced improved progression-free survival but not overall survival in recent trial of trastuzumab-refractory MBC); platinum salts may be effective in triple-negative patients.

  - Recent phase III trial of paclitaxel and bevacizumab demonstrated improved progression-free survival compared to paclitaxel alone in treatment-naïve MBC patients.

  - Patients with hormone-positive MBC should receive endocrine therapy as first-line treatment unless vital organs are involved ("visceral crisis"), with response rates and disease-control rates of 30–40% and 50–70%, respectively; premenopausal patients should be treated with tamoxifen and ovarian ablation via oophorectomy and GnRH analogues should be strongly considered; postmenopausal patients should receive an AI in doses listed above; patients who progress on first-line therapy can be offered an alternative AI, fulvestrant (pure estrogen-antagonist), progestins, or high-dose estradiol.

○ Adjuncts to treating MBC include bisphosphonates (zoledronic acid 4 mg IV monthly [or dose-adjusted for renal dysfunction] or pamidronate 60–90 mg IV monthly) for bone metastases to improve pain and decrease risk of fracture or surgical intervention; narcotic analgesic for pain; palliative radiation to symptomatic sites of disease; resection or stereotactic radiation for solitary brain metastasis; intrathecal methotrexate (via Ommaya reservoir preferred) for leptomeningeal metastasis; hematopoietic growth factors (darbopoietin 500 mcg subcutaneous every 4 weeks, erythropoietin 40,000–60,000 Units weekly, pegfilgrastim 6 mg following myelosuppresive chemotherapy) for chemotherapy-induced cytopenias.

COMPLICATIONS OF TREATMENT

- Surgery: complications include infection, seroma formation, nerve injury, postmastectomy pain syndromes, poor cosmesis, chronic lymphedema, infection/cellulitis, angiosarcoma (rare) following ALND, and psychologic issues.
- Radiation: acute complications include fatigue, nausea, moist skin desquamation, edema, pain; long-term complications include skin telangiectasia, lymphedema, and increased risk of angiosarcoma.
- Chemotherapy: typical side-effects for each agent will not be discussed; however, some unique chemotherapy-related complications in BC patients include:
  ○ Cardiotoxicity: anthracyclines (cumulative dose >350–400 mg/m^2 doxorubicin), trastuzumab (3–4% as monotherapy, 10–15% with concurrent anthracycline).
  ○ Chemotherapy-related myelodysplastic syndrome: early onset (2–3 years) following anthracyclines and later onset (5–7 years) following cyclophosphamide.
  ○ Peripheral neuropathy: taxanes (especially paclitaxel), vinorelbine, cisplatin.
  ○ Hand-foot syndrome: capecitabine, liposomal doxorubicin, docetaxel.
  ○ Premature menopause: especially alkylating agents.
- Estrogen-deprivation therapy, dependent on drug class:
  ○ Tamoxifen: hot-flushes, vaginal dryness and/or discharge, edema, emotional lability, fatigue, uterine cancer (<2%), cataracts, thromboembolic complications; tumor-flare phenomenon in patients with bulky disease (bone pain, hypercalcemia, urine retention, spinal cord compression).
  ○ Aromatase inhibitors: asthenia, nausea, diarrhea, hot-flushes, dry skin, arthralgia/myalgias (20–30%), edema, flulike symptoms, carpal tunnel syndrome, osteopenia, increased fracture risk.
- Bisphosphonates: flulike illness (myalgias, fevers, fatigue), hypocalcemia, hypophosphatemia, renal dysfunction (zoledronic acid), and ONJ.

Table 7–2 Regimens for BC*

Adjuvant

HER2/*neu*-negative

Dose-dense AC→paclitaxel: doxorubicin 60 mg/m² IV day 1 and cyclophosphamide 600 mg/m² IV day 1 every 14 days × 4 cycles followed by paclitaxel 175 mg/m² IV every 14 days × 4 cycles; all cycles followed by filgrastim support; alternative weekly dosing of paclitaxel (without growth-factor support): 80 mg/m² IV weekly × 12 cycles

TAC: docetaxel 75 mg/m² IV day 1, doxorubicin 50 mg/m² IV day 1, cyclophosphamide 500 mg/m² IV day 1 every 21 days × 6 cycles with filgrastim support

AC: doxorubicin 60 mg/m² IV day 1 and cyclophosphamide 600 mg/m² IV day 1 every 21 days × 4 cycles

TC: docetaxel 75 mg/m² IV day 1 and cyclophosphamide 600 mg/m² IV day 1 every 21 days × 4–6 cycles

AC→docetaxel: doxorubicin 60 mg/m² IV day 1 and cyclophosphamide 600 mg/m² IV day 1 every 21 days × 4 cycles followed by docetaxel 100 mg/m² IV day 1 every 21 days × 4 cycles

CMF: cyclophosphamide 100 mg/m² by mouth days 1–14, methotrexate 40 mg/m² IV days 1,8, 5-FU 600 mg/m² IV days 1,8 every 28 days × 6 cycles

HER2/*neu*-positive

AC→weekly paclitaxel with trastuzumab: doxorubicin 60 mg/m² IV day 1 and cyclophosphamide 600 mg/m² IV day 1 every 21 days × 4 cycles followed by paclitaxel 80 mg/m² IV weekly × 12 weeks with trastuzumab 4 mg/kg IV with first dose paclitaxel then 2 mg/kg IV weekly for total of 52 weeks; alternatively, 6 mg/kg IV every 3 weeks after weekly paclitaxel/trastuzumab

Dose-dense AC→paclitaxel with trastuzumab: doxorubicin 60 mg/m² IV day 1 and cyclophosphamide 600 mg/m² IV day 1 every 14 days × 4 cycles followed by paclitaxel 175 mg/m² IV day 1 every 14 days × 4 cycles (with filgrastim support) and trastuzumab 4 mg/kg IV with first dose paclitaxel then 2 mg/kg IV weekly for total of 52 weeks; alternatively, 6 mg/kg IV every 3 weeks after paclitaxel

TCH: docetaxel 75 mg/m² IV day 1 and carboplatin AUC 6 IV day 1 every 21 days × 6 cycles with trastuzumab 4 mg/kg IV week 1 then 2 mg/kg IV weekly × 17 weeks then 6 mg/kg IV every 3 weeks to complete 52 weeks

Neoadjuvant

HER2/*neu*-negative

AC→docetaxel (NSABP B-27): doxorubicin 60 mg/m² IV and cyclophosphamide 600 mg/m² IV day 1 every 21 days × 4 cycles followed by docetaxel 100 mg/m² IV day 1 every 21 days × 4 cycles followed by surgery several weeks later

HER2/*neu*-positive

Paclitaxel→FEC with trastuzumab : trastuzumab 4 mg/kg IV prior to first paclitaxel dose then 2 mg/kg weekly × 23 weeks; paclitaxel 225 mg/m² IV via 24-hour infusion every 21 days × 4 cycles OR paclitaxel 80 mg/m² IV weekly × 12 weeks followed by 5-FU 500 mg/m² IV days 1,4, epirubicin 75 mg/m² IV day 1, cyclophosphamide 500 mg/m² IV day 1 every 21 days × 4 cycles

(continued)

Table 7–2 Continued

Metastatic BC

Combination regimens (shown to increase survival in phase III trials)

Gemcitabine 1250 mg/m^2 IV days 1,8 and paclitaxel 175 mg/m^2 IV day 1 every 21 days

Docetaxel 75 mg/m^2 IV day 1 and capecitabine 950 mg/m^2 by mouth twice a day on days 1–14 every 21 days

Regimens for HER2/*neu*-positive MBC*

Paclitaxel 175 mg/m^2 IV day 1 every 21 days or 80 mg/m^2 IV weekly and trastuzumab

Docetaxel 75–100 mg/m^2 IV every 21 days and trastuzumab

Vinorelbine 25 mg/m^2 IV weekly and trastuzumab

Capecitabine 1000 mg/m^2 by mouth twice a day on days 1–14 every 21 days and trastuzumab

Trastuzumab-resistant MBC: capecitabine 1000 mg/m^2 by mouth twice a day on days 1–14 and lapatanib 1250 mg by mouth daily every 21 days

Bevacizumab-containing regimens for HER2/*neu*-negative MBC

Paclitaxel 90 mg/m^2 IV days 1,8,15 and bevacizumab 10 mg/kg IV days 1,15 every 28 days

Single-agent regimens

Doxorubicin 60–75 mg/m^2 IV day 1 every 21 days (if no prior doxorubicin)

Paclitaxel 80 mg/m^2 IV days 1,8,15 every 28 days or 175 mg/m^2 IV day 1 every 21 days

Docetaxel 60–100 mg/m^2 IV every 21 days

Albumin-bound paclitaxel 100–150 mg/m^2 IV days 1,8,15 every 28 days

Gemcitabine 800–1200 mg/m^2 IV days 1,8,15 every 28 days

Vinorelbine 25 mg/m^2 weekly or days 1,8,15 every 28 days

Ixabepilone 40 mg/m^2 IV every 21 days

Capecitabine 1000–1250 mg/m^2 by mouth twice a day on days 1–14 every 21 days

*Trastuzumab component: 4 mg/kg IV day 1 followed by 2 mg/kg IV weekly or 8 mg/kg IV day 1 followed by 6 mg/kg IV every 3 weeks with chemotherapy; can also administer trastuzumab as monotherapy.

FOLLOW-UP

- There are approximately 2.3 million BC survivors in the United States; varying degrees of follow-up are required in these patients to assess for locoregional or distant recurrence, which may be early (within 2 to 3 years) with aggressive tumor phenotypes as triple-negative and HER-2 positive and late (>10 years) in ER-positive tumors.
- History and physical examination every 3 to 6 months for the first 3 years following primary treatment, every 6 months years 4 and 5, and then annually.
- Mammogram 6 months following completion of radiation and then annually.

- In patients with nonmetastatic BC, routine laboratory studies, tumor markers, or imaging tests are NOT indicated for routine follow-up, because this practice does not improve survival; all imaging and laboratory tests should be symptom- or sign-directed.
- Follow-up for complications of treatment, both acute and delayed.
  - Patients on adjuvant AIs should be monitored for osteoporosis/osteopenia with periodic DEXA scans and prescribed vitamin D/calcium supplements and weight-bearing exercise; chemotherapy-induced menopause may also contribute to loss of bone density.
  - Patients on adjuvant tamoxifen should receive yearly gynecologic exams and endometrial biopsy if vaginal bleeding develops; symptomatic treatment of vaginal dryness with nonestrogen lubricants and hot flashes with non-CYP2D6-inhibiting serotonin uptake inhibitors (e.g., venlafaxine) or gabapentin.
  - Post-ALND and postradiation lymphedema should be treated with compression sleeves, occupational therapy, and avoidance of infection; rare patients may develop angiosarcoma, and suspicious lesions should be biopsied.
  - Monitoring of cardiac function should be considered in patients treated heavily with anthracyclines and/or trastuzumab.
  - Peripheral neuropathy from taxanes may be complicated by digital injury, ulceration, or infection; as such, careful instruction regarding hand and foot care is essential.
  - Encouragement of healthy lifestyle and general cancer screening.

PROGNOSIS

- DCIS has excellent long-term survival following mastectomy or BCS.
- Prognosis of BC is multifactorial, with nodal status being most important predictor of long-term survival.
  - 50–70% of node-positive patients relapse without adjuvant systemic therapy, whereas only 25–30% of node-negative patients relapse after locoregional treatment.
  - As a general rule, each additional positive node increases risk of recurrence by several percentage points; patients with >10 nodes have a risk of recurrence and/or metastasis exceeding 80%.
  - Macrometastasis (>2 mm) and micrometastasis (0.2–2.0 mm) carry negative prognostic significance.
- Patients with triple-negative BC have a worse short-term prognosis (3 to 4 years) than ER-positive tumors, which, despite having excellent short-term prognosis, may present with metastatic disease and cause death a decade or more later.
- Young age (<35 years), black race, and triple-negative tumors are adverse prognostic features.
- Patients with CNS metastasis have a median survival of 4 to 6 months; some patients with resectable solitary lesions may survive longer than a year with aggressive treatment.

REFERENCES

Ann Oncol 2002;13:1531.
Ann Oncol 2009;20:1771.
Br J Cancer 1982;45:361.
Clin Cancer Res 2007;13:228.
JAMA 2006;295:2492.
Lancet 2005;365:1687.
N Engl J Med 2004;351:2817.
N Engl J Med 2005;353:1659.
N Engl J Med 2005;353:1673.
N Engl J Med 2005;353:2747.
N Engl J Med 2006;355:2733.
N Engl J Med 2008;358:1663.
Oncol Rev 2009;3:237.
Prim Care Rep 2009;15:69.
Prim Care Rep 2009;15:81.

8 ■ OVARIAN CANCER

BACKGROUND

- Ovarian cancer (OC) is the sixth most common female malignancy, with 21,500 cases and 14,600 deaths estimated in 2009.
- OC is the most common fatal genital malignancy in women, with >90% of cases being epithelial histology.
- The mean age at diagnosis of OC is 60 years, with 80% of cases occurring after age 40.
- Risk factors: family history (one first-degree relative with OC increases risk three to four times), BRCA1/2 mutation, nulliparity, >35 years old at first pregnancy.
- Due to lack of adequate screening tests, OC is often diagnosed at an advanced and incurable stage; despite aggressive treatment, <40% of women are cured.

PATHOBIOLOGY

- Over 80% to 90% of cases of OC are of epithelial histology, arising from the surface of the ovary; other histologies will not be discussed.
  - Clear-cell and mucinous carcinoma epithelial subtypes portend poor prognosis.
- Chronic ovarian epithelial inflammation from years of ovulation may result in cumulative DNA damage and acquisition of the malignant phenotype, although this is not a proven.
- Hereditary syndromes, including mutation/loss of tumor-suppressor BRCA1 and BRCA2 genes and Lynch syndrome due to loss of mismatch DNA repair genes with increased susceptibility to colon, uterus, and ovarian cancer, account for a minority of cases but provide insight into the genetics of the disease.
- OC not only invades local pelvic structures, but characteristically involves all peritoneal surfaces, leading to ascites, bowel obstruction, malnutrition, and pain; transdiaphragmatic migration of malignant ascites results in pleural effusion.

CLINICAL PRESENTATION

- Early stage OC is generally asymptomatic, but pelvic discomfort, urinary symptoms, irregular periods, or constipation may occur; vaginal bleeding is rare.

- Population screening with transvaginal ultrasound and CA-125 levels does not detect disease earlier or reduce mortality from OC.
- Advanced/metastatic OC: pain, increased abdominal girth, tighter-fitting clothing, early satiety, bloating, vomiting, constipation, anorexia, or dyspnea.

PHYSICAL FINDINGS

- Early stage OC patients typically have a normal examination; pelvic mass may be present.
- Advanced/metastatic OC: pelvic mass, rectal mass, palpable mass in cul-de-sac on rectal examination (Blummer shelf), abdominal distention, ascites (umbilical eversion, shifting dullness), dullness to lung percussion (pleural effusion), supraclavicular adenopathy.

DIAGNOSTIC TESTING AND STAGING

- Pelvic ultrasound: complex cystic-solid adnexal mass common; uterine/rectal invasion, hydronephrosis, and ascites may be present.
- Abdomino-pelvic CT: may reveal masses, adenopathy, peritoneal implants, ascites, liver capsule/parenchymal metastases, small bowel obstruction, or pleural effusion; does NOT substitute for surgical staging.
- Chest radiograph: may reveal pleural effusion in stage IV OC.
- Serum CA-125: elevated in 80–85% of cases of OC, although not specific; may be elevated in other conditions that irritate the peritoneum.
- Surgery: laparotomy by a gynecologic-oncologist with a subxiphoid to pubic symphysis incision is standard of care for staging (and treatment) in surgically fit patients.
  - Hysterectomy, bilateral salpingo-oophorectomy, examination/biopsy of pelvic/aortic nodes, examination/biopsy of diaphragm and paracolic gutters, omentectomy, peritoneal washing cytology, and maximal resection of all macroscopic disease to <1–2 cm.
    - Studies reveal patients staged by specialty surgeons have improved surgical staging compared to general surgeons/gynecologists (97% vs. 35%/52%).
  - After surgical staging: 23% stage I, 13% stage II, 47% stage III, 16% stage IV.

Table 8–1 TNM Staging Criteria

Primary tumor (T)
T1: tumor limited to ovary(ies); one ovary, intact capsule, no surface tumor, negative peritoneal washing (1a); both ovaries, intact capsule, no surface tumor, negative peritoneal washing (1b); one or both ovaries with one of the following: ruptured capsule, surface tumor, positive peritoneal washing (1c); **T2:** tumor of one or both ovaries with pelvic involvement; involvement of uterus/tube(s), negative peritoneal washing (2a); involvement of other pelvic tissue, negative peritoneal washing (2b); pelvic involvement (2a or 2b) with positive peritoneal washing (2c); **T3:** tumor involves one or both ovaries with extra-pelvic, peritoneal metastases; microscopic extra-pelvic peritoneal metastases (3a); macroscopic extra-pelvic peritoneal metastases (3b); extra-pelvic peritoneal metastases >2cm in greatest dimension (3c)

Regional lymph nodes (N)
N0: absent; **N1:** present

Distant metastasis (M)
M0: absent; **M1:** present (excludes peritoneal disease)
Note: liver capsule metastases are T3; liver parenchyma metastases are M1; malignant pleural effusion is M1

Stage grouping
Stage I: IA: T1a N0 M0; **IB:** T1b N0 M0; **IC:** T1c N0 M0
Stage II: IIA: T2a N0 M0; **IIB:** T2b N0 M0; **IIC:** T2c N0 M0
Stage III: IIIA: T3a N0 M0; **IIIB:** T3b N0 M0; **IIIC:** T3c N0 M0, Tany N1 M0
Stage IV: Tany Nany M1

TREATMENT

- Surgery: staging surgery as outlined above by a gynecologic-oncologist is the cornerstone of OC management, with attempted maximal debulking of tumor implants to <1 cm.
  - Patients initially inoperable may be rendered operable with three cycles of neoadjuvant taxane/platinum chemotherapy ("interval cytoreduction").
- Chemotherapy.
  - Adequately staged stage IA/B, grade 1 tumors do not require adjuvant chemotherapy; observation may be considered for IA/B, grade 2 tumors; stage IA/B, grade 3 and stage IC should receive adjuvant chemotherapy.
  - Stage II: intravenous carboplatin and paclitaxel for three to six cycles is the most widely used regimen.
  - Stage III/IV: systemic chemotherapy with carboplatin and paclitaxel or carboplatin and docetaxel for six to eight cycles are accepted regimens based on level I data.
  - Stage III patients with minimal disease after debulking who are fit and motivated benefit from intraperitoneal (IP) therapy with cisplatin and paclitaxel.

- GOG 172 demonstrated a 16-month survival advantage to IP therapy (65 vs. 49 months), although had more adverse effects than IV therapy and only 42% completed all six cycles; IV therapy can be offered in patients intolerant to the IP route.
- Maintenance chemotherapy: patients with complete remission after initial treatment may be offered monthly paclitaxel (175 mg/m^2 IV) based on GOG 178, although this is not universally accepted.
- Recurrent disease: most patients with advanced OC will relapse and are categorized according to the duration of the chemotherapy-free interval; there is no standard regimen.
  - Less than 6 months until relapse—platinum-resistant: many of these patients can be treated with single-agent regimens, such as paclitaxel, gemcitabine, topotecan, ifosfamide, capecitabine, oxaliplatin, or liposomal doxorubicin; bevacizumab is being studied; none of these drugs are category 1.
  - More than 6 to 12 months until relapse—platinum-sensitive: phase III data demonstrate improved outcomes with platinum-based combinations with taxanes or gemcitabine; carboplatin/paclitaxel is category 1.
- Palliative therapy: patients with end-stage OC may experience a variety of complications that require palliation.
  - Paracentesis for ascites; thoracentesis/pleurodesis for pleural effusion; nephrostomy/stents for hydronephrosis; gastric tubes/surgery for bowel obstruction; octreotide for vomiting/bowel obstruction.

Table 8–2 Regimens for OC

Initial treatment regimens
Paclitaxel 175 mg/m^2 IV and carboplatin AUC 5–7.5 IV every 21 days × 6 cycles (category 1)
Docetaxel 60–75 mg/m^2 IV and carboplatin AUC 5–6 IV every 21 days × 6 cycles (category 1)
Intraperitoneal (GOG 172) regimen: paclitaxel 135 mg/m^2 IV over 24 hrs day 1; cisplatin 100 mg/m^2 IP day 2; paclitaxel 60 mg/m^2 IP day 8; every 21 days × 6 cycles (category 1)

Recurrent disease
>6-month platinum-free interval: carboplatin/paclitaxel regimen above (category 1); Gemcitabine 1000–1250 mg/m^2 IV day 1,8 and carboplatin AUC 5–6 IV every 21 days
<6-month platinum-free interval: single-agent nonplatinum regimen (e.g., liposomal doxorubicin, gemcitabine, topotecan) although no standard category 1 regimen

COMPLICATIONS OF TREATMENT

- Surgery: ileus, wound infection, venous thromboembolism, myocardial infarction.
- Intraperitoneal chemotherapy: cisplatin-related: nausea, vomiting, neuropathy, renal failure, electrolyte wasting, cytopenia, infection;

catheter-related: infection, abdominal pain, adhesions/bowel obstruction, catheter failure, diarrhea.
- Systemic chemotherapy: all agents cause nausea, vomiting, myelosuppresion, infection; carboplatin: hypersensitivity reactions; cisplatin (IV or IP): renal failure, electrolyte wasting, tinnitus, hearing loss, neuropathy; paclitaxel/docetaxel: myalgia, arthralgia, neuropathy, hypersensitivity reactions, edema; pegylated doxorubicin: stomatitis, hand-foot syndrome; congestive heart failure (uncommon).

FOLLOW-UP CARE

- History, physical, pelvic examination, and CA-125 every 3 months for 2 years, every 3 to 6 months for 3 years, then annually.
- Ultrasound and CT if symptoms indicate recurrence or if CA-125 is rising on serial tests.
- Patients with clinical/radiographic remission with rising CA-125 after initial treatment will typically experience symptoms and/or radiographic disease within 6 months; immediate therapy based on biochemical relapse only does not improve survival.

PROGNOSIS

- 5-year survival correlates with initial surgical staging: stage I, 90% to 95%; stage II, 70% to 80%; stage III, 25% to 50%; stage IV, <5%.
- Extent of residual disease following initial surgical staging affects survival; tumor deposits >2 cm after debulking markedly decrease survival (<18 month survival).
- Tumor grade affects prognosis: 5-year survival for poor-, moderately-, and well-differentiated cancers is 88%, 58%, 27%, respectively.

REFERENCES

Anticancer Res 2009;29:2803.
Curr Oncol 2007;14:195.
Int J Gynecol Cancer 2008;18:943.
J Clin Oncol 1996;14:1552.
J Clin Oncol 2001;19:1901.
J Clin Oncol 2003;21:3194.
J Natl Cancer Inst 2003;95:105.
N Engl J Med 2006;354:34.
Semin Oncol 1995;22(Suppl 15):1–6.

BACKGROUND

- Melanoma is an aggressive malignant tumor of epithelial surfaces, typically the skin, and is increasing in incidence more rapidly than any solid tumor.
- Approximately 62,000 cases and 8000 deaths annually, with melanoma ranking only second to acute leukemia in terms of loss of potential life years.
- Leading cause of death amongst skin cancers, accounting for 1% to 2% of all cancer deaths.
- Median age at diagnosis is 59 years, with males having a 1 in 53 and females a 1 in 78 lifetime risk.
- Risk factors: family history, BRCA2 mutation carrier, previous melanoma, numerous atypical moles/dysplastic nevi, ultraviolet light, severe/blistering sunburns early in life, intermittent/ intense sun exposure, fair skin/freckles/blue eyes/red hair, immunosuppression or solid organ transplantation.

PATHOBIOLOGY

- Melanoma results from neoplastic transformation of epidermal pigment-producing melanocytes that derive from embryologic neural crest cells.
- Mutations of various genes affecting cell growth/proliferation may occur, including p16/CDKN2A, BRCA2, N-RAS, and B-RAF; targets of emerging treatments.
- Predilection for hematogenous dissemination to any organ, most commonly brain, lungs, bone, and liver; small bowel, bronchus, and eye not infrequent.
- Early micrometastases (even with stage I) may remain dormant and emerge years to decades later.

CLINICAL PRESENTATION

- Patients may notice a new skin, nail, or mucosal lesion, note a change in preexisting mole, or have physician discover at annual skin examination.
- Patient may report adenopathy or symptoms of metastatic disease, such as headache, seizures, weight loss, cough, dyspnea, melena, or abdominal pain.

PHYSICAL FINDINGS

- "ABCDE" of melanoma: <u>A</u>symmetry, <u>B</u>order (typically irregular), <u>C</u>olor (varying shades of brown, black, purple, blue, or pink; may have mixed color); <u>D</u>iameter (>6 mm more likely to be melanoma); <u>E</u>volution (change in appearance of lesion or development of itching or bleeding).
- Four subtypes based on appearance (and histology), in order of frequency:
  - Superficial spreading: accounts for 70% of melanomas; can occur anywhere but often on trunk and extremities; ABCDE rule applies commonly.
  - Nodular: rapidly enlarging, nodular lesion; often blue or black; the ABCDE rule does NOT apply to nodular melanoma; may not produce pigment—"amelanotic" melanoma.
  - Lentigo maligna: more common in elderly; manifests as hyperpigmented macule on sun-exposed skin, especially head, neck, distal extremities.
  - Acral lentiginous: more common in blacks, Hispanics, and Asians; manifests as discolored, irregular plaque/macule on palm, sole, or nail bed.
- Metastatic melanoma: focal neurologic findings with brain metastases; hepatomegaly/tenderness with liver metastases; pleural effusion with lung metastases; supraclavicular adenopathy.

DIAGNOSTIC TESTING AND STAGING

- Adequate biopsy of any suspicious skin lesion is mandatory and should follow several principles.
  - Biopsy deep enough (to the dermis) by either a punch tool or scalpel with careful attention to orient the incision longitudinal to the limb; shave biopsy should generally be avoided; excisional biopsy with 1–3 mm margins is acceptable for small lesions.
- The biopsy report should include the following:
  - Accurate T stage with reporting of Breslow level (I–V) for stage 1 tumors (<1 mm) and margin status
  - Mitotic rate: more than six mitoses per high-power field is negative prognosticator.
  - Presence or absence of ulceration is a negative prognosticator.
  - Miscellaneous features: vertical growth phase, presence of tumor-infiltrating lymphocytes, and regression
- SLNB is recommended if tumor >1 mm and is most important risk-stratifying procedure; <5% false-negative rate.
  - Number of positive nodes, total number of nodes, extracapsular extension, size of tumor in sentinel node(s).
  - 5% to 30% of clinical stage I–II melanoma (no palpable nodes) patients having SLNB will be upstaged to stage III based on presence of micrometastases (better prognosis than macrometastases).
- For lesions <1 mm thick, imaging is unnecessary (especially PET scan).

- Routine blood studies such as CBC and LDH and chest radiography are of low diagnostic yield in patients with stage I–II melanoma but are typically obtained in node-positive patients (stage III) to screen for metastatic disease.
- CT imaging studies are not routinely indicated in stage I and II melanoma; <5% of patients with clinically negative nodes and a positive SLNB (stage IIIA) will have evidence of metastases on CT imaging; 4% to 16% of patients with clinically positive nodes with positive SLNB have metastases on CT imaging.
- PET imaging is not indicated for stage I and most cases of stage II node-negative melanoma, but may be considered in stage IIC–III patients with worrisome symptoms, palpable adenopathy, or abnormal labs; 98% sensitivity for detection of lymph node metastases in some series and accurate to detect bone metastases.
- FNA is suggested in a patient presenting with clinical stage III disease (palpable adenopathy); if tumor is present, complete node dissection is warranted without SLNB.
- Cerebral imaging, preferably with MRI, should be considered in patients with headache or neurologic symptoms due to the propensity of melanoma to metastasize to the CNS.

Table 9–1 TNM Staging Criteria

Primary tumor (T)
T1: tumor ≤1 mm thick (Clark II/III) without ulceration (1a) or ≤1 mm thick (Clark IV/V) with ulceration (1b); **T2:** tumor 1.01–2.0 mm thick without ulceration (2a) or with ulceration (2b); **T3:** tumor 2.01–4.0 mm thick without ulceration (3a) or with ulceration (3b); **T4:** tumor >4 mm thick without ulceration (4a) or with ulceration (4b)

Regional lymph nodes (N)
N0: none involved; **N1:** metastasis in one node microscopic (1a) or macroscopic (1b); **N2:** metastases in 2–3 nodes microscopic (2a) or macroscopic (2b); satellite or in-transit metastases without nodal metastases (2c); **N3:** metastases in ≥4 regional nodes, matted nodes, in-transit metastasis, or satellite metastasis

Distant metastases (M)
M0: none; **M1:** metastases to skin, subcutaneous tissue, or distant nodes (1a) or lung (1b) or all other visceral sites or any site with elevated LDH (1c)

Stage grouping
Stage IA: T1a, N0 M0
Stage IB: T1b/T2a N0 M0
Stage IIA: T2b/3a N0 M0
Stage IIB: T3b/4a N0 M0
Stage IIC: T4b N0 M0
Stage IIIA: T1–4a N1a–2a M0
Stage IIIB: T1–4b N1a–2a M0 T1–4a N1b–2b M0 T1–4a/b N2c M0
Stage IIIC: T1–4b N1b–2b M0 Tany N3 M0
Stage IV: Tany Nany M1

TREATMENT

- Wide local excision with margin depending on tumor thickness:
  - ≤1.0 mm: 1-cm margin.
  - 1.01–2.0 mm: 1- to 2-cm margin.
  - 2.01–4 mm (and >4 mm): 2-cm margin.
- SLNB (as described) for tumors >1 mm thick or <1 mm thick with adverse features such as high mitotic rate and young age; if positive, a complete anatomic nodal dissection in regional basin; immediate lymphadenectomy confers survival benefit over delayed lymphadenectomy.
- Adjuvant interferon (IFN): recent meta-analyses have shown disease-free and overall survival benefit of 7% and 3%, respectively, in patients with stage IIB/C and III melanoma treated for 1 year with high-dose IFN.
  - 20 million units/m² IV 5 days per week for 4 weeks followed by 10 million units/m² subcutaneously three times per week for 48 weeks.
- Radiation therapy to nodal basin may be considered if significant nodal disease (IIIC).
- Brain metastases: surgical resection or stereotactic radiosurgery for one to three metastases followed by whole-brain radiation may prolong survival and improve quality of life; diffuse metastases derive limited benefit from radiation, with survival often measured in weeks.
- Dacarbazine considered standard reference drug, but temozolomide has similar response rates of 10% to 20% and duration of response of 3 months; temozolomide crosses blood–brain barrier.
- Other agents with activity include carboplatin, cisplatin, vinblastine, and paclitaxel, although benefit is modest.
- No proven survival benefit and added toxicity with combination drug regimens.
- Metastatic melanoma is incurable, although a few patients may achieve a durable, prolonged remission with high-dose interleukin (IL)-2; 720,000 IU/kg IV every 8 hours for up to 14 doses on days 1 through 5 and 15 through 19; repeat at 6- to 12-week intervals.

Table 9–2 Regimens for Metastatic Melanoma (Category 2b)

High dose IL-2: 720,000 Units/kg IV every 8 hours for up to 14 doses days 1–5 and 15–19; may repeat at 6- to 12-week intervals
Dacarbazine 250 mg/m² IV days 1–5 every 21 days or 850 mg/m² IV day 1 every 4–6 weeks
Temozolomide 150–200 mg/m² by mouth days 1–5 every 28 days

COMPLICATIONS OF TREATMENT

- IFN: fever, headache, myalgia, arthralgia, anorexia, nausea, vomiting, fatigue, depression, suicide, transaminitis, anemia, leucopenia, thrombocytopenia, hypothyroidism, hypertriglyceridemia.
- High-dose IL-2: fever, chills, myalgias, anorexia, vomiting, headache, capillary-leak syndrome (hypotension, edema, effusions, tachycardia, oliguria, acute renal failure), myelosuppression, hepatitis, delirium/confusion, rash, hypothyroidism/hyperthyroidism.
- Chemotherapy: fatigue, nausea, vomiting, alopecia, cytopenia, febrile neutropenia, infection, neuropathy.

FOLLOW-UP CARE

- History and physical examination most important components of surveillance after primary treatment; interval not well defined, but consider every 3 to 6 months for 5 years, then annually.
  - Attention to scar for recurrence; restaging and excision appropriate.
  - Attention to proximal lymphatic drainage pattern for in-transit recurrence; restaging with excision should be considered.
  - Attention to regional nodal basins for recurrence; FNA or node biopsy and restaging indicated with excision of recurrence or complete node dissection if not done previously; radiation should be considered.
  - Total skin examination annually to detect new lesions.
- No proven benefit for routine laboratory monitoring, but reasonable to consider periodic chest radiograph and LDH if >1 mm tumor.
  - Imaging studies (e.g., CT, PET, MRI) should be based on symptoms and/or signs of recurrence or considered in patients at high risk for recurrence (e.g., higher than stage IIB), but no data to show impact on survival.
- Patient education: skin self-examination, sun avoidance, sunscreens, long sleeves, hats, sunglasses.

PROGNOSIS

- Prognosis correlates with stage/tumor thickness at diagnosis: tumors <1 mm thick, 5-year survival of >90%; presence of regional node metastases, 5-year survival of 20% to 70%; stage IV disease, 5-year survival of <10%.
- Prognosis affected by primary site: favorable sites include forearm and leg; unfavorable sites include scalp, hands, feet, trunk, and mucous membranes.
- Brain metastases portend very poor prognosis with survival typically in the range of 2 to 6 months.

REFERENCES

Ann Oncol 2009;20S:14.
Cancer Chemotherap Rep 1970;54:119.
Cancer Control 2009;16:248.
J Clin Oncol 1996;14:7.
J Clin Oncol 1999;17:2105.
J Clin Oncol 2000;18:158.
J Clin Oncol 2004;22:53.
N Engl J Med 2006;355:1307.

BACKGROUND

- Carcinoma of unknown primary (CUP) is a biopsy-proven epithelial malignancy for which no obvious site of origin can be identified after a comprehensive evaluation, including history, physical examination, blood testing, and various imaging procedures, such as CT, ultrasonography, and endoscopy.
  - A primary tumor is discovered in <50% of patients at autopsy.
- CUP is one of the 10 most common malignancies, accounting for approximately 3% to 5% of all cancer diagnoses and approximately 31,000 annual cases.
- CUP is more common in males, with a mean age of 60 years.
- Excluding histologies such as melanoma, lymphoma, and germ cell cancer is important, because these malignancies have stage- and histology-based therapies that often portend a different prognosis.

PATHOBIOLOGY

- CUP is a biologically heterogeneous group of malignancies that generally follow an aggressive and fatal course.
- 50% to 60% of cases of CUP consist of moderately or well-differentiated adenocarcinomas; 30% poorly differentiated/undifferentiated carcinomas; and the remainder squamous cell or neuroendocrine carcinomas.
- The reason some cancers manifest as CUP is unclear, but proposed mechanisms include regression or immune destruction of the primary cancer after metastatic seeding, dominance of an early metastatic clone, or the presence of a very small undetectable primary tumor mass.
- CUP has metastatic affinity for the liver, bones, lungs, and nodes; over 50% of patients have multiple metastatic sites.
- CUP tumors possess several chromosomal abnormalities and/or overexpression of certain tumor-promoting genes, such as RAS, BCL-2, and p53.
- The presence of isochomosome 12p, i(12)p, occurs in approximately 25% of patients with poorly differentiated CUP involving midline structures and has a more favorable prognosis.
- Other favorable histologic subsets of CUP include:
  - Female with papillary adenocarcinoma of peritoneal cavity.
  - Female with adenocarcinoma of axillary nodes.
  - Squamous carcinoma of neck nodes or inguinal nodes.

- Male with adenocarcinoma and blastic bone metastases.
- Poorly differentiated neuroendocrine carcinoma.
- Immunohistochemistry plays a vital role in diagnosis of CUP subtypes; a detailed discussion is beyond the scope of this text, but salient points include:
    - Most CUP tumors are positive for anticytokeratin antibody CAM5.2 and epithelial membrane antigen (EMA) and negative for S-100 (melanoma) and LCA (lymphoma).
    - Immunostaining for various cytokeratins (CK), most often CK7 and CK20, may assist in narrowing the primary site.
        - CK7-positive: lung, ovary, uterus, breast, stomach, pancreas, biliary tree.
        - CK20-positive: colon, stomach, pancreas, biliary, Merkel cell, urothelial.
        - Combinations of CK7 and CK20 are often used to narrow the primary site (e.g., lung typically CK7+/CK20– and colon CK7–/CK20+), although no pattern is diagnostic.
        - Prostate, liver, and kidney cancer are CK7–/CK20–.
- Thyroid transcription factor (TTF-1) is positive in approximately 50% to 60% of lung cancers and most thyroid cancers.
- Gross cystic disease fibrous protein (GCGFP)-15 is found in most breast cancers; ER and PR receptors suggest breast or endometrial primary CUP.
- Thyroglobulin is specific for thyroid cancers (follicular and papillary).

CLINICAL PRESENTATION

- Patients with metastatic CUP may present with fatigue, weight loss, anorexia, back pain, abdominal pain, gastrointestinal bleeding, dyspnea, hematuria, or cough.

PHYSICAL FINDINGS

- Physical examination of the CUP patient should focus on excluding a favorable prognostic primary site by evaluating for the presence of isolated cervical, axillary, or inguinal adenopathy, adnexal mass, or ascites.

DIAGNOSTIC TESTS AND STAGING

- A thorough history and physical examination with attention to the breasts, prostate, testes, vagina, cervix, adenxa, anus, rectum, skin, oral cavity, and thyroid is mandatory to exclude a known primary site that would affect treatment decisions.

- Radiographic studies: chest radiography and CT scan of the chest, abdomen, and pelvis are indicated in most patients; mammography and/or breast MRI in women with axillary adenopathy without breast mass; PET scan may be useful in select patients and identify a primary site in up to 50% of cases.
- Endoscopy (generally limited to symptomatic patients or those with abnormal laboratory tests that predict a high yield): bronchoscopy, esophagogastroduodenoscopy, colonoscopy.
  - Patients with isolated squamous cell CUP should undergo nasopharyngoscopy, laryngoscopy, bronchoscopy, and random biopsies of the base of the tongue, the tonsils, and the pyriform sinus.
- Tumor markers are generally nonspecific, but ones that may be considered include CA 27–29 (breast), CEA (colorectal), CA 19–9 (pancreatic/biliary), and CA 125 (ovary/peritoneal); an elevated PSA is specific for prostate cancer and increased levels of LDH, β-HCG, and AFP suggest a germ cell cancer.
- There is no specific staging system for CUP.

TREATMENT

- Patients with favorable subtypes benefit from disease-specific treatment.
  - Midline poorly differentiated CUP: treat as metastatic testicular cancer.
  - Female with papillary adenocarcinoma of peritoneal cavity: treat as advanced ovarian cancer.
  - Female with isolated axillary adenocarcinoma: treat as node-positive breast cancer.
  - Squamous cell cancer of cervical nodes: treat as locally advanced head and neck cancer.
  - Male with high PSA and blastic bone lesions: treat as metastatic prostate cancer.
  - Isolated inguinal nodes: inguinal node dissection and cisplatin-based chemotherapy.
- Patients with disseminated adeno-CUP may have prolonged survival and improved quality of life with platinum and taxane- or gemcitabine-based chemotherapy regimens, although no level I data exist because most data are based on institutional phase II trials; metastatic squamous CUP may benefit from fluorouracil–platinum, with or without taxane.
- Poorly differentiated neuroendocrine CUP often responds favorably to etoposide and cisplatin/carboplatin; hepatic transarterial chemoembolization (TACE) may be of benefit if significant liver metastases are present; patients with diarrhea may respond to depot-octreotide.

Table 10–1 Regimens for CUP (Typically Based on Category 3 Evidence)

Paclitaxel 200 mg/m^2 IV day 1 and carboplatin AUC 5–6 IV day 1 +/– etoposide 100 mg^2 IV days 1–3 every 21 days
Cisplatin 100 mg/m^2 IV day 1 and etoposide 100 mg/m^2 IV days 1–5 every 21 days
Gemcitabine 1000 mg/m^2 IV day 1 and 8 and cisplatin 75–100 mg/m^2 IV day 1 every 21 days

COMPLICATIONS OF TREATMENT

- In most cases, long-term complications are not a significant issue due to the short median survival.
- Acute complications of chemotherapy include cytopenia and infection (all agents); peripheral neuropathy (taxanes and cisplatin); tinnitus/hearing loss (cisplatin); renal failure/electrolyte-wasting (cisplatin); edema/capillary-leak syndrome (gemcitabine).

FOLLOW-UP CARE

- History and physical every 3 months for the first 3 years in surviving patients; diagnostic testing is based on symptoms and abnormal physical findings.

PROGNOSIS

- Median survival for CUP is 6 to 9 months in most series; progression after first-line chemotherapy is dismal, with survival typically measured in weeks.
- Patients with the above favorable subsets (especially those with midline cancers) may enjoy a prolonged survival; however, most patients remain incurable and ultimately die of their disease.

REFERENCES

Ann Oncol 2003;14:191.
Cancer 2004;100:1257.
Cancer 2000;89:2655.
Cancer 1982;50:2751.
Crit Rev Oncol Hematol 2009;69:271.
J Clin Oncol 1997;15:2385.

BACKGROUND

- Pancreatic carcinoma (PC) arises from the ductal epithelium of the pancreas and is the most aggressive visceral neoplasm.
- Approximately 33,700 cases and 33,200 deaths annually in the United States, with most deaths occurring within 2 years of diagnosis; 5-year survival only 5%.
- Median age at diagnosis 72 years; more common in males and blacks.
- Risk factors: smoking, chronic pancreatitis, first-degree relative with PC, familial syndromes (BRCA2, melanoma-mole syndrome, von Hippel Lindau, Lynch II syndrome, Gardner syndrome), perhaps diabetes (may be a manifestation of PC rather than a risk factor).

PATHOBIOLOGY

- Mutation of the KRAS oncogene found in majority of cases of PC; results in malignant transformation/proliferation.
- Loss of function of tumor-suppressor genes p53, CDKN2A, and BRCA2.
- Anatomic proximity of the pancreas to celiac trunk, portal vein, celiac plexus, and bile ducts responsible for clinical manifestations and determinants of resectability.

CLINICAL PRESENTATION

- Tumors involving pancreatic head present with painless jaundice and may be resectable.
- Tumors involving body and tail present after disease is unresectable with symptoms of abdominal or back pain.
- Adenocarcinoma cells may liberate procoagulants, resulting in disseminated intravascular coagulation (DIC), venous thrombosis, and cardiac valve vegetations.
- Weight loss, fatigue, dark urine, pruritis, nausea, vomiting, and anorexia are common.

PHYSICAL FINDINGS

- Icterus common with pancreatic head tumors; wasting, supraclavicular adenopathy (Virchow node), abdominal mass, palpable gallbladder

(Courvoisier sign), hepatosplenomegaly, or ascites may occur in some patients.

DIAGNOSTIC TESTS AND STAGING

- Abdominal ultrasound: useful initial test; may reveal pancreatic mass, biliary dilation, ascites, or hepatosplenomegaly.
- CT scan: more accurate than ultrasound but requires oral and IV contrast; modern helical multislice scanners improve diagnosis.
  - Pancreatic mass, biliary dilation, vascular invasion (portal, splenic, or mesenteric veins and/or celiac or superior mesenteric arteries), adenopathy, ascites, liver metastases.
  - CT-guided tissue biopsy; concern for seeding of needle tract exists.
- Endoscopic retrograde cholangiopancreatography (ERCP): invasive test that injects contrast into pancreatic duct via side-arm endoscope—typical finding in PC is stricture/filling defect; allows brushing for cytology and placement of palliative stent.
- Magnetic resonance cholangiopancreatography (MRCP): similar sensitivity to ERCP; noninvasive; does not allow tissue sampling.
- PET/CT: perhaps most useful to assess for distant metastases.
- Endoscopic ultrasound (EUS): emerging as diagnostic test of choice for T and N staging with accuracy of 78% to 94% and 64% to 82%, respectively, assessing for vessel invasion, and FNA of mass or nodes (less risk of needle-tract seeding than CT biopsy); more accurate than CT for smaller tumors (<3 cm).
- Diagnostic laparoscopy: often used to exclude peritoneal, liver, or other intraabdominal disease that would preclude morbid surgery.
- Serum tumor markers: CA 19–9, 70% to 80% sensitivity and specificity; higher levels portend worse prognosis; declining values suggestive of treatment response.

Table 11–1 TNM Staging Criteria

Primary tumor (T)
T1: tumor limited to pancreas, <2 cm; **T2:** tumor limited to pancreas, >2cm; **T3:** tumor extends beyond pancreas but not involving celiac axis or superior mesenteric artery; **T4:** tumor involves celiac axis and/or superior mesenteric artery (unresectable)

Regional lymph nodes (N)
N0: node metastases absent; **N1:** node metastases present

Distant metastases (M)
M0: absent; **M1:** present

Stage grouping
Stage I: T1–2 N0 M0
Stage II: T3 N0 M0; T1–3 N1 M0
Stage III: T4 Nany M0
Stage IV: Tany Nany M1

TREATMENT

- Surgery: the only chance for cure of PC is aggressive surgical resection, but only 10% to 20% of patients are candidates (stages I/II); the Whipple procedure, or pancreaticoduodenectomy, is procedure of choice for head/uncinate lesions and consists of resection of:
  - Proximal pancreas, duodenum, proximal jejunum, common bile duct, gallbladder, partial gastrectomy with creation of gastrojejunostomy and biliary anastomosis.
- Adjuvant treatment: somewhat controversial; different approaches in Europe and United States, with Europe favoring chemotherapy alone and the United States favoring combined chemotherapy and radiation following resection.
  - Phase III German trial showed adjuvant gemcitabine superior to surgery alone even with R1 resection; favored among European oncologists.
  - Phase III U.S. trials have shown benefit (mainly for head tumors) for neoadjuvant gemcitabine followed by 5-FU and radiation followed by gemcitabine compared to 5-FU and radiation; median survival of 20.5 months and 3-year survival of 31%; favored among U.S. oncologists.
- Chemoradiation for locally advanced/unresectable (stage III) PC: continuous-infusion 5-FU and radiation is most commonly utilized regimen, although recent data supports gemcitabine and radiation combinations.
- Chemotherapy for metastatic PC: palliative gemcitabine improves quality of life and survival in many patients with PC.
  - Several randomized trials have established monotherapy with nucleoside analogue, gemcitabine, to be reference standard; landmark 1997 trial of gemcitabine vs. 5-FU showed median survival of 5.7 vs. 4.4 months and 1-year survival of 18% vs. 2%, respectively; although few clinical responses, less pain and more weight gain in gemcitabine group.
  - Recent randomized trials have shown addition of the tyrosine kinase inhibitor erlotonib or capecitabine may increase survival when added to gemcitabine, albeit to a small degree.
- Palliative procedures: biliary stent to relieve pruritus and prevent cholangitis; celiac plexus block/ablation via CT or EUS guidance; duodenal stent for obstruction; intestinal bypass in fit patients.

COMPLICATIONS OF TREATMENT

- Surgery: wound infection, bile leak, gastrojejunal anastomosis leak, thromboembolism, heart failure.
- Chemoradiation: nausea, vomiting, diarrhea (radiation enteritis), weight loss, fatigue, cytopenia, hand-foot syndrome.
- Gemcitabine: cytopenia (especially thrombocytopenia), edema, capillary-leak syndrome (hypotension, edema, body cavity effusions), nausea, vomiting, diarrhea, flulike syndrome, pneumonitis, thrombotic microangiopathy (rare).

Table 11–2 Regimens for PCNSL

Adjuvant
Gemcitabine 1000 mg/m^2 IV day 1,8,15 every 28 days for 6 cycles
5-fluorouracil 250 mg/m^2/day by continuous infusion prior to radiation; 1–2 weeks later, same dose daily during radiation 50.4 Gy; followed 3–5 weeks later by same infusional dose 4 weeks off 2 weeks on 2 weeks off for 2 cycles
RTOG 9704: gemcitabine 1000 mg/m^2 IV weekly for 3 weeks prior to radiation; 1–2 weeks later, 5-FU 250 mg/m^2/day IV continuous infusion during radiation 50.4 Gy; followed 3–5 weeks later by gemcitabine 1000 mg/m^2 IV day 1,8,15 every 28 days for 3 cycles

Chemoradiation/chemotherapy for unresectable PC
5-FU as continuous infusion (200–250 mg/m^2 IV daily) during radiation treatment
Gemcitabine 1000 mg/m^2 IV weekly for 7 weeks followed by 1 week rest then day 1,8,15 every 28 days

Palliative/metastatic
Gemcitabine 1000 mg/m^2 IV weekly for 7 weeks; 1 week rest then day 1,8,15 every 28 days
Gemcitabine and capecitabine (GEM-CAP): gemcitabine 1000 mg/m^2 by mouth days 1,8,15 and capecitabine 830 mg/m^2 by mouth days 1–21 every 28 days
Gemcitabine and erlotinib: gemcitabine monotherapy regimen above and erlotonib 100 mg by mouth daily

- Fluoropyrimidines: diarrhea, mucositis, hand-foot syndrome, cytopenias, nausea, vomiting, cerebellar toxicity, hyperbilirubinemia, angina (rare).
- Erlotinib: acneiform rash, dry skin, diarrhea, nausea, pneumonitis (cough, fever, infiltrates, rare but may be fatal), anorexia, conjunctivitis.

FOLLOW-UP CARE

- Following resection, PC has a 50% to 85% relapse rate, usually locoregionally or in the liver.
- History, physical examination, bilirubin, liver enzymes, and CA 19–9 should be performed every 3 months after adjuvant treatment.
- CT scans should be considered every 3 to 6 months for the first 2 years.

PROGNOSIS

- 5-year survival for resected patients is 5% to 25%; patients with tumors <3 cm, negative surgical margins (R0), and negative nodes have best prognosis.
- Median survival of approximately 4 to 7.5 months for unresectable or metastatic disease treated with gemcitabine-based regimens; 1-year survival of 18% for stage IV treated with gemcitabine.
- 5-year survival <5%.

REFERENCES

Cancer Treat Rev 2009;35:335.
JAMA 2008;299:1019.
JAMA 2007;297:267.
J Clin Oncol 2005;23:16S.
J Clin Oncol 1997;15:2403.
Proc ECCO 2005;15:abstract II.

12 ■ CHOLANGIOCARCINOMA

BACKGROUND

- Cholangiocarcinoma (CC) is a highly malignant neoplasm arising from the intrahepatic and/or extrahepatic biliary ductal system (this does not include the gallbladder and ampulla of Vater, which will not be discussed).
- CC is rare, with 9200 cases and 3300 deaths annually.
- CC is most common in females >50 years of age.
- Risk factors: primary sclerosing cholangitis associated with inflammatory bowel disease, primary biliary cirrhosis, choledochal cysts (Caroli disease), chronic biliary infection, liver flukes, hepatitis B and C infection, choledocholithiasis, toxins (e.g., dioxin, thorotrast, asbestos), obesity.

PATHOBIOLOGY

- Chronic biliary obstruction and/or inflammation induce local release of cytokines that cause malignant transformation of biliary epithelium.
- Malignant transformation is a multistep process of proliferative stimuli, escape from apoptosis, and response to angiogenesis resulting from mutations in oncogenes and tumor-suppressor genes such as K-RAS, c-MYC, BCL-2, and p53.
- >90% of CC are adenocarcinomas, often mucin-producing and expressing cytokeratin (CK) 7.
- CC may develop within the liver (intrahepatic CC, 10%), the hilum/bifurcation of right and left hepatic ducts (Klatskin tumor, 50% to 60%), or distal extrahepatic ducts (20% to 30%).
- CC results in early invasion of adjacent organs such as the liver, nodes, portal vein, hepatic artery, or neural plexi.

CLINICAL PRESENTATION

- Most patients present with jaundice and abdominal pain; nausea, vomiting, fatigue, pruritis, acholic stools, and weight loss are common.
- Bleeding into the bile ducts (hemobilia) may result in silver-colored stools.

PHYSICAL FINDINGS

- Cachexia, jaundice, abdominal tenderness, hepatomegaly, supraclavicular adenopathy, skin excoriation from itching.

DIAGNOSTIC TESTS AND STAGING

- Serum chemistries: alkaline phosphatase, bilirubin, liver transaminases often elevated.
- Ultrasound: >90% sensitivity to detect biliary obstruction; may reveal mass and/or portal adenopathy.
- Abdominal triple-phase helical CT scan: can detect CC >1 cm and invasion of vasculature and adjacent organs—features that may preclude resection (60% accurate).
  - CT-guided biopsy of mass for diagnosis.
- ERCP and percutaneous transhepatic cholangiography (PTC): acquisition of cytologic specimens and insertion of stent for drainage.
- MRCP: noninvasive and as accurate as ERCP, but cannot obtain biopsy.
- MRI: perhaps best overall imaging study for CC; can identify vessel invasion and liver metastases.
- PET: may detect metastases as small as 1 cm, especially when fused with CT images.
- Laparoscopy: tissue diagnosis and to exclude metastases that preclude resection.
- CA 19–9 and CEA are often elevated but nonspecific; CA 19–9 >100 U/mL is very suggestive of CC.

Table 12–1 TNM Staging Criteria (Intrahepatic Bile Ducts)

Primary tumor (T): **T1:** solitary tumor, no vascular invasion; **T2:** solitary tumor with vascular invasion or multiple tumors <5 cm; **T3:** multiple tumors >5cm or invasion of major branch of portal vein or hepatic vein(s); **T4:** Tumor(s) with invasion of adjacent organs other than gallbladder of perforation of visceral peritoneum
Regional lymph nodes (N): N0: node metastases absent; **N1:** node metastases present
Distant metastases (M): M0: absent; **M1:** present
Stage grouping
Stage I: T1 N0 M0
Stage II: T2 N0 M0
Stage III: **IIIA:** T3 N0 M0; **IIIB:** T4 N0 M0; **IIIC:** Tany N1 M0
Stage IV: Tany Nany M1

TREATMENT

- Surgical resection is only potential for cure; however, radiologic criteria that preclude surgery include: bilateral hepatic duct invasion to secondary radicles; encasement of proximal portal vein; hepatic lobe atrophy; invasion of superior mesenteric artery or both hepatic arteries; and distant metastases.
- Resectability should be determined by a multidisciplinary team consisting of a radiologist, hepatobiliary surgeon or surgical oncologist,

Table 12-2 TNM Staging Criteria (Extrahepatic Bile Ducts)

Primary tumor (T): T1: tumor histologically confined to bile duct; **T2:** tumor invades beyond bile duct; **T3:** tumor invades liver, gallbladder, pancreas, ipsilateral branches of portal vein or hepatic artery; **T4:** tumor invades any of these: main portal vein/branches, common hepatic artery, adjacent organs (colon, stomach, duodenum)

Regional lymph nodes (N): N0: node metastases absent; **N1:** node metastases present

Distant metastases (M): M0: absent; **M1:** present

Stage grouping

Stage I: IA: T1 N0 M0; **IB:** T2 N0 M0
Stage II: IIA: T3 N0 M0; **IIB:** T1-3 N1 M0
Stage III: T4 Nany M0
Stage IV: Tany Nany M1

gastroenterologist, and oncologist; in addition to imaging studies, respectability may require laparoscopy to exclude liver or peritoneal metastasis.

- Adjuvant fluoropyrimidine-based chemoradiation or chemotherapy (e.g., 5-FU or gemcitabine) is often administered because gross residual disease (R2), positive nodes, and positive surgical margins (R1) are often present, and, even with an R0 resection, local recurrence is common; however, no proven benefit for adjuvant chemotherapy.
- Unresectable CC can be treated with fluoropyrimide-based chemoradiation (although no proof of benefit exists), gemcitabine-based chemotherapy, fluoropyrimidine-based chemotherapy, or supportive care, such as stent placement for patients with poor performance status.
- There is no well-accepted standard-of-care chemotherapy regimen for advanced or metastatic CC, although a 2009 study will likely change this. Valle *et al.* reported a randomized phase II/III trial showing a 3.5-month survival benefit with gemcitabine and cisplatin compared to gemcitabine alone.

Table 12-3 Chemotherapy Regimens for CC

Gemcitabine 1000 mg/m^2 IV day 1,8 and cisplatin 25 mg/m^2 IV day 1,8 every 21 days
Gemcitabine 1000 mg/m^2 IV day 1,8,15 every 28 days
Gemcitabine 1000 mg/m^2 IV day 1,8 and capecitabine 650 mg/m^2 by mouth twice a day on days 1-14 every 21 days
Gemcitabine 1000 mg/m^2 IV day 1 and oxaliplatin 100 mg/m^2 IV day 1 every 14 days
Capecitabine 825-1000 mg/m^2 by mouth twice a day on days 1-14 every 21 days

COMPLICATIONS OF TREATMENT

- Surgery: death, infection, bleeding, myocardial infarction, venous thromboembolism, visceral fistulae, ileus.

- Chemotherapy: nausea/vomiting (all agents), neuropathy (cisplatin), electrolyte wasting/acute renal failure (cisplatin), diarrhea/mucositis (fluoropyrimidines), cytopenias (all agents), edema/capillary leak (gemcitabine), pneumonitis (gemcitabine).

FOLLOW-UP CARE

- Patients treated with resection with or without chemoradiation, should be followed every 3 to 6 months for 2 to 3 years with history, physical examination, and measurement of CA19–9; abdominal CT every 6 months for 2 years may be considered; no evidence supports any specific follow-up.
- Rising CA 19–9 and/or CEA often indicate local or metastatic recurrence.

PROGNOSIS

- The 5-year survival is 5% to 10%; patients with an R0 resection of early stage disease may experience prolonged survival.
  - 75% of patients die within 1 year of diagnosis, often due to biliary sepsis.
- Median survival is 18 to 30 months for intrahepatic CC and 12 to 24 months for hilar CC.
- Survival correlates with tumor grade: 10 months for well-differentiated and 2 months for anaplastic/undifferentiated cancers.

REFERENCES

Ann Oncol 2004;15:1339.
Cancer 2004;101:578.
Cancer Lett 2007;250:155.
Crit Rev Hematol Oncol 2009;69:259.
J Clin Oncol 2009;27(15suppl):Abstr 4503.
J Clin Oncol 2005;23:2332.
J Gastrointest Surg 2004;8:90.
Oncologist 2008;13:415.

13 ■ HEPATOCELLULAR CARCINOMA

BACKGROUND

- Hepatocellular carcinoma (HCC) is the leading global cause of cancer mortality, resulting in over 1 million annual deaths.
  - Endemic hepatitis B infection causes most cases in Asia and Africa, and hepatitis C is the leading cause in the North America, Europe, and Japan.
- Approximately 19,000 cases and 17,000 deaths in United States annually; most U.S. cases result from hepatitis C, alcohol, or nonalcoholic steatohepatitis (NASH), most often in the setting of cirrhosis or abnormal liver histology.
- Most cases occur in men > 55 years with chronic liver disease; 3:1 male to female ratio.
- <25% of HCC are resectable; screening with biannual AFP and hepatic ultrasound in at-risk patients has shown earlier detection and improved outcomes in some studies.
- Risk factors: cirrhosis of any cause, hepatitis B/C infection, alcohol, hemochromatosis, androgenic steroids, smoking, thorotrast, autoimmune hepatitis, NASH, primary biliary cirrhosis, α-1-antitrypsin deficiency, Wilson disease, porphyria, aflatoxins.

PATHOBIOLOGY

- Excluding fibrolamellar variant is vital, because this occurs in young patients without cirrhosis and has better prognosis than typical HCC.
- May be multifocal or unifocal; angiotrophic neoplasm with invasion of hepatic veins or vena cava common.
- Chronic liver inflammation from infections, toxins, or metabolic disorders may result in DNA damage, hepatocyte transformation, and acquisition of malignant phenotype.
- HCC may produce growth factors and cytokines that result in paraneoplastic syndromes such as erythrocytosis, hypoglycemia, hyperglycemia, hyperlipidemia, and thrombocytosis.

CLINICAL PRESENTATION

- Symptoms of cirrhosis may predominate and make diagnosis difficult; common symptoms of HCC include abdominal pain, anorexia, weight loss, vomiting, and worsening ascites.

- Acute tumor necrosis and rupture may lead to hemoperitoneum with acute abdomen, shock, and death.

PHYSICAL FINDINGS

- Hepatomegaly or palpable liver mass, bruit, splenomegaly.
- Stigmata of liver disease/cirrhosis: gynecomastia, spider angiomata, ascites, edema, skin excoriation, jaundice, palmar erythema, dilated abdominal wall veins.

DIAGNOSTIC TESTS AND STAGING

- Ultrasound: excellent initial study to identify mass, hypervascularity, portal vein invasion, tumor thrombus.
- Helical/triphasic CT scan: rapid-contrast bolus; perhaps best imaging test to asses vascularity and vascular invasion.
  - Three contrast phases: arterial, portal venous, and delayed venous phase; intense arterial enhancement followed by contrast washout in delayed venous phase is highly suggestive of HCC.
  - Typical enhancement pattern of >2 cm mass on triphasic CT with AFP >200 ng/mL diagnostic of HCC without biopsy.
- MRI: similar accuracy to CT for staging and assessing vessel involvement.
- Biopsy: not necessary if classic CT findings and elevated AFP; CT-guided biopsy may be necessary in some.

Table 13–1 TNM Staging Criteria

Primary tumor (T)
T1: solitary tumor without vessel invasion; **T2:** solitary tumor with vessel invasion or multiple tumors <5cm; **T3:** multiple tumors >5 cm or tumor invading major branch of portal/hepatic vein(s); **T4:** tumor(s) directly invading organs other than gallbladder or with perforated visceral peritoneum

Regional lymph nodes (N)
N0: node metastases absent; **N1:** node metastases present

Distant metastases (M)
M0: absent; **M1:** present

Stage grouping
Stage I: T1 N0 M0
Stage II: T2 N0 M0
Stage III: IIIA: T3 N0 M0; **IIIB:** T4 N0 M0; **IIIC:** Tany N1 M0
Stage IV: Tany Nany M1

- Liver enzymes, bilirubin, alkaline phosphatase, albumin, prothrombin time, creatinine, BUN, CBC/platelet count, AFP (elevated in 50% of HCC in United States).
- Hepatitis B and C serologies, ferritin/transferrin saturation, and genetic testing if hemochromotosis is suspected; specific tests for other uncommon etiologies as indicated.
- Chest radiograph or CT and bone scan if metastases suspected.
- Evaluation of hepatic reserve in surgical candidates.
  - Model for End Stage Liver Disease (MELD) score: objective scoring equation based on bilirubin, creatinine, INR.
- The TNM system is shown in Table 13–1; however, other staging systems such as the CLIP and Okuda are often utilized.

TREATMENT

- Surgical resection is treatment of choice for stage I/II HCC with adequate liver function; most cases unresectable due to invasion of portal vein, celiac artery, severe cirrhosis, or multifocal tumor.
- Liver transplantation considered in setting of unilobar or bilobar HCC or cirrhosis in suitable patients (stage I/II HCC); therapeutic for cirrhosis.
- Transarterial chemoembolization (TACE): arterial catheter inserted into hepatic artery for delivery of chemotherapy (e.g., doxorubicin, cisplatin) and embolizing agent; may result in prolonged survival in some patients with >5 cm unresectable HCC; occluded main portal vein or decompensated liver disease are contraindications.
- Radiofrequency ablation (RFA): percutaneous/laparascopic placement of heat probe into tumor generates high local temperatures and necrosis of tumors <4–5 cm.
- Percutaneous ethanol injection: may benefit some patients with solitary tumor <3–5 cm.
- Cytotoxic chemotherapy without benefit for vast majority of patients; single-agent doxorubicin most widely used without demonstrated survival benefit.
- Sorafenib: an oral tyrosine kinase inhibitor of vascular endothelial growth factor receptor is new standard therapy for advanced/metastatic HCC based on phase III data.
  - 400 mg orally twice a day: 46-week versus 34-week survival versus placebo (p=0.00058).
  - Avoid with hyperbilirubinemia or severe liver dysfunction.

COMPLICATIONS OF TREATMENT

- Hepatectomy: 5% to 10% mortality; liver failure, infection, bleeding, thromboembolism.
- TACE: fever, abdominal pain, nausea, vomiting, cholecystitis, portal vein occlusion, bone marrow suppression.

- "Postembolization syndrome" common: fever, abdominal pain, ileus.
- Sorafenib: hypertension, rash, hand-foot syndrome, diarrhea, bleeding, epistaxis, fatigue, cytopenia, hypophosphatemia.

FOLLOW-UP CARE

- No standard regimen; history, physical examination, serum AFP, and imaging studies every 3 to 6 months is reasonable.

PROGNOSIS

- Patients with advanced tumors exhibiting unfavorable features (vascular invasion, extrahepatic disease, symptoms) have a median survival of 4 months.
- Underlying liver disease makes survival data difficult to interpret because many patients die of cirrhosis.
- Some patients with resectable tumors or liver transplant may enjoy prolonged survival (50% to 70% 5-year survival).
- Properly selected TACE patients may have 1 and 2 year survival of 82% and 63%, respectively.
- 5-year survival of up to 50% in patients with solitary HCC treated with ablation therapies.

REFERENCES

Am J Med 2007;120:194.
Hepatology 2005;42:1208.
Lancet 2002;359:1734.
N Engl J Med 2008;357:378.
N Engl J Med 1996;334:693.
Radiology 2008;247:260.

14 ■ ESOPHAGEAL CANCER

- Esophageal cancer (EC) is a virulent malignancy that consists of adeno-carcinoma and squamous cell carcinoma.
- Often presents in advanced or metastatic stage due to lack of serosa, which normally serves to contain tumor.
- Adenocarcinoma is increasing in incidence more rapidly than any solid-organ neoplasm in the United States, especially among middle-aged white males; squamous cell is less common and predominantly affects elderly black males with significant exposure to alcohol and/or smoking.
  - The most common site of adenocarcinoma is the lower-third of the esophagus or the gastroesophageal (GE) junction.
  - Incidence rates vary geographically; EC is especially common in Asia, southern/eastern Africa, and Northern France.
- There are approximately 16,500 cases and 14,000 deaths annually in the United States due to EC.
- Risk factors for adenocarcinoma: chronic gastroesophageal reflux, Barrett's esophagus, obesity.
  - Barrett's most important risk; defined as presence of metaplastic glandular epithelium involving distal esophagus; >50% to 60% of adenocarcinomas have evidence of Barrett's.
- Risk factors for squamous cell carcinoma: smoking, alcohol, tylosis, lye/caustic injury, Plummer-Vinson syndrome, achalasia, radiation, nitrates, long-term very hot tea.

PATHOBIOLOGY

- Chronic irritation from alcohol, very hot tea, or smoking plays a role in squamous cell EC pathogenesis; prior caustic injury may induce scar formation and later malignant squamous transformation.
- Long-term reflux of gastric contents leads to glandular metaplasia, dysplasia, and malignant transformation; aneuploidy and p53 mutations are common.

CLINICAL PRESENTATION

- Dysphagia (initially for solids) and weight loss very common; odynophagia or choking may occur.

- Vomiting, nausea, chest/upper abdominal pain, hematemesis, cough and fever (if tracheoesophageal fistula [TEF]).

PHYSICAL FINDINGS

- Normal with early stage disease.
- Metastatic disease: supraclavicular/cervical adenopathy, pallor, cachexia, ascites, hepatomegaly.

DIAGNOSTIC TESTS AND STAGING

- Endoscopy to determine tumor location and type of GE junction EC: type I, infiltrates GE junction from above; type II, arises from GE junction; type III, infiltrates GE junction from below, typically the cardia.
  - Biopsy or brushing for tissue diagnosis.
- Nasopharyngoscopy and bronchoscopy in patients with squamous cell EC because of significant risk of cancer in these areas ("field cancerization").
- Barium esophagram: stricture, intraluminal filling defect with irregular margins, or tracheoesophageal fistula; may miss small cancers; if concern for TEF, utilize gastrograffin to avoid barium aspiration.
- CT scan of chest and upper abdomen: determination of node involvement, local invasion, or metastases.
- PET/CT: more accurate than CT at determining respectability and excluding metastases.
- Endoscopic ultrasound (EUS): very accurate at determining T and N stage; can be used to obtain biopsy of adjacent nodes.

Table 14–1 TNM Staging Criteria

Primary tumor (T)
T1: tumor invades lamina propria or submucosa; **T2:** tumor invades muscularis propria; **T3:** tumor invades adventitia; **T4:** tumor invades adjacent structures/organs

Regional lymph nodes (N)
N0: node metastases absent; **N1:** node metastases present

Distant metastases (M)
M0: absent; **M1:** present
Lower thoracic tumors: M1a: celiac node metastases; **M1b:** other distant metastases
Mid-thoracic tumors: M1a: N/A; **M1b:** nonregional node and/or distant metastases
Upper thoracic tumors: M1a: cervical node metastases; **M1b:** other distant metastases

Stage grouping
Stage I: T1 N0 M0
Stage II: IIA: T2–3 N0 M0; **IIB:** T1–2 N1 M0
Stage III: T3 N1 M0; T4 Nany M0
Stage IV: IVa: Tany Nany M1a; **IVb:** Tany Nany M1b

TREATMENT

- Historically, surgery alone was standard care; recently, meta-analyses support routine use of combined-modality treatment in fit patients.
  - Optimal surgery depends on surgeon's experience; better survival when >11 nodes resected.
- Principles of combined treatment: radiation for preoperative tumor shrinkage; chemotherapy to treat micrometastases; surgery for optimal local control.
- Combined chemoradiation (typically 5-FU and cisplatin) can be utilized as definitive therapy in patients not fit for surgery, administered adjuvantly, or utilized preoperatively (neoadjuvant) to down-stage and treat micrometastases early (trimodality treatment) in patients with stage II/III EC.
  - Meta-analysis (*Lancet Oncol* 2007) showed trimodality treatment improved 2-year survival (HR=0.81, *p*=0.002) and reduced local recurrence compared to surgery alone; this is the preferred method amongst most oncologists.
  - Squamous EC more sensitive to chemoradiation and may not benefit from surgery if adequately treated with chemoradiation; if esophagectomy performed, no chemotherapy indicated if R0 margin resection, regardless of node status.
- Preoperative and postoperative ECF (epirubicin, cisplatin, 5-FU) has shown survival benefit in subgroup of GE junction EC; adjuvant chemotherapy only given if neoadjuvant was administered for GE junction cancers; if margins contain cancer (R1, R2), postoperative chemoradiation may be considered.
- Radiation alone can be considered in very ill patients for palliation, but does not increase survival.
- Metastatic EC is treated with chemotherapy, often with two- or three-drug regimens depending on patient's performance status; response rates may approach 50%.
  - European phase III REAL2 study compared four regimens in patients with advanced esophagogastric cancer (squamous and adenocarcinoma): epirubicin, cisplatin, 5-FU (ECF) or capecitabine (ECX); or epirubicin, oxaliplatin, 5-FU (EOF) or capecitabine (EOX): longer OS with EOX, which was less toxic and more convenient.
  - Unfit patients may receive single-agent taxanes or capecitabine, brachytherapy, stents or laser fulgration for dysphagia, or external-beam radiation.
  - Although palliative chemotherapy does not improve survival, it often improves quality of life.
- Palliative maneuvers: opiate pain control, endoscopic dilation, esophageal stent, or laser fulgration for malignant dysphagia, feeding gastrostomy/jejunostomy.

Table 14–2 Regimens for EC

Neoadjuvant/perioperative

MAGIC trial, GE junction subgroup: (ECF) epirubicin 50 mg/m^2 IV day 1, cisplatin 60 mg/m^2 IV day 1, 5-fluorouracil 200 mg/m^2/day IV continuous infusion on days 1–21; every 21 days for 3 cycles before and after surgery

CALGB 9871: cisplatin 100 mg/m^2 IV day 1 and 5-FU 1000 mg/m^2/day by continuous infusion days 1–4 during weeks 1 and 5 of concurrent radiation (50.4 Gy, 1.8 Gy per fraction); patients with squamous cell carcinoma can be treated with additional chemotherapy during weeks 9 and 13 without surgery with similar outcome

Adjuvant

5-FU 425 mg/m^2 IV day and leucovorin 20 mg/m^2 IV day for 5 days, followed by 4500 cGy radiation with modified doses on first 4 and last 3 days of radiation

Palliative/metastatic

DCF regimen (category 1): docetaxel 75 mg/m^2 IV day 1, cisplatin 75 mg/m^2 IV day 1, 5-FU 750 mg/m^2/day by continuous infusion days 1–4 every 21 days

EOX regimen (category 1): epirubicin 50 mg/m^2 IV day 1, oxaliplatin 130 mg/m^2 IV day 1, capecitabine 625 mg/m^2 by mouth twice a day on days 1–14, every 21 days

FLO regimen: 5-FU 2600 mg/m^2 IV by continuous infusion day 1, leucovorin 200 mg/m^2 IV day 1, oxaliplatin 85 mg/m^2 IV day 1, every 14 days

CapeOx: capecitabine 1000 mg/m^2 by mouth twice a day on days 1–14, oxaliplatin 130 mg/m^2 IV day 1, every 21 days

COMPLICATIONS OF TREATMENT

- Esophagectomy: anastomotic fistula/leak, mediastinitis, empyema, subphrenic abscess, pneumonia, wound infection, sepsis, venous thromboembolism, death (5% to 10%).
- Radiation: esophagitis, oral mucositis, malnutrition, stricture, pneumonitis, dermatitis, fatigue.
- Chemotherapy: cytopenias (all agents), mucositis, neuropathy (platinums, taxanes), electrolyte wasting (cisplatin), deafness (cisplatin), hypersensitivity reactions/rashes (taxanes), diarrhea (taxanes, fluoropyrimidines), hand-foot syndrome (capecitabine).

FOLLOW-UP CARE

- No standard regimen but history, physical examination, and CBC reasonable every 3 months following multimodal treatment; imaging studies such as CT and endoscopy as clinically indicated.

PROGNOSIS

- Overall prognosis for EC is poor, with most patients (>90%) dying of their disease.
- Some studies have shown 5-year survival of 40% with trimodality therapy and median OS of 4.5 years.

REFERENCES

Br J Cancer 2007;96:1348.
Curr Treat Option Oncol 2008;9:375.
J Clin Oncol 2008;26:1435.
Lancet Oncol 2007;8:226.
N Engl J Med 2006;355:11.
N Engl J Med 2001;345:725.
N Engl J Med 1992;326:1593.

15 ■ GASTRIC CANCER

BACKGROUND

- Gastric cancer (GC) is an aggressive cancer with significant worldwide variation—being most common in Japan and China—and is the second leading cause of cancer death in the world.
- Approximately 21,500 cases and 11,000 annual deaths in the United States; incidence has decreased significantly over the last 75 years, possibly due to advancement in food preservation with refrigeration.
- Surgery is the mainstay of curative therapy; only 30% to 50% of patients are resection candidates.
- Risk factors: *Helicobacter pylori* infection, smoking, obesity, dietary nitrates, smoked/salted foods, atrophic gastritis, blood group A, germline mutation of E-cadherin gene (associated with hereditary diffuse gastric cancer).

PATHOBIOLOGY

- Over 80% of GC are adenocarcinomas: divided into two types:
  - Diffuse type: absent cell cohesion, diffusely thickened gastric wall without mass (*linitis plastica*); due to mutation of E-cadherin gene, which codes for cell adhesion protein.
  - Intestinal type: ulcerative, mass-like areas of neoplastic glandular epithelium.
- Loss of gastric acidity (atrophic gastritis, gastrectomy) may lead to overgrowth of bacteria such as *H. pylori* that convert dietary nitrates to carcinogenic nitrites, resulting in cellular/DNA damage and acquisition of malignant phenotype.

CLINICAL PRESENTATION

- Early tumors may be asymptomatic, which allows for unhindered growth and often advanced disease at presentation.
- Abdominal pain, early satiety, nausea, vomiting, hematesis, melena, weight loss, and fatigue are common with advanced/metastatic disease.

PHYSICAL FINDINGS

- Metastatic GC: icterus, supraclavicular nodes, hepatomegaly, ascites, periumbilical mass (Sister Mary Joseph node), palpable ovarian masses (Kruckenberg tumors), mass in cul-de-sac on rectal exam (Blumer's shelf).
- Uncommon findings include acanthosis nigricans and superficial phlebitis.

DIAGNOSTIC TESTS AND STAGING

- Endoscopic evaluation of stomach with biopsy; GC may manifest as a gastric ulcer, which mandates histologic evaluation of any gastric ulcer to exclude neoplasia.
- Determination of respectability with CT or PET scan and EUS; 70% to 80% of resected cases have nodal metastases.
  - CT and/or PET/CT to determine nodal involvement, local organ or vascular invasion, or metastases; PET/CT more accurate than CT alone to detect distant disease; CT is insensitive for detection of peritoneal metastases.
  - EUS is more accurate (65% to 92%) than CT for T and N staging; distinction between T2 and T3 tumors difficult and highly operator dependent.
  - Diagnostic laparoscopy may identify intraabdominal/peritoneal metastases that preclude curative surgery.

Table 15–1 TNM Staging Criteria

Primary tumor (T)
T1: tumor invades lamina propria or submucosa; **T2:** tumor invades muscularis propria (T2a) or subserosa (T2b); **T3:** tumor penetrates visceral peritoneum but not adjacent structures; **T4:** tumor invades adjacent structures (e.g., spleen, colon, liver, diaphragm, pancreas, kidney, etc.)

Regional lymph nodes (N)
N0: node metastases absent; **N1:** metastases in 1–6 nodes; **N2:** metastases in 7–15 nodes; **N3:** metastases in >15 nodes

Distant metastases (M)
M0: absent; **M1:** present

Stage grouping
Stage I: IA: T1 N0 M0; **IB:** T1 N1 M0; T2a/b N0 M0
Stage II: T1 N2 M0; T2a/b N1 M0; T3 N0 M0
Stage III: IIIA: T2a/b N2 M0; T3 N1 M0; T4 N0 M0; **IIIB:** T3 N2 M0
Stage IV: T4 N1–3 M0; T1–3 N3 M0; Tany Nany M1

TREATMENT

- Gastrectomy: goal is R0 resection with adequate resection of regional lymphatics; at least 15 nodes should be harvested; D1 resection should be performed (resection of stomach, omentum, and N1 nodes along the lesser and greater curvatures).
- Perioperative chemotherapy with ECF (epirubicin, cisplatin, 5-FU) before and after surgery (category 1) for resectable GE junction and gastric

cancers improves survival (MAGIC trial); similar regimens based on
REAL2 study also acceptable [epirubicin, oxaliplatin, fluorouracil (EOF),
epirubicin, oxaliplatin, capecitabine (EOX), or epirubicin, cisplatin,
capecitabine (ECX)].
- Postoperative chemoradiation with *fluoropyrimidine*-based regimen
  increases survival and locoregional control demonstrated in INT-0116
  trial (category 1): 5-FU infusion 1 month prior to combined chemoradiation and for 2 months after.
- Traztuzumab: the TOGA trial reported at 2009 American Society of Clinical
  Oncology (ASCO) meeting showed benefit for traztuzumab for HER-2/*neu*
  positive GC; further data awaited.
- Palliative chemotherapy: improves quality of life and survival; category
  1 regimens include DCF (docetaxel, cisplatin, 5-FU), ECF, EOF, ECX, and
  EOX; many other category 2 regimens based on phase II trials; single-
  agent paclitaxel, docetaxel, irinotecan, or capecitabine may induce 10%
  to 25% response rates and be more suitable for frail patients.
- Palliative procedures: gastric bypass and gastrojejunostomy may help
  obstruction; venting gastrostomy; pyloric stent.

Table 15-2 Regimens for GC

Perioperative/neoadjuvant
MAGIC trial: ECF: epirubicin 50 mg/m^2 IV day 1, cisplatin 60 mg/m^2 IV day 1, fluorouracil 200 mg/m^2 IV by continuous infusion days 1–21, every 21 days for 3 cycles before and after surgery (can also consider regimens from REAL2 trial, NEJM, 2008)

Adjuvant
INT 0116: 5-FU 425 mg/m^2/day IV and leucovorin 20 mg/m^2/day IV for 5 days before radiation, followed by 4500 cGy radiation, and bolus 5-FU 400 mg/m^2 IV and LV 20 mg/m^2 IV on first 4 and last 3 days of radiation

Palliative/metastatic
DCF: Docetaxel 75 mg/m^2 IV day 1, cisplatin 75 mg/m^2 IV day 1, 5-FU 750 mg/m^2/day IV by continuous infusion days 1–4, every 21 days
EOX: epirubicin 50 mg/m^2 IV day 1, oxaliplatin 130 mg/m^2 IV day 1, capecitabine 625 mg/m^2 by mouth twice daily days 1–14, every 21 days

COMPLICATIONS OF TREATMENT

- Surgery: anastomotic leak, intraabdominal abscess, wound infection,
  sepsis, respiratory failure, thromboembolism, myocardial infarction.
- Chemoradiation: distal esophagitis/gastritis, stricture, fatigue, myelosuppression.

- Chemotherapy: cytopenias (all agents), vomiting (all agents), neuropathy (cisplatin, oxaliplatin, taxanes), hypersensitivity reactions (taxanes), mucositis (fluoropyrimidines), heart failure (epirubicin), hand-foot syndrome (capecitabine), tumor perforation (rare).

FOLLOW-UP CARE

- There is no standard follow-up protocol following curative-intent surgery or chemoradiation; however, a reasonable approach is history, physical examination, and basic laboratory tests (e.g., CBC, serum chemistries) every 3 to 6 months; imaging with CT or PET/CT should be considered if concern for recurrence exists; endoscopy should be considered if symptoms of local recurrence develop.

PROGNOSIS

- 5-year survival for resected stage I and II GC is 60% and 34%, respectively.
- Survival is better at any stage following R0 resection and when >14 nodes are resected.
- Patients with advanced/metastatic GC treated with ECF, ECX, EOF, or EOX have median survivals of 9.9, 9.9, 9.3, and 11.2 months, respectively.

REFERENCES

Crit Rev Hematol Oncol 2009;70:216.
J Clin Oncol 2007;25:3205.
J Clin Oncol 2006;24:4991.
N Engl J Med 2008;358:36.
N Engl J Med 2006;355:11.
N Engl J Med 2001;345:725.

16 ■ COLORECTAL CANCER

BACKGROUND

- Overall, colorectal cancer (CRC) is the fourth most common cancer and the second leading cause of cancer death in the United States; colon cancer (CC) and rectal cancer (RC) account for approximately 106,000 and 41,000 cases, respectively, with 50,000 annual deaths.
- CRC typically affects patients >50 years, but it may occur in younger patients, in whom diagnosis is often delayed.
- One-third of patients have a relative with CRC; familial syndromes account for a small percentage of patients, but are vital to recognize.
  - Polyposis syndromes: familial adenomatous polyposis (FAP): 0.5% to 1% of CC, dominant inheritance, mutated APC gene on chromosome 5, thousands of colon polyps at young age, 100% incidence of CC if colectomy not performed.
    - Variants: Gardner syndrome (FAP with ampullary cancer, desmoids, and soft tissue/bone tumors); Turcot syndrome (FAP with brain tumors).
  - Nonpolyposis syndromes: hereditary nonpolyposis CC (HNPCC or Lynch syndrome): 5% of CC in patients <50 years of age, CC develops quickly often without polyps, proximal colon predominance, dominant inheritance, mutations in DNA mismatch repair genes (MSH2, MLH1, PMS1, PMS2, MSH6), increased risk for cancers of uterus, small bowel, urothelium, stomach, and bile ducts.
- Risk factors: colon polyps, inflammatory bowel disease, diet high in animal fat and calories, smoking.

PATHOBIOLOGY

- Sporadic CC and RC result from prolonged accumulation of genetic mutations that ultimately result in the cancer phenotype (tumor); this often takes years, which forms the basis of periodic screening colonoscopy.
- Adenocarcinoma accounts for >90% of cases of CC/RC; signet ring and mucinous variants may occur; stain positive for cytokeratin (CK) 20 and usually CDX-2.
- The "adenoma–atypia–carcinoma" sequence is characterized by sequential genetic loss of 5q (APC gene), 18q (K-ras activation, DCC gene inactivation), 17p (p53 inactivation), and 8p; the development of an adenoma may take decades, with invasive cancer often occurring 2 to 5 years later.

- Cyclooxygenase pathway may lead to tumorigenesis—studies of cyclooxygenase inhibitors decrease adenomas in some studies.
- Adenomatous polyps are premalignant, but only 1% become cancerous; synchronous polyps in one-third of patients; prior adenoma increases risk of CC.
- Risk of malignant degeneration of adenomatous polyp related to sessile growth, villous histology, size (1.5–2.5 cm, 2% to 10% risk, >2.5 cm, >10% risk).
- Inflammatory bowel disease (especially ulcerative colitis) patients with pancolitis have higher risk due to continuous inflammation/proliferation leading to DNA damage.
- Detection of tumor KRAS mutation occurs in 40% of patients; renders tumor unresponsive to cetuximab and tanezumab.
- Dietary factors such as high fat intake may increase carcinogenic bile acids, causing cell damage; no evidence that high-fiber diet prevents adenoma recurrence.
    - Obesity increases circulating insulin-like growth factor (IGF-I), which stimulates mucosal proliferation.
- Metastatic spread of CC involves portal vein to the liver as the initial site of distant disease; RC may metastasize to the lungs or supraclavicular nodes bypassing the liver via the paravertebral venous (Batson's) plexus.

CLINICAL PRESENTATION

- Many cases are asymptomatic, discovered on screening colonoscopy or prompted by iron deficiency anemia or detection of occult fecal blood.
- Symptoms of advanced cancer: fatigue, dyspnea, angina, (especially for right-sided cancers because stool is liquid and bleeding often intermittent and slow), abdominal pain, changes in stool caliber, tenesmus, constipation/diarrhea for left-sided/rectosigmoid lesions, which are often obstructing; occasionally, symptoms of obstruction (vomiting, distention) or perforation (acute pain) may be presenting manifestation.

PHYSICAL FINDINGS

- Pallor, smooth tongue, or koilonychia may occur with iron deficiency.
- Abdominal distention/tenderness (obstruction) or rebound tenderness/guarding (perforation).
- Rectal mass may be palpated with low-lying RC.
- Hepatomegaly, jaundice, supraclavicular adenopathy, or ascites may be present with metastatic disease.

DIAGNOSTIC TESTS AND STAGING

- Colonoscopy: ideal test for diagnosis of asymptomatic CC/RC—allows visualization and biopsy; average-risk patients should commence screening at age 50; patients with hereditary syndromes or strong family history should commence screening earlier.

- Presence of adenomatous polyp(s) mandates periodic colonoscopy (every 3 to 5 years since >5 years necessary for cancer to develop).
- Advanced CC/RC may be diagnosed based on symptom-prompted colonoscopy (e.g., pain, weight loss, rectal bleeding, constipation) or iron deficiency anemia.

- Barium enema (air contrast): useful for diagnosis of annular/obstructing cancers; not sensitive for sessile adenomas; biopsy cannot be performed.
- Carcinoembryonic antigen (CEA): although not diagnostic of CC/ RC, elevated levels of CEA preoperatively predict recurrence; rising levels during/after therapy suggest active disease.
- Chest radiograph: may detect lung metastases, especially with RC.
- CT scan of abdomen/pelvis: useful for detection of metastatic disease, bowel obstruction, fistula formation, or perforation.
- PET/CT: increasingly used for preoperative staging to exclude nodal/ systemic metastases; assess for treatment response to neoadjuvant chemotherapy for liver metastasis; postoperative setting to localize site of recurrence with rising CEA level and after radiofrequency ablation (RFA) of liver metastases to assess tumor viability; complete metabolic response shortly after starting chemotherapy may be predictive of favorable outcome.
- EUS: most accurate modality to ascertain T (87% accuracy) and N (74% accuracy) stage for RC, which influences neoadjuvant therapy (≥T3 or node positive receives chemoradiotherapy).
- MRI: useful in staging RC; may reveal involvement of nodes, vessels, mesorectal fascia; predictive of circumferential resection margin (CRM) status.

Table 16–1 TNM Staging Criteria

Primary tumor (T)
T1: tumor invades submucosa; **T2**: tumor invades muscularis propria; **T3**: tumor invades through muscularis propria into subserosa or nonperitonealized tissues; **T4**: tumor perforates visceral peritoneum and/or adjacent organs (other colon segments, bladder, pancreas, stomach)
Regional lymph nodes (N)
N0: node metastases absent; **N1**: metastases in 1–3 nodes; **N2**: metastases in ≥4 nodes
Distant metastases (M)
M0: absent; **M1**: present
Stage grouping
Stage I: T1–2 N0 M0
Stage II: IIA: T3 N0 M0; IIB: T4 N0 M0
Stage III: IIIA: T1–2 N1 M0; IIIB: T3–4 N1 M0; IIIC: Tany N2 M0
Stage IV: Tany Nany M1

TREATMENT

- Colon cancer: surgery is only curative modality for CC—typically subtotal colectomy; resection of >12 nodes vital for adequate staging and also improves prognosis; laparoscopic technique yields similar results to laparotomy, with less blood loss and shorter hospitalization.
  - Although adjuvant chemotherapy for stage II CC is controversial, providing an absolute survival benefit of 2% to 4% (with mortality of 0.5% to 1%), patients with high-risk features may benefit: perforated tumor, lymphovascular invasion, T4 tumor, <12 nodes harvested, or obstruction.
  - Adjuvant chemotherapy demonstrated to benefit patients with stage III CC in several phase III trials; for example, the MOSAIC trial solidified FOLFOX (infusional 5-FU, leucovorin, oxaliplatin) every 2 weeks for 6 months as the standard of care for stage III CC, with an absolute survival benefit of 8% to 10%; although effective in stage IV CRC, irinotecan provides no benefit in adjuvant setting and should NOT be used.
- Rectal cancer: patients with T1 RC may undergo endoscopic mucosal resection (EMR) if an experienced endoscopist available, but local recurrence a concern; patients with stage II/III should receive neoadjuvant chemoradiation, followed by total mesorectal excision (TME), and adjuvant chemotherapy due to higher risk of local recurrence than CC.
  - Preoperative radiation dose of 50.4 Gy in conjunction with infusional 5-FU decreased risk of local recurrence (6% vs. 13%, $p=.006$) and higher sphincter preservation (39% vs. 19%, $p=004$) compared to postoperative chemoradiation (German Rectal Cancer Trial); does not improve survival; surgery should follow chemoradiation by 4 to 8 weeks to allow maximal effect.
    - Current studies investigating role of neoadjuvant treatment with oxaliplatin and cetuximab.
  - TME is standard of care for RC: sharp dissection and removal of rectum *en bloc* with enveloping mesorectal fascia and contents (rectum, nodes, vessels, fat) decreases local recurrence rate to approximately 10%.
  - Patients with complete pathologic response to neoadjuvant chemoradiation (approximately 10% to 15% of patients) have improved prognosis; pathologic involvement of CRM poor prognosticator.
  - Adjuvant chemotherapy for 4 to 6 months administered by many oncologists after surgery; FOLFOX regimen widely utilized.
- Metastatic disease (CC/RC).
  - Approximately 50% to 60% of patients with CRC develop metastases.

- Metastatic CRC is incurable, but survival rates have increased over the last decade from <12 months to approximately 22 to 24 months with modern drugs.
- A variety of drugs are available in the metastatic setting: 5-FU, capecitabine (oral 5-FU prodrug), oxaliplatin (platinum analogue), irinotecan (CPT-11, topoisomerase I inhibitor), bevacizumab (VEGF antibody), cetuximab and panitumumab (both EGFR antibodies); exposure to all drug classes increases median survival.
- FOLFOX and bevacizumab improves survival; FOLFIRI (infusional 5-FU, leucovorin, irinotecan) and bevacizumab provides similar benefit; both regimens can be used first-line, with switch to other at progression; capecitabine substituted for 5-FU may be more convenient without significant decrease in efficacy.
- Cetuximab (chimeric IgG antibody) is only effective for KRAS wild-type tumors; clinicians should consider testing tumor at diagnosis.
  - CRYSTAL trial showed benefit of cetuximab in patients with wild-type KRAS cancers; cetuximab can be used as monotherapy or with irinotecan, even with prior irinotecan use.
  - Panitumumab (human IgG antibody) is indicated for monotherapy only for KRAS wild-type tumors and provides increase in progression-free survival.
- Patients with poor performance status can be treated with single-agent capecitabine; bolus 5-FU is not indicated.
- Mitomycin-C has shown some activity in phase II trial in patients previously treated with 5-FU, oxaliplatin, and irinotecan.
- Resectable liver metastases: patients with liver metastasis can often undergo primary resection or resection following several cycles of "conversion" chemotherapy (e.g., FOLFOX, FOLFIRI), often in conjunction with bevacizumab, if resection status is questionable; although there is no specific number of lesions that precludes resection, preservation of postresection hepatic function is required, as is controlled extrahepatic disease; prolonged chemotherapy can lead to hepatic injury, increasing perioperative complications; bevacizumab should be discontinued several weeks prior to hepatic resection to avoid hemorrhage; postresection chemotherapy should be considered.
- RFA of liver metastases can be considered in patients with severe comorbidity, unfavorable location, or inadequate liver volume for resection.
- Resection of lung metastases should be considered if R0 resection can be performed, there are no widespread metastases, and overall disease is controlled.

Table 16–2 Regimens for CRC

Adjuvant
Modified FOLFOX6: 5-FU 400 mg/m^2 IV day 1, followed by 1200 mg/m^2/day IV continuous infusion for 2 days; leucovorin 400 mg/m^2 IV day 1; oxaliplatin 85 mg/m^2 IV over 2 hours day 1; every 2 weeks for 6 months (may require reduction or cessation of oxaliplatin for severe neuropathy)
XELOX: capecitabine 1000 mg/m^2 by mouth twice a day on days 1–14 and oxaliplatin 130 mg/m^2 IV day 1 every 21 days for 6 months

Neoadjuvant RC
5-FU 225 mg/m^2/day IV continuous infusion during 50.4 Gy radiation
5-FU 1000 mg/m^2/day IV continuous infusion days 1–5 during week 1 and 5 of 50.4 Gy radiation
Capecitabine 825 mg/m^2 by mouth twice daily during 50.4 Gy radiation

Metastatic
Modified FOLFOX6 and bevacizumab: see above + bevacizumab 5 mg/kg IV every 2 weeks
FOLFIRI +/– bevacizumab: 5-FU 400 mg/m^2 IV day 1, followed by 5-FU 1200 mg/m^2/day continuous infusion for 2 days; leucovorin 400 mg/m^2 IV day 1; irinotecan 180 mg/m^2 IV day 1; bevacizumab 5 mg/kg IV; every 2 weeks
CapeOX +/– bevacizumab: capecitabine 850–1000 mg/m^2 by mouth twice daily on days 1–14 and oxaliplatin 130 mg/m^2 IV day 1; bevacizumab 7.5 mg/kg IV day 1; every 3 weeks
Capecitabine: 1000–1250 mg/m^2 by mouth twice daily days 1–14 every 21 days
Irinotecan: 300–350 mg/m^2 IV every 21 days or 180 mg/m^2 IV every 14 days (monotherapy or with cetuximab in KRAS wild-type)
Cetuximab: 400 mg/m^2 IV loading dose then 250 mg/m^2 IV weekly (wild-type KRAS only; monotherapy or with above regimens)
Panitumumab: 6 mg/kg IV every 2 weeks (wild-type KRAS only; monotherapy only)

COMPLICATIONS OF TREATMENT

- Besides surgical complications (e.g., infection, heart failure, thromboembolism), systemic therapy of metastatic CRC may cause several toxicities.
  - 5-FU: mucositis, diarrhea, angina, cytopenia (uncommon), hand-foot syndrome (uncommon), liver dysfunction.
  - Capecitabine: mucositis, diarrhea, hand-foot syndrome, liver dysfunction.
  - Oxaliplatin: cold-induced dysthesia/parasthesia (acute), peripheral neuropathy (dose-limiting symptom; data suggest that IV calcium and magnesium may prevent or ameliorate symptoms), cytopenias, infusion reactions (bronchospasm, chills, hypotension).

- Irinotecan: acute cholinergic diarrhea (prevented with atropine), late diarrhea (may be life-threatening), sepsis, cytopenia (patients with UGT1A1*28 polymorphism have increased risk of severe neutropenia and require dose reduction).
- Bevacizumab: venous/arterial thrombotic events, bleeding, impaired wound healing, hypertension, proteinuria/nephrotic syndrome, reversible posterior leukoencephalopathy.
- Cetuximab/panitumumab: skin rash (scaly or acne-like), infusion reaction such as urticaria, hypotension, bronchospasm, or anaphylaxis, may occur in 1% to 3% of patients; cetuximab infusion reaction more common in Appalachian states (environmental exposure), pulmonary toxicity/interstitial pneumonitis, hypomagnesemia, paronychia.

FOLLOW-UP CARE

- History, physical examination, and CEA every 3 to 6 months for 2 to 3 years and then every 6 months until year 5.
- CT scan of abdomen and pelvis annually for 3 years.
- Colonoscopy at 1 year and then every 3 to 5 years or as clinically indicated.

PROGNOSIS

- Node status (not tumor size) is related to survival; patients with <12 nodes harvested have an inferior prognosis compared to those with >12 nodes harvested.
- Majority of recurrences occur in first 4 years; 5-year survival predictive of cure.
- Poor prognostic factors: perforation, poorly differentiated tumor, aneuploidy, venous invasion, and elevated preoperative CEA; microsatellite instability (MSI) associated with better prognosis; females better prognosis.
- Positive CRM (tumor <1–2 mm from margin) negative prognostic factor for local and distant recurrence and survival for RC; positive CRM, 9% 3-year disease-free survival (DFS) and negative CRM, 52% 3-year DFS.
- 5-year survival rates: stage I, 93%; stage IIA, 85%; stage IIB, 72%; stage IIIA, 83%; stage IIIB, 64%; stage IIIC, 44%; stage IV, 8%.
- Some studies reveal 5- and 10-year survival of 50% to 60% and 25%, respectively, following resection of hepatic metastases.
- Median survival for stage IV CRC approaches 22 to 24 months with modern pharmacologic agents.

REFERENCES

Ann Surg 2006;244:1024.
Crit Rev Hematol Oncol 2009;70:160.
Curr Oncol Rep 2009;11:167.
Eur J Cancer 2009;45:1748.
J Clin Oncol 2005;23:4866.
J Clin Oncol 2004;22:229.
J Nucl Med 2009;50:43S.
N Engl J Med 2004;350:2335.
N Engl J Med 2004;350:2343.
N Engl J Med 2004;351:337.

BACKGROUND

- Anal cancer (AC) is a curable malignancy with multimodality chemotherapy and radiation.
- Approximately 6000 cases and 700 deaths annually in the United States; slightly more common in females; mean age 58 to 65 years, earlier in HIV patients.
- Risk factors: human papillomavirus (HPV-16 or -18 found in 72% of cases), history of anal genital warts, sexually transmitted disease, or anal-receptive intercourse; multiple sexual partners, HIV infection, history of cervix cancer, immunosuppression for solid-organ transplants, smoking.
- Screening for AC in high-risk groups (e.g., HIV patients, history of cervix cancer) includes digital rectal exam (DRE) and anal pap smear; anoscopy if pap smear abnormal.

PATHOBIOLOGY

- Basic anal anatomy: only anal canal/verge cancers will be discussed; cancer of involved perianal skin treated in disease-specific manner.
  - Anal canal is a 4-cm structure surrounded by sphincter muscles, lies distal to rectum from the transition zone (consists of rectal, urothelial, modified nonkeratinized squamous histology) extending to anal verge—area where modified hair-bearing, keratinized, squamous epithelium begins.
    - Tumors may develop from transitional or distal nonkeratinized squamous tissue (anal canal cancer) or perianal skin (anal margin cancer).
    - The pectinate or dentate line is an area of anal valves/sinuses at the transition zone where mucosa changes to exclusive nonkeratinized squamous epithelium.
    - Lymphatic drainage of AC below dentate line involves inguinal nodes; AC above dentate line involves internal iliac node system.
    - AC can spread to the lungs via systemic circulation; metastasis at presentation uncommon (<20%).
- Majority of AC is squamous cell carcinoma, keratinizing and nonkeratinizing, which are treated the same; adenocarcinoma may arise from gland mucosa; rare types include melanoma, small cell carcinoma, sarcoma, and lymphoma.

- Most AC results from HPV infection (types 16, 18, 31, 33, 35) of squamous epithelium; causes metaplasia and neoplasia in multistep process from HPV integration into host genome.
- HIV infection or immunosuppression following organ transplant may prevent host eradication of HPV, allowing chronic infection and malignant transformation.
- Most cases of non-HPV AC harbor *p53* mutation.

CLINICAL PRESENTATION

- Bleeding most common symptom; anal pain, sensation of mass, fecal soilage, loose stools, not uncommon; treatment delay frequent because benign anal problems such as hemorrhoids or fissures common.

PHYSICAL FINDINGS

- Mass lesion protruding from anus may be evident on inspection; often verruciform.
- DRE may detect mass; anoscopy may visualize mass or ulceration.
- Palpable inguinal nodes indicate node involvement or reactive hyperplasia.

DIAGNOSTIC TESTS AND STAGING

- Anoscopy/proctoscopy of anal canal under sedation/anesthesia.
- Incisional biopsy of anal mass; needle aspiration/biopsy of palpable nodes.

Table 17–1 TNM Staging Criteria (Anal Canal)

Primary tumor (T)
T1: tumor ≤2 cm; **T2:** tumor >2 cm but ≤5 cm; **T3:** tumor >5 cm; **T4:** tumor invades adjacent organ(s), (e.g., vagina, urethra, bladder, prostate)
Regional lymph nodes (N)
N0: none; **N1:** metastasis in perirectal nodes; **N2:** metastasis in unilateral internal iliac and/or inguinal node(s); **N3:** metastasis in perirectal and inguinal nodes and/or bilateral internal iliac and/or inguinal nodes
Distant metastasis (M)
M0: absent; **M1:** present
Stage grouping
Stage I: T1 N0 M0
Stage II: T2–3 N0 M0
Stage III: IIIA: T1–3 N1 M0; T4 N0 M0; IIIB: T4 N1 M0; Tany N2–3 M0
Stage IV: Tany Nany M1

- CT of pelvis and abdomen to assess nodal enlargement or invasion of adjacent structures; PET useful for detecting node metastases.
- Chest radiograph to exclude lung metastases, although uncommon at presentation.
- HIV testing if risk-factors.

TREATMENT

- T1 N0 M0 lesions can be treated with wide local excision alone; if sphincter compromised, definitive radiation (or chemoradiation) can be considered.
- Standard-of-care for locally advanced AC is chemoradiation therapy; Nigro *et al.* reported sentinel study of high rate of complete pathologic response with infusional 5-FU/mitomycin-C (MMC) regimen combined with 45 Gy radiotherapy.
  - Chemoradiation decreases local recurrences, cancer-specific mortality, and colostomy-free survival.
  - Treatment interruption for toxicity compromises treatment efficacy; aggressive supportive care for skin, anal, systemic effects vital.
- Salvage therapy for recurrent or progressive disease: locoregional failure reported in up to 40% of patients—correlated with higher T and N stage.
  - Abominoperineal resection (APR) (requires colostomy) with or without platinum–fluorouracil; inguinal node dissection performed if nodes palpable.
  - Clinical relapse isolated to inguinal nodes can be treated with inguinal dissection or inguinal radiation.
  - Systemic metastases treated with cisplatin–flourouracil chemotherapy.

Table 17–2 Chemotherapy Regimens for AC

Localized AC: 5-FU 1000 mg/m^2/day IV by continuous infusion days 1–4, 29–32 and mitomycin-C 10 mg/m^2 IV days 1, 29 of daily radiation to 45 Gy
Metastatic AC: 5-FU 1000 mg/m^2/day IV by continuous infusion days 1–5 and cisplatin 100 mg/m^2 IV day 2; every 28 days

COMPLICATIONS OF TREATMENT

- Acute radiation toxicity: perianal moist desquamative dermatitis, diarrhea, dysuria, hematuria, fatigue, nausea/vomiting, vaginal irritation.
- Late radiation toxicity: fecal incontinence (may require colostomy), rectal/vaginal stricture, fistula formation, telangiectasia, hematochezia, hematuria, vaginal bleeding, anal pruritis, skin ulcers, perianal skin atrophy,

genital/extremity edema, osteoradionecrosis of femoral head(s), second malignancy.
- Mitocycin C toxicity: Myelotoxicity is dose limiting, cumulative, and delayed; nausea/vomiting, vesicant with skin necrosis, thrombotic microangiopathy/thrombotic thrombocytopenic purpura (TTP), interstitial pneumonitis.
- 5-FU toxicity: stomatitis, diarrhea, hand-foot syndrome, angina, cytopenia.
- Cisplatin toxicity: fatigue, nausea/vomiting, tinnitus/hearing loss, neuropathy, electrolyte wasting, cytopenia.

FOLLOW-UP CARE

- DRE 8 to 12 weeks after treatment; if mass palpated or visualized, biopsy indicated; however, early false-positive biopsy may occur because tumor regression may continue for several months following chemoradiation.
  - If biopsy shows residual tumor without clinical progression, close clinical follow-up (4 weeks) indicated: if progression noted, salvage therapy with APR with or without platinum-based chemotherapy; if regression noted, continued frequent monitoring.
- Patients with complete remission should undergo DRE, anoscopy, and inguinal node palpation every 3 to 6 months for 5 years.
- Annual pelvic CT and chest radiography considered for T3/T4 tumors or node-positive disease.

PROGNOSIS

- Primarily related to tumor size and presence of node metastases.
  - <2 cm tumors cured in 80% of patients; >5 cm tumors cured in approximately 50% of patients.
  - 5-year survival of 18% in patients with inguinal node involvement at presentation.
- Most local recurrences occur in 2 years, treated with salvage APR; 5-year survival of 39% to 64% reported, but toxicity high.

REFERENCES

Bull Cancer 1999;86:861.
Cancer 1983;51:1826.
J Clin Oncol 1996;14:2527.
JAMA 2008;299:1914.
Oncol Rev 2009;3:27.
Surg Gynecol Obstet 1985;161:509.

18 ■ GASTROINTESTINAL STROMAL TUMOR

BACKGROUND

- Gastrointestinal stromal tumor (GIST), once classified as leiomyosarcoma of the GI tract, is a distinct neoplasm, characterized by a unique cell phenotype and resistance to cytotoxic chemotherapy.
- GIST is the most common mesenchymal tumor of the GI tract, with approximately 3500 annual cases in the United States.
- Median age at diagnosis 60 years; infrequent before age 40, without gender predilection.

PATHOBIOLOGY

- Recent data suggest GIST arises from mesenchymal stem cells or the interstitial cells of Cajal, pacemaker cells of the GI tract; rarely GIST can arise from mesentery or omentum; may reach extreme size (>20 cm).
- Spindle-shaped histology typical; increased mitoses (>5 per 50 high-power fields [HPF]), hypercellularity, necrosis, nuclear atypia, and mucosal invasion predict more aggressive/malignant behavior.
- GISTs have characteristic immunohistochemistry profile: positive staining for CD117 (*c-kit* proto-oncogene, member of receptor tyrosine kinase family) and CD34 (stem cell marker); negative for S-100 and desmin.
- 85% of GISTs harbor activating mutation of *c-kit* proto-oncogene, which leads to increased cell proliferation; 3% to 5% have mutation in PDGFRα gene; mutation of exon-11 involving *c-kit* confers increased response to imatinib (see below) compared to exon-9 mutation or wild-type *c-kit*.
- GIST location: 65% gastric, 25% small intestine, 10% esophagus, colon, rectum, or extraintestinal.
- 50% of GISTs metastatic at diagnosis; liver and peritoneum most commonly involved sites.

CLINICAL PRESENTATION

- Small (<2 cm) GIST tumors may be asymptomatic or diagnosed incidentally during upper endoscopy.
- GIST may present with hematochezia or melena due to hemorrhagic tendency of these neoplasms.
- Large tumors may result in vomiting, abdominal pain, early satiety, weight loss, fatigue, bowel obstruction, or, rarely, perforation.

PHYSICAL FINDINGS

- Metastatic GIST may manifest with hepatomegaly or abdominal mass; adenopathy is rare.

DIAGNOSTIC TESTS AND STAGING

- GIST often diagnosed during endoscopy for other reasons; may appear "benign" or ulcerated; biopsy for diagnosis with staining for CD117.
- EUS useful for biopsy; preferable to percutaneous biopsy.
- Percutaneous biopsy of GIST should be avoided, because it carries risk of peritoneal seeding or tumor rupture.
- CT scan may show intraabdominal mass or liver metastases; intraabdominal mass without adenopathy suggestive of GIST.
- Chest radiograph to exclude lung metastases.
- PET scan useful to assess for metastasis or response to treatment; decreased flourodeoxyglucose (FDG) uptake may be noted as soon as 24 hours after commencing therapy.

TREATMENT

- Surgical resection for localized GIST is therapy of choice; goal is *en bloc* resection with R0 margins; incomplete resection for palliation if curative resection not possible.
  - Lymphadenectomy unnecessary because node metastases uncommon.
  - Resection of limited metastatic deposits may benefit some patients.
- Imatinib, an oral inhibitor of tyrosine kinases, including *c-kit* and PDGFRα, is drug of choice for metastatic/unresectable GIST.
- Imatinib demonstrated significant activity in patients with metastatic GIST (70% to 80% partial response or stable disease with clinical improvement in 88% to 89% of patients in phase I–II trials); symptomatic improvement may occur within days.
  - Starting dose of 400 mg orally daily with food; patients with exon-9 *c-kit* mutations respond better to 800 mg.
  - Decreased metabolic activity may be noted on PET scan within several days of starting therapy—predictive of CT response at 8 weeks; CT may show necrosis or cystic degeneration without change in size.
- Phase II trials showed benefit with neoadjuvant imatinib 400 mg orally daily in patients with primary or resectable metastatic GIST; consider if tumor reduction would reduce surgical morbidity or if borderline resectability.
- Phase III trial of adjuvant imatinib 400 mg orally daily for 1 year following complete resection of primary GISTs >3 cm demonstrated improved recurrence-free survival compared to placebo (98% vs. 83%, HR=0.35, *p*<.0001); no survival benefit noted thus far.
- GIST may develop imatinib resistance; options include dose escalation to 800 mg orally daily or sunitinib, a multikinase inhibitor (50 mg orally

daily, 28 days on, 14 days off showed benefit compared to placebo in phase III trial).
- GIST tumors radioresistant and unresponsive to conventional chemotherapy, with response rates of <5% to doxorubicin.

COMPLICATIONS OF TREATMENT

- Rarely, tumor rupture and spillage during resection.
- Imatinib: edema (periorbital, extremity), fatigue, nausea, vomiting, diarrhea, myalgias, rash, fluid retention (ascites, pleural effusion, weight gain), myelosuppression, hepatic dysfunction, hypothyroidism, drug interactions.
  - Life-threatening GI or intraabdominal hemorrhage reported in patients with bulky tumor (5% incidence in some series).
- Sunitinib: hypertension, rash, diarrhea, stomatitis, yellow skin, fatigue, bleeding, proteinuria/nephrotic syndrome, cytopenia, hypothyroidism, left ventricle dysfunction, reversible posterior leukoencephalopathy syndrome (RPLS).

FOLLOW-UP CARE

- Most GISTs recur within 3 to 5 years after resection.
- History, physical, and abdominopelvic CT every 3 to 6 months for resected or unresectable disease.
- PET scan may be useful if CT findings equivocal of recurrence.

PROGNOSIS

- Complete (R0) resection of primary GIST has 5-year survival of 48% to 65%.
- Esophageal and gastric GIST have better prognosis than small intestinal GIST.
- Tumors ≤5 cm and < 2 mitoses per 50 HPF have better prognosis; >5 mitoses per HPF, >10 cm tumor, or gastric GIST are independent predictors of postoperative recurrence—adjuvant imatinib for 1 year should be considered.
- Median survival of metastatic and recurrent GIST is 20 and 9 to 12 months, respectively.
- Exon-11 mutation predicts recurrence and shorter 5-year survival (86% vs. 49%).

REFERENCES

Br J Surg 2003;90:1178.
Cancer Res 1999;59:4297.
Lancet 2009;373:1097.
Lancet 2001;358:1421.
N Engl J Med 2002;347:472.

19 ■ THYROID CANCER

BACKGROUND

- For ease of discussion, thyroid cancer (TC) is classified as differentiated (papillary and follicular), medullary, and anaplastic.
- There are approximately 31,000 cases and 1500 deaths annually in the United States; median age at diagnosis and death is 45 and 75 years, respectively.
  - Anaplastic TC more common in females (55% to 77%) in the sixth and seventh decades.
  - Medullary TC may be sporadic (70%) or familial (30%).
- Differentiated cancers account for 90% (80% papillary, 10% follicular), medullary for 5% to 9%, and anaplastic for 1% to 2% of cases of TC.
- The majority of TC are small, <2 cm, and often diagnosed incidentally during imaging studies or thyroid surgery for other indications.
- The only well-established risk factor is radiation exposure, especially during childhood (e.g., Hodgkin's therapy, nuclear accidents); adenomatous polyposis, Cowden's disease, and Gardner's syndrome have increased incidence of differentiated TC.

PATHOBIOLOGY

- Differentiated TC (papillary and follicular): neoplasms of thyroid hormone-producing follicular cells; mutations of BRAF gene and RAS–RAF–MAP kinase signal pathway common; papillary TC tends to spread to local nodes and follicular TC tends to spread to lungs and bone; produce thyroglobulin, which is useful in diagnosis and surveillance of recurrence.
- Medullary TC: neoplasm of neuroendocrine calcitonin-producing parafollicular C-cells; mutation in RET proto-oncogene common; autosomal-dominant familial cases (30%) associated with MEN 2A syndrome (medullary TC, pheochromocytoma, parathyroid hyperplasia), MEN 2B syndrome (medullary TC, pheochromocytoma, ganglioneuromas, marfanoid habitus), or non-MEN familial form (70%).
- Anaplastic TC: often occurs in setting of differentiated TC; histology: numerous mitoses, necrosis, hemorrhage, vessel invasion; does not stain with thyroglobulin; loss of tumor suppressor *p53* common; cells do not uptake iodine; lungs/pleura/bone most common metastatic sites; may be confused histologically with lymphoma.

CLINICAL PRESENTATION

- Differentiated TC: most present as incidental mass during imaging procedures or thyroid resection for other indications; nontender neck mass noted by some patients; metastatic symptoms such as dyspnea or bone pain rare at presentation.
- Medullary TC: painless thyroid/neck mass most common with non-MEN type; adenopathy common; hypercalcitoninemia may cause diarrhea or flushing; adrenocorticotropin hormone (ACTH) production may produce Cushing's syndrome (weight gain, polyuria, weakness); if MEN 2A/B present, symptoms of pheochromocytoma may predominate (paroxysmal tachycardia, headaches, sweating).
- Anaplastic TC: rapid-onset lower neck pain, swelling, erythema; may produce stridor, dysphagia, dyspnea, hemoptysis, or dysphonia due to invasion of local structures.

PHYSICAL FINDINGS

- Well-differentiated TC: nontender thyroid nodule; adenopathy more common with papillary TC.
- Medullary TC: thyroid mass/adenopathy; MEN 2A/B: hypertension if pheochromocytoma present; MEN2B: Marfanoid features, mucosal neuromas (lips and mouth); rare Cushing's syndrome (moon faces, striae, truncal obesity).
- Anaplastic TC: large (3–20 cm), tender, firm, warm, lower neck mass; adenopathy common; vocal cord paralysis often noted on laryngoscopy.

DIAGNOSTIC TESTS AND STAGING

- FNA initial procedure of choice for all types of TC; high sensitivity/specificity.
  - Follicular TC is indistinguishable from follicular adenoma on FNA; definitive diagnosis of follicular TC requires biopsy or thyroidectomy which demonstrate capsular and vascular invasion.
- Neck ultrasound typically reveals isolated thyroid nodule; nuclear thyroid scans not indicated routinely at initial diagnosis.
- Chest imaging (radiograph or CT) if respiratory symptoms present.
- Medullary TC: CT of neck; PET scan to assess for metastases (no role for I^{131} scan); serum calcitonin and CEA; serum/urine catecholamines to screen for pheochromocytoma; serum calcium to screen for hyperparathyroidism; testing for RET oncogene in patient and family if familial syndrome suspected (prophylactic thyroidectomy should be considered for family members with RET mutation).
- Anaplastic TC is typically clinical diagnosis confirmed by FNA/biopsy; stage IV by definition.
  - Thyroid scan is of no value; no iodine uptake by anaplastic cells.

- CT of neck/chest to determine local extent and structure invasion; PET scan accurate to detect distant metastases (present in 50% at presentation).

Table 19–1 TNM Staging Criteria

Primary tumor (T)
T1: tumor <2 cm limited to thyroid; T2: tumor >2 cm but <4 cm limited to thyroid; T3: tumor >4 cm limited to thyroid or any size tumor with extension to sternohyoid or perithyroid soft tissues; T4a: tumor of any size extending beyond capsule invading soft tissue, larynx, trachea, esophagus, or recurrent laryngeal nerve; T4b: tumor invading prevertebral fascia or encasing carotid artery or mediastinal blood vessels Anaplastic TC (all considered stage IV): IVa: intrathyroidal tumor—resectable; IVb: extrathyroidal tumor—unresectable

Regional lymph nodes (N)
N0: no nodal metastases; **N1a:** metastases involving pretracheal, paratracheal, prelaryngeal/Delphinian nodes); **N1b:** metastases involving unilateral, bilateral, or contralateral cervical or superior mediastinal nodes

Distant metastasis (M)
M0: absent; **M1:** present

Stage grouping

Papillary/follicular <45 years
Stage I: Tany Nany M0
Stage II: Tany Nany M1
Papillary/follicular ≥45 years
Stage I: T1 N0 M0
Stage II: T2 N0 M0
Stage III: T3 N0 M0; T1–3 N1a M0
Stage IV: IVa: T4a N0–1a M0; T1–3 N1b M0; T4a N1b M0; IVb: TIVb Nany M0; IVc: Tany Nany M1
Medullary TC
Stage I: T1 N0 M0
Stage II: T2 N0 M0
Stage III: T3 N0 M0; T1–3 N1a M0
Stage IV: IVa: T4a N0–1a M0; T1–3 N1b M0; T4a N1b M0; IVb: T4b Nany M0; IVc: Tany Nany M1
Anaplastic TC: all considered stage IV
Stage IV: IVa: T4a Nany M0; IVb: T4b Nany M0; IVc: Tany Nany M1

TREATMENT

- Differentiated TC.
  - Surgery mainstay: most oncologists recommend total thyroidectomy, although hemithyroidectomy/ismuthectomy may be considered in

young patients with small solitary tumor (<1 cm); postoperative thyrotropin (TSH) suppression with L-thyroxine to minimize tumor growth with goal TSH of <0.1 mU/L.

- Postresection I^{131} ablation: single dose of 100–150 mCi I^{131} to ablate any residual cancer and normal thyroid tissue (removes source of thyroglobulin which aids in surveillance) in patients with tumors >1 cm and/or extrathyroidal involvement; iodinated contrast, high-iodine diet, and inadequate thyrotropin (TSH) suppression with thyroxine diminish efficacy of ablation; repeat dosing for late metastatic disease if lesions concentrate iodine on diagnostic scan.
- Chemotherapy for metastatic palliation: single-agent doxorubicin best-studied drug, with response rates of 15% to 20%; addition of cisplatin increases response rate but not survival.
- Sorafenib (oral VEGF and BRAF inhibitor) being studied for radioactive iodine-refractory disease.
- Radiation therapy for palliation of painful bone metastases.
- Resection of brain metastases improves survival in some patients.

- Medullary TC.
  - Total thyroidectomy with bilateral central compartment node with or without lateral neck dissection for local disease; adjuvant radiation considered for T4 disease; widespread metastases can be treated with sorafenib 400 mg orally twice a day, which may lead to stable disease, symptom improvement, or decreased calcitonin, or chemotherapy (e.g., doxorubicin, cisplatin, dacarbazine), but durable responses uncommon; small molecules being studied; diarrhea from hypercalcitoninemia treated with octreotide or diphenoxylate; no role for radioactive iodine treatment.

- Anaplastic TC.
  - Patients with stage IVa disease may benefit from surgical resection followed by radiation and chemotherapy, although this is not feasible in most patients.
  - Airway management crucial for palliation, because death often occurs by tracheal compression, intraluminal obstruction, or bilateral vocal cord paralysis; immediate radiation to preserve airway; prophylactic tracheostomy does not improve survival and delays radiation; emergent cricotomy may be needed on occasion.
  - Chemotherapy: palliative single-agent doxorubicin is drug of choice with responses of 20%; platinum may increase response but not survival.
  - Multimodal treatment: chemoradiation alone or followed by resection may improve outcome in some patients; optimal regimen unknown.

Table 19–2 Regimens for Anaplastic/Metastatic TC

Doxorubicin 60 mg/m^2 IV day 1 every 21 days
Doxorubicin 60 mg/m^2 IV day 1 and cisplatin 40 mg/m^2 IV day 1, every 21 days

COMPLICATIONS OF TREATMENT

- Thyroidectomy: hypocalcemia from parathyroid loss, hoarseness from recurrent laryngeal nerve injury.
- I^{131} treatment: sialodentitis, thyroiditis, oligospermia, late malignancy.
- Radiation for anaplastic TC: pharyngitis, stomatitis, dermatitis, tracheitis, myelopathy.

FOLLOW-UP CARE

- Medullary TC: serum calcitonin and CEA every 2 to 3 months initially, then yearly; neck and chest imaging with CT can be considered yearly.
- Differentiated TC: periodic thyroglobulin measurements and neck ultrasound; at 1 year, check thyroglobulin after administration of recombinant human thyrotropin—if >2 ng/mL, diagnostic whole-body imaging obtained to search for metastases; if negative, PET scan can detect residual disease in many patients.
  - Metastases that concentrate iodine are treated with I^{131}, with responses of up to 45%.

PROGNOSIS

- Overall, 10-year survival for differentiated TC is 90% and medullary carcinoma 75% to 85%, but 40% if metastases are present; anaplastic TC has a median survival of 4 to 12 months; 5-year survival is essentially nil—most deaths result from airway failure.
- Poor prognostic features for well-differentiated TC include age >45 years, male gender, larger tumor, and extrathyroid extension; regional node metastasis does not decrease survival.
- Patients with metastatic well-differentiated TC may survive for decades with palliative I^{131} and supportive treatment.

REFERENCES

Arch Intern Med 1996;156:2165.
Cancer 1985;56:2155.
Cancer Control 2006;13:119.
Eur J Endocrinol 1998;138:249.
Eur J Surg Oncol 2001;27:260.
Lancet 2003;361:501.
Oncologist 2008;13:539.

- Carcinoid tumors (CT) are a heterogeneous group of malignant neoplasms arising from neuroendocrine cells from a variety of organ systems that are characterized by production, storage, and release of biogenic amines and other regulatory hormones.
- Although CT can arise from obscure sites such as the thymus or ovary, the majority arise from the gastrointestinal (GI) tract (55%) and bronchopulmonary (BP) tract (30%)—these two sites will be the focus of this chapter.
- CT are the most common neuroendocrine neoplasm, with an incidence of approximately two cases per 100,000 persons in the United States annually (2500 cases annually); the incidence has recently increased due to improved diagnosis, although they are frequently noted incidentally at autopsy (up to 1% of autopsies).
- CT are more common in women prior to age 50, but in the elderly there is a higher incidence in males; age-adjusted incidence for CT at any sites is highest for black males (4.5 cases per 100,000 persons).
- Although most CT are asymptomatic or present with localized symptoms, carcinoid syndrome (CS) occurs in only 5% to 10% of patients and depends on tumor location and whether hepatic metastases are present; CS may be confused with other more common disease syndromes and requires a high index of suspicion to diagnose.
- Risk factors: multiple endocrine neoplasia (MEN) type I, neurofibromatosis type I, and first-degree relative with CT.

PATHOBIOLOGY

- CT are often characterized with regards to their anatomic embryologic origin because tumors of similar embryonic origin share biochemical and clinical characteristics; overall, 70% of CT originate from the bronchus, the jejunoileum, or the colorectum.
  - Foregut: thymus, BP tract, stomach, duodenum.
    - Foregut CT typically have low serotonin content and uncommonly cause CS with liver metastases, but are prone to metastasize to bone.
  - Midgut: jejunum, ileum, appendix, Meckel's appendage, ascending colon.
    - Midgut CT synthesize large amounts of serotonin and are especially prone to produce CS with liver metastases; uncommonly metastasize to bone.

- Hindgut: transverse colon and rectum.
  - Hindgut CT rarely synthesize serotonin and do not cause CS with liver metastases; bone metastasis not uncommon.
- CT arise from *enterochromaffin* (Kulchitsky) cells located throughout the epithelium of the GI and BP tracts.
  - *Enterochromaffin* refers to cells that stain with chrome salts, which is typical of serotonin-containing cells; CT cells also silver stain-avid.
  - Immunohistochemical stains are useful in the diagnosis of CT of any site and typically stain positive for one or more of the following: chromagranin A (CgA), neuron specific enolase (NSE), and synaptophysin.
  - Electron microscopy reveals dense-core granules that contain various biogenic amines (e.g., serotonin [5-hydroxytrypatamine, 5-HT], dopamine, histamine), peptides (e.g., atrial natriuretic peptide, CgA, vasoactive intestinal polypeptide [VIP], substance P), and tachykinins (e.g., kallikrein).
    - Serotonin is the most biologically active and predominant substance secreted by CT cells and is synthesized from tryptophan; usurpation of tryptophan into serotonin synthesis leads to depletion of niacin resulting in pellagra.
    - Tryptophan is converted to serotonin (5-HT) by two enzymatic steps that include tryptophan hydroxylase and aromatic L-amino acid decarboxylase; serotonin is then stored in granules and released into the circulation where monoamine oxidase and aldehyde dehydrogenase convert it into the dominant urinary metabolite 5-HIAA (5-hydroxyindoleacetic acid); measurement of urinary 5-HIAA is important in the diagnosis and monitoring of treatment response in patients with CT.
- Some general pathologic principles apply to CT of any anatomic origin: also known as APUDomas (**a**mine **p**recursor **u**ptake **d**ecarboxylation), ultrastructurally contain dense core granules that store biologically active compounds, are histologically similar, the presence/absence of symptoms cannot be predicted based on immunocytochemistry, histologic classifications do not always predict biologic aggressiveness—only tissue invasion or distant metastasis establishes malignancy.
- The CS typically occurs in the presence of liver metastases; normally, the liver inactivates serotonin and its metabolites; however, in the presence of metastatic involvement, hepatic dysfunction and direct release of serotonin into the systemic circulation via the hepatic veins leads to CS; uncommonly, direct release of biogenic compounds into the circulation, bypassing the liver, occurs with foregut (typically bronchial) CT.
- Serotonin interacts with various 5-HT receptors that induce intestinal smooth muscle motility and fluid secretion resulting in diarrhea, a hallmark symptom of CT and CS.
- Serotonin is a fibrogenic amine and may result in significant tissue desmoplasia/fibrosis, which may lead to small bowel obstruction or esenteric vascular encasement and bowel infarction; additionally, tumoral release

of fibrogenic factors, such as transforming growth factor-β and basic fibroblast growth factor, contribute to fibrogenesis.
- Carcinoid heart disease (CHD) may occur in later stages of metastatic CT and typically affects the right-sided cardiac valves and results from deposition of serotonin-induced fibrotic plaques on the tricuspid and pulmonary valves; left-sided cardiac valves are typically not involved because biogenic amines are inactivated in the lungs.
    - The carcinoid plaque consists histologically of smooth muscle cells, myofibroblasts, and elastic tissue and are typically located on the endocardium of the tricuspid and pulmonary valves as well as the right atrium and ventricle.
- Neuroendocrine tumors are classified pathologically into three categories: well-differentiated/indolent (typical CT), moderately differentiated/low-grade malignancy (atypical CT), poorly differentiated tumors/aggressive malignancy (small cell or large cell neuroendocrine tumors).

CLINICAL PRESENTATION

- Although many CT are asymptomatic and discovered incidentally during radiologic procedures, endoscopy, or appendectomy, it is important for the clinician to consider the diagnosis because symptoms can be nonspecific.
- Symptoms of CT can be related to local tumor mass-effect, tumor-induced fibrosis, or release of serotonin and/or other bioactive compounds resulting in CS.
- Tumor-related symptoms include hemoptysis and cough (bronchial CT); abdominal pain, distention, vomiting, melena/hematochezia (gastric, small intestinal, appendiceal, colorectal CT).
    - Small bowel obstruction can occur due to mass causing luminal blockage or intussusceptions.
- Tumor-induced fibrosis symptoms can include vomiting and abdominal pain/distention due to bowel obstruction or abdominal pain, diarrhea, hematochezia, and weight loss due to mesenteric ischemia.
- CS symptoms include paroxysmal skin flushing (typically involving the face, neck, and torso) that may be spontaneous or provoked by alcohol, exercise, emotion, or serotonin-rich foods (e.g., avocado, banana, kiwi, cheese); wheezing; abdominal cramping; and diarrhea, which is often watery and large-volume.
- Carcinoid heart disease occurs in 20% to 70% of patients with metastatic CT and may result in fatigue, dyspnea, and peripheral edema.
- Bone metastases may result in back or extremity pain.
- Pellagra resulting from niacin deficiency may present with confusion, depression, tongue pain, anorexia, fatigue, diarrhea, and a pruritic rash affecting sun-exposed skin.

PHYSICAL FINDINGS

- Bronchial CT may present with wheezing or rhonchi.
- Abdominal distention and tenderness may occur in cases of midgut CT-induced bowel obstruction or mesenteric ischemia from mesenteric fibrosis.
- Cardiac manifestations include a holosystolic murmur of tricuspid regurgitation, right ventricular lift/heave, jugular venous distention, pulsatile hepatomegaly, ascites, and peripheral edema; picture of *cor pulmonale* is common with advanced disease.
- Findings related to CS include cutaneous flushing, which is often well-demarcated over the face, neck, and/or torso, and telangiectasia.
- Pellagra related to niacin deficiency manifests as a scaly rash (often around the sun-exposed neck—known as Casal's necklace), erythematous and swollen tongue, and delirium.

DIAGNOSTIC TESTS AND STAGING

- Generally, neuroendocrine tumors, including CT, should be diagnosed biochemically before pursuing anatomic localization; however, patients presenting with symptoms related to mass effect or tissue-related symptoms, even in the absence of neurohormonal excess, are an exception; additionally, it is not uncommon for CT to be diagnosed incidentally during evaluation for another problem (e.g., appendectomy revealing asymptomatic CT).
- Radiographic and endoscopic techniques are frequently necessary for the evaluation of localized BP and GI tract CT.
  - Bronchoscopy required if endobronchial CT suspected; biopsy can be performed, but significant hemorrhage may occur.
  - Esophagogastroduodenoscopy (EGD) for gastric and duodenal CT.
  - Colonoscopy for colorectal CT.
  - EUS may be useful for evaluation of foregut and hindgut carcinoids and surrounding lymph node involvement.
  - Video capsule endoscopy has been suggested by some authors for detecting small bowel CT.
  - Chest radiography is the typical initial diagnostic test for BP CT and typically reveals a solitary hilar area mass lesion.
  - Computed tomography is useful if concern for bowel obstruction exists and may reveal an intraluminal mass, intussusceptions, dilated bowel loops, and/or air-fluid levels; typically the imaging study of choice to detect liver metastasis.
  - MRI may be useful for assessing liver metastasis or vascular encasement.
  - Selective angiography is an invasive procedure in which a catheter is inserted into a mesenteric vessel of interest for biochemical measurements.

- Somatostatin-receptor scintigraphy ("octreotide scan") is a useful tumor localization study for the primary site as well as metastatic foci.
    - CT cells frequently express high-affinity somatostatin receptors that bind radiolabeled octreotide with a sensitivity of 73% to 89% for localization of CT; a positive octreotide scan should be followed by an anatomic imaging study such as computed tomography or MRI for precise size measurement; false-positive studies may occur with granulomatous diseases, thyroiditis, wound infections, and lymphoma.
- Radionuclide bone scan is very sensitive at detecting skeletal metastasis.
- Biochemical testing should be performed prior to anatomic localization studies if a CT or CS is suspected; several modalities may be useful.
    - 24-hour urine collection for measurement of 5-HIAA is very sensitive but less specific for the diagnosis of CS; false-positive elevation of urinary 5-HIAA may occur with ingestion of banana, kiwi, avocado, pineapple, pecans, walnuts, or medications, including acetaminophen, guaifenesin, antihistamines, warfarin, or aspirin.
    - Serum CgA levels are elevated in 60% to 100% of patients with CT, with or without evidence of CS, and correlate with burden of tumor.
    - Pentagastrin stimulation test may be considered if the index of suspicion for CT persists despite negative or equivocal biochemical and imaging studies; this test should occur in a monitored environment with intravenous octreotide available if carcinoid crisis develops.
- Echocardiography with Doppler evaluation is important for diagnosis and follow-up of CHD; right atrial and ventricular enlargement, tricuspid valve thickening, and insufficiency are the most common findings.

TREATMENT

- Surgical resection is the only curative treatment for CT; specific procedures are beyond the scope of this text, but general principles of surgery for CT include:
    - BP tract CT: surgical resection and lymphadenectomy is suggested.
    - Gastric/small bowel CT: gastric CT <1 cm can be endoscopically removed; surgical resection is suggested for those >1–2 cm; small bowel carcinoids are treated with *en-bloc* bowel/mesentery resection with regional lymphadenectomy.
        - Prophylactic cholecystectomy should be considered during small bowel resection if octreotide therapy is anticipated, because this drug increases risk of gallstone formation.
    - Appendiceal CT: <1 cm, simple appendectomy; 1–2 cm, simple appendectomy or hemicolectomy and lymph node dissection if patient young or if adverse histologic features present; >2 cm, hemicolectomy

with lymph node dissection; indications for aggressive cancer surgery also include lymphatic invasion, lymph node metastasis, involvement of mesoappendix, positive resection margins at initial appendectomy, cellular pleomorphism, and/or high mitotic index.

- Colorectal CT: colonic CT can be approached in a manner similar to colon cancer with colectomy and lymphadenectomy; rectal CT require low anterior resection or abdominoperineal resection in a manner similar to rectal cancer.
- Metastatic CT: GI CT typically metastasize to the liver, where significant disease bulk may occur, resulting in symptomatic CS; surgical debulking should be considered to decrease tumor load, which can lead to significant disease improvement and, perhaps, increased survival; patients with bowel obstruction or mesenteric ischemia resulting from tumor-induced fibrosis may benefit from surgical resection.

- **Medical management for symptomatic CS.**
  - General treatment measures include avoidance of conditions or foods (e.g., avocado, banana, kiwi) that induce flushing; treatment of diarrhea with loperamide or diphenoxylate; niacin supplements to avoid pellagra; diuretics for volume overload from carcinoid heart disease; and treatment of wheezing with beta-agonists.
  - Octreotide, an analogue of somatostatin that blocks hormone secretion, cell growth, and smooth muscle contraction, is useful in controlling symptoms related to overproduction of serotonin and related peptides and may have some antitumor effect; tumoral uptake on octreotide scan is predictive of therapeutic response to octreotide administration.
    - Long-acting injectable octreotide (octreotide-LAR 30 mg) administered every 4 weeks is effective in ameliorating symptoms in up to 70% to 80% of patients with CS.

- **Medical/invasive management for metastatic CT.**
  - Transarterial chemoembolization (TACE) with cisplatin, doxorubicin, and mitomycin-C may result in disease improvement and benefit patients who are not surgical candidates; radiofrequency ablation (RFA) is another option for hepatic cytoreduction.
  - Interferon-α has a tumoristatic effect that may slow growth of metastatic CT, but has significant side-effects; biochemical responses of up to 70% have been noted.
  - Cytotoxic chemotherapy has minimal activity for metastatic CT, with response rates of <20%; chemotherapy is typically not indicated in most patients with metastatic CT because no agent has been demonstrated to improve overall survival.
  - Radiation therapy to symptomatic bone metastasis may provide palliation.
  - Supplementation with niacin should be provided to prevent pellagra.

- Treatment of CHD involves loop diuretics, digoxin, and octreotide to decrease circulating serotonin; valvular replacement may benefit some patients.

- Carcinoid crisis is an uncommon but life-threatening complication of CT that most often results from stressful conditions such as chemotherapy, sepsis, anesthesia, or surgical manipulation of tumor tissue during resective surgery; manifestations include tachycardia, flushing, and cardiovascular instability/shock, which may be fatal.
  - Treatment of carcinoid crisis includes aggressive crystalloid and plasma resuscitation and octreotide; prophylaxis against this syndrome with octreotide 150–200 µg subcutaneously every 6 to 8 hours should commence 24 to 48 hours prior to surgery or anesthesia.

COMPLICATIONS OF TREATMENT

- Octreotide: injection site pain, nausea, dyspepsia, diarrhea, cholelithiasis, steatorrhea, hyperglycemia, gastroparesis.
- TACE: "embolization" syndrome (right upper quadrant pain, hepatitis, fever, chills, leukocytosis), nausea, vomiting, hepatic infarction/abscess, renal failure, carcinoid crisis, and death (7%).

FOLLOW-UP CARE

- Patients with localized CT can be followed every 3 to 6 months with history, physical examination, and, possibly, serum CgA; chest radiography for BP tract CT should be considered.
- Patients with metastatic CT and/or CS should be monitored periodically for urinary serotonin and/or CgA, especially if symptoms fail to respond to treatment.
- Assessment for CHD in patients with metastatic CT or CS should be performed once or twice yearly with history, cardiovascular examination, and echocardiography; measurement of serum B-natriuretic peptide may be useful.
- Second malignancies are common in patients with CT with one study revealing a 52% incidence of a second cancer—this may result from tumorigenic properties of CT-released compounds; as such, lifelong cancer screening is suggested and may include: mammography, colonoscopy (colon cancer is the most common second primary cancer), chest radiography, pelvic examination, and pap smear.

PROGNOSIS

- The presence and extent of liver metastasis is the single most important prognostic factor for survival.
- Other adverse prognostic factors for CT include: male gender, older age, presence of carcinoid syndrome, tumor size (>75% incidence of liver metastasis with primary tumor >2 cm), lymph node involvement, tumor depth, histologic features (e.g., differentiation, increased mitoses,

vascular/perineural invasion), markedly elevated CgA, and development of second primary cancer.
- Foregut carcinoids without metastasis have a 5-year survival of 95% and with metastasis, only 20%.
- CT of the appendix has the best prognosis, with a 5-year survival approaching 100% for localized tumors.
- Patients with CHD have a poor prognosis (median survival <2 years) but may benefit from tricuspid valve replacement.

REFERENCES

Ann Surg 2005;241:839.
Cancer 2008;113:5.
Circulation 2007;116:2860.
Cleve Clin J Med 2008;75:849.
J Clin Oncol 2007;25:1967.
J Surg Oncol 2000;75:310.
N Engl J Med 1999;340:858.
Oncologist 2008;13:1255.
Oncologist 2005;10:123.
Tumori 2007;93:587.

BACKGROUND

- Head and neck cancer (HNC) consists of a heterogeneous group of epithelial carcinomas, typically squamous cell carcinoma (SCC), that arise from mucosal surfaces of head and neck structures: nasopharynx, oral cavity, oropharynx, hypopharynx, and larynx; tumors of the paranasal sinuses and salivary glands are uncommon and will not be discussed.
- There are approximately 45,000 cases and 11,000 deaths in the United States annually; worldwide, nasopharyngeal carcinoma (NPC) is endemic in the Far East and parts of the Mediterranean basin.
- More common in males and blacks; mean age 60 years; 2.5:1 male:female ratio; 7:1 for larynx cancer, however.
- Risk factors: chronic alcohol and smoking predominant risk factors for all sites of HNC in United States; smokeless tobacco and betel nut in India for oral cavity cancers; marijuana; sexually acquired human papilloma virus (HPV; types 16, 18, 31, 33) responsible for increasing incidence of oral cavity and tonsil cancers in young patients without typical risk factors; Epstein-Barr virus (EBV) infection major risk for NPC; salted fish and NPC; low consumption of fruits and vegetables.
- Increased risk for subsequent HNC and other aerodigestive cancers in smokers: "field cancerization" effect.

PATHOBIOLOGY

- Smoking/alcohol-related HNC: carcinogen-containing smoke and alcohol "bathe" at-risk mucosal surfaces; invasive SCC results after a stepwise progression of hyperplasia, dysplasia, and *in situ* disease due to an accumulation of genetic events such as loss of *p53* or 9p21.
  - Oral SCC preceded by intraepithelial neoplasia that, with genetic "hits" (e.g., loss of tumor suppressor genes on 3p and 9p), presents as leukoplakia, and then cancer.
  - Activation of EGFR common in squamous HNC, leading to increased cell proliferation, invasion, survival, and decreased apoptosis.
  - Metastasis is a late feature, with lungs, liver, and bone typical sites.
- HPV-related HNC: HPV (types 16, 18, 31, 33) acquired by sexual contact associated with verrucous SCC of tongue and tonsils; HPV types 16/18 isolated from 60%; viral proteins E6 and E7 inactivate *p53* and *Rb* tumor suppressor genes, causing loss of cell cycle regulation, cell proliferation, and chromosomal instability; HPV-induced HNC often presents with large

neck mass and small primary; better prognosis than smoking/alcohol-related HNC.

- Epstein-Barr-related NPC: not associated with smoking/ETOH; latent EBV infection; World Health Organization (WHO) subtypes of NPC: type I, keratinizing SCC; type II, nonkeratinizing SCC; type III, undifferentiated cancer (lymphoepithelioma, which contains infiltrates of lymphocytes); EBV oncogenes LMP-1 and EBNA-1 integrate into host genome causing malignant transformation; prone to early metastasis.

CLINICAL PRESENTATION

- Symptoms often localize HNC to a general or specific anatomic site; metastasis affect 10% of patients at presentation (exception NPC).
  - Oral cavity: pain, ulcer/mass, sore gums, ill-fitting dentures, halitosis, bleeding, trismus, painless neck mass (typically submental/submandibular area [level I nodes]).
  - NPC: facial pain, epistaxis, nasal obstruction, ear fullness/otalgia/impaired hearing, double vision (invasion of carotid sinus and segments of cranial nerves III, IV, VI), painless neck mass (typically upper neck [level I nodes] or posterior triangle [level V nodes]).
  - Oropharynx/hypopharynx/larynx: sore throat, dysphagia, hoarseness (vocal cord or laryngeal nerve involvement), painless neck mass (larynx/pharynx typically upper neck [levels II, III nodes]), dyspnea or stridor for advanced laryngeal cancers.

PHYSICAL FINDINGS

- Oral cavity SCC: leukoplakia is a white, nonscrapeable plaque on mucosal surface; erythroplakia is a red, velvety lesion (higher malignant risk than leukoplakia); ulcerative or mass lesion over any surface; tongue fixation; loose teeth.
- Other sites: tonsillar mass, neck adenopathy, pharyngeal erythema/ulcer/mass.

DIAGNOSTIC TESTS AND STAGING

- Patients with suspected HNC of any site require thorough head and neck examination with attention to all mucosal surfaces by inspection and bimanual palpation where possible, cranial nerve examination (especially for NPC), and examination of all surrounding lymph node areas.
- Referral to a head and neck surgeon for direct laryngoscopy and endoscopic assessment of the oral cavity, nasopharynx, oropharynx, hypopharynx, and larynx is appropriate.
- In cases of metastatic neck disease without obvious primary, triple endoscopy (laryngopharyngoscopy, esophagoscopy, bronchoscopy) with

able 21–1 TNM Staging Criteria (Oral Cavity, Oropharynx, Hypopharynx, Larynx)

Primary tumor (T)

Lip/oral cavity: T1: tumor ≤2 cm; **T2:** tumor >2 cm but <4 cm; **T3:** tumor >4 cm; **T4a (lip):** tumor invades bone, inferior alveolar nerve, mouth floor, facial skin; **T4a (oral cavity):** tumor invades bone, deep tongue musculature, maxillary sinus, facial skin; **T4b:** tumor invades masticator space, pterygoid plates, skull base and/or encases carotid artery

Oropharynx: T1: tumor ≤2 cm; **T2:** tumor >2 cm but <4 cm; **T3:** tumor >4 cm; **T4a:** tumor invades larynx, deep tongue musculature, medial pterygoid, hard palate, or mandible; **T4b:** tumor invades lateral pterygoid, pterygoid plates, lateral nasopharynx, skull base, and/or encases carotid artery

Hypopharynx: T1: tumor limited to one subsite and <2 cm; **T2:** tumor invades more than one subsite or adjacent site or >2cm but <4 cm without fixation of hemilarynx; **T3:** tumor >4 cm or fixation of hemilarynx; **T4a:** tumor invades thyroid/cricoid cartilage, hyoid, thyroid, esophagus, or central compartment tissue; **T4b:** tumor invades prevertebral fascia, encases carotid artery, or mediastinal structures

Larynx—supraglottis : T1: tumor limited to one subsite with normal vocal cord mobility; **T2:** tumor invades mucosa of >1 adjacent subsite of supraglottis or glottis or region outside supraglottis (e.g., mucosa of tongue, vallecula, pyriform sinus) without fixation of larynx; **T3:** tumor limited to larynx with vocal cord fixation and/or invades any: postcricoid area, pre-epiglottic tissues, paraglottic space, and/or erosion of inner cortex of thyroid cartilage; **T4a:** tumor invades through thyroid cartilage and/or invades tissue beyond larynx (e.g., trachea, soft tissue of neck, deep tongue musculature, strap muscles, thyroid, or esophagus); **T4b:** tumor invades prevertebral space, encases carotid artery, or mediastinal structures

Glottis: T1: tumor limited to vocal cords with normal mobility; **T2:** tumor extends to supraglottis and/or subglottis, and/or with impaired vocal cord mobility; **T3:** tumor limited to larynx with vocal cord fixation and/or invades paraglottic space, and/or erosion of inner cortex of thyroid cartilage; **T4a:** tumor invades through thyroid cartilage and/or invades tissues beyond larynx (e.g., trachea, soft tissue of neck, deep tongue musculature, strap muscles, thyroid, or esophagus); **T4b:** tumor invades prevertebral space, encases carotid artery, or mediastinal structures

Regional lymph nodes (N)

N0: no nodal metastases; **N1:** metastasis in single ipsilateral node <3 cm; **N2a:** metastasis in single ipsilateral node >3 cm but <6 cm; **N2b:** metastasis in multiple ipsilateral nodes, all <6 cm; **N2c:** metastasis in bilateral or contralateral nodes, all <6 cm; **N3:** metastasis in any node >6 cm

Distant metastasis (M)

M0: absent; **M1:** present

Stage grouping

Stage I: T1 N0 M0
Stage II: T2 N0 M0
Stage III: T3 N0 M0; T1–3 N1 M0
Stage IVA: T4a N0–1 M0; T1–3 N2 M0; T4a N2 M0
Stage IVB: T4b Nany M0; Tany N3 M0
Stage IVC: Tany Nany M1

Table 21–2 TNM Staging Criteria (Nasopharynx)

Primary tumor (T)

T1: tumor confined to nasopharynx; **T2:** T2a: tumor extends to oropharynx and/or nasal cavity; **T2b:** any tumor with parapharyngeal extension; **T3:** tumor involves bone and/or paranasal sinuses; **T4:** tumor with intracranial extension and/or involvement of cranial nerves, infratemporal fossa, hypopharynx, orbit, or masticator space

Regional lymph nodes (N)

N1: unilateral nodal metastases <6 cm, above supraclavicular fossa; **N2:** bilateral nodal metastasis <6 cm, above supraclavicular fossa; **N3:** N3a: >6 cm node; N3b: extension to supraclavicular fossa

Distant metastasis (M)

M0: absent; **M1:** present

Stage grouping

Stage I: T1 N0 M0
Stage IIA: T2a N0 M0
Stage IIB: T1–2 N1 M0; T2a N1 M0; T2b N0–1 M0
Stage III: T1–2b N2 M0; T3 N2 M0
Stage IVA: T4 N0–2 M0
Stage IVB: Tany N3 M0
Stage IVC: Tany Nany M1

mucosal biopsies of the nasopharynx, base of tongue, tonsils, and pyriform sinuses may reveal primary tumor.

- CT or MRI of the neck can identify nodal metastases with reasonable accuracy: large, centrally necrotic, irregular, matted nodes are usually malignant; patchy enhancement may occur.
- Screening for widespread metastases usually low yield because <10% of HNC patients present with distant disease (chest radiograph reasonable and may detect primary lung cancer); exception may be hypopharynx cancer, which spreads early due to rich lymphatic network in this area; incidence of metastasis approximately 60% in patients with node-positive NPC.
- PET/CT scan generally not indicated in patients with non-NPC T1/T2 tumors and/or negative or N1 nodes; useful in patients presenting with neck metastases of unknown origin; false-positive PET may complicate local inflammation or dental disease.
- Recent data show that patients achieving complete clinical and radiologic response (e.g., CT, PET) have <5% incidence of isolated neck recurrence; PET/CT has shown sensitivity, specificity, and negative predictive values after chemoradiation of 98%, 92%, and 100%, respectively, in some studies.

- Histologic diagnosis via endoscopic biopsy of primary site, FNA of neck node, or excisional biopsy (typically unnecessary unless NPC type III or lymphoma suspected).

TREATMENT

- HNC can be divided into early stage (T1/T2) without positive nodes (N0) or single ipsilateral node <3 cm (N1) and locally advanced stage (T3/T4) and/or large, multiple, or contralateral nodes (N2/N3).
- Criteria for unresectable tumor: base of skull invasion, fixation to prevertebral fascia, encasement of carotid artery, pterygoid muscle involvement.
- Early stage oral cancers surgically resected; early stage laryngeal cancers treated with laryngectomy or larynx-sparing definitive radiation (70 Gy in 1.8–2 Gy daily fractions over 7 weeks)—both as unimodality treatment.
- Locally advanced HNC requires multimodality treatment: resection followed by radiation/chemoradiation or organ-sparing chemoradiation; high-risk tumors at significant risk for locoregional relapse.
  - Absolute benefit of 8% for concurrent chemoradiation compared to radiation alone.
  - Indications for postoperative chemoradiation (cisplatin 100 mg/m^2 IV every 21 days during radiation improves locoregional control and disease-free survival): positive surgical margins, extracapsular node spread, perineural invasion, lymphovascular invasion, and multiple positive nodes.
  - Cisplatin 100 mg/m^2 IV every 3 weeks during radiation standard regimen for oropharynx, pharynx, and hypopharynx cancers; weekly cisplatin at lower dose or weekly carboplatin and paclitaxel options if cisplatin contraindicated, but no randomized comparisons.
  - Concurrent chemoradiation with cisplatin improves larynx preservation (88% at 2 years) compared to radiation or induction chemotherapy and is standard for larynx preservation in lieu of laryngectomy in stage III/IV larynx cancer; intensity modulated radiotherapy (IMRT) minimizes toxicity to area tissues.
  - Concurrent radiation and weekly cetuximab an option for patients with a contraindication to platinum.
- Historically, patients with locally advanced HNC with node involvement treated with primary modified neck dissection (MND) receive adjuvant radiation therapy; however, primary treatment with chemoradiation has increased in popularity, with neck dissection reserved for patients with large pretreatment nodes or a clinically positive neck following chemoradiation.
  - Bulky prepharynx nodes >6 cm (N3) associated with high incidence of microscopic posttherapy cancer; planned neck dissection following radiation (approximately 8 to 12 weeks later) may improve local

Table 21–3 Regimens for HNC and NPC

Primary treatment

Organ-sparing chemoradiation

Cisplatin 100 mg/m^2 IV every 21 days (days 1,22,43) of radiotherapy with 70 Gy in daily 2 Gy fractions

Cetuximab 400 mg/m^2 IV once followed 1 week later by 250 mg/m^2 IV weekly during radiotherapy; limited to patients with contraindication to cisplatin

Induction regimens for locally advanced disease

TPF: docetaxel 75 mg/m^2 IV, cisplatin 100 mg/m^2 IV, 5FU 1000 mg/m^2/day IV by continuous infusion for 4 days, every 21 days for 3 cycles (dexamethasone and prophylactic antibiotic or G-CSF support) followed 4–8 weeks later by weekly carboplatin AUC 1.5 IV concurrent with 70–74 Gy radiation to primary tumor; nodes irradiated as well with dose dependant (typically 50 Gy) on whether posttreatment neck dissection planned (surgery indications: ≥N2 nodes with partial response, N3 nodes, or residual disease following chemoradiotherapy)

PF: cisplatin 100 mg/m^2 IV and 5FU 1000 mg/m^2/day IV by continuous infusion for 4 days, every 21 days for 3 cycles

Adjuvant chemoradiation

Cisplatin 100 mg/m^2 IV every 21 days (days 1,22,43) during radiation with 60 Gy in high-risk postoperative patients (positive margin, ≥2 positive nodes, extracapular tumor extension)

Nasopharyngeal carcinoma

Cisplatin 100 mg/m^2 IV every 21 days (days 1,22,43) during daily radiotherapy with 70 Gy in 2 Gy daily fractions followed by adjuvant cisplatin 80 mg/m^2 IV day 1 and 5FU 1000 mg/m^2/day IV by continuous infusion for 4 days every 21 days for 3 cycles

Metastatic/recurrent disease

Cisplatin 100 mg/m^2 (or carboplatin AUC 5) IV day 1 and 5FU 1000 mg/m^2/day IV for 4 days every 21 days; can be utilized with or without cetuximab (see below for dosing)

Cetuximab 400 mg/m^2 IV week 1 then 250 mg/m^2 IV weekly; premedication with acetaminophen and diphenhydramine; patients living in North Carolina and surrounding states experience much higher risk of allergic infusion reaction

    control and survival if disease remains, albeit at a higher cost of operative morbidity.

- Selective neck dissection of prior bulky nodes after chemoradiation is better tolerated and been shown to control local disease.
- N1 or N2 nodes preradiation with clinical response do not typically need neck dissection.

- Primary chemoradiation may be combined with induction chemotherapy, which may allow organ preservation for laryngeal/hypopharyngeal tumors and increase survival in some patients.

  - Docetaxel, cisplatin, and 5-FU (TPF) for three to four cycles prior to radiation or chemoradiation with weekly carboplatin (AUC 1.5

for 7 weeks) improves progression-free survival and overall survival (71 vs. 30 months, $p=0.006$) in patients with locally advanced, unresectable HNC (TAX 323 and 324) compared to platinum/5FU induction; early administration of TPF felt to eradicate systemic micrometastases.

- Recurrent/metastatic disease: addition of the monoclonal anti-EGFR antibody, cetuximab, to cisplatin or carboplatin and 5-FU improves overall survival (10.1 vs. 7.4 months, $p=0.04$), disease-free progression, and disease control rate in patients with recurrent/metastatic HNC; single-agent weekly cetuximab may benefit patients with recurrent platinum-resistant disease (response rate 13%, disease control rate 46%); cisplatin and 5FU widely utilized for metastatic HNC, but cetuximab option if contraindication to platinum; taxanes (paclitaxel, docetaxel) and methotrexate have low response rates.
- NPC: standard regimen based on Intergroup 0099 trial is concurrent chemoradiation with cisplatin followed by adjuvant cisplatin and 5-FU (5-year overall survival 67% vs. 37%, $p<0.001$).

COMPLICATIONS OF TREATMENT

- Chemoradiation/radiation: stomatitis, pharyngitis, esophagitis, weight loss, stricture, xerostomia, dental caries, skin discoloration, hypothyroidism, vascular stenosis, second late malignancies (rare), Lhermitte's phenomenon, mandibular osteonecrosis.
- Neck dissection: wound infection, pain, deformity, decreased range of motion.
- Postchemoradiation neck dissection: higher complication rate due to radiation effect on wound healing (e.g., vessel and tissue sclerosis).
- Cisplatin: nausea/vomiting, fatigue, peripheral neuropathy, ototoxicity, optic neuritis, vascular thrombosis, microangiopathy, renal failure, electrolyte wasting.
- Docetaxel: stomatitis, pharyngitis, edema, malaise, cytopenia, febrile neutropenia, diarrhea, hand-foot syndrome.
- Cetuximab: acneiform rash, diarrhea, fatigue/asthenia, allergic infusion reactions (hypotension, urticaria, wheezing, anaphylaxis), interstitial pneumonitis (<1%), paronychia, hypomagnesemia, sepsis/infection.

FOLLOW-UP CARE

- Patients with N1/N2 nodes prechemoradiation with no posttreatment palpable adenopathy can be observed with frequent follow-up: neck palpation, ultrasound, neck CT; salvage surgery can reserved for patients who have neck relapse.
  - Neck examination should follow chemoradiation by 6 to 8 weeks after local edema, inflammation, and induration subside.

- Patients with locally advanced HNC treated with chemoradiation may undergo PET scan 8 to 12 weeks following therapy; endoscopic assessment by head and neck surgeon several weeks after treatment; history and physical examination with attention to regional nodes every 3 to 6 months for 2 to 3 years; chest radiograph to assess for lung metastases.
- Periodic thyroid measurements and consideration of carotid ultrasonography due to risk of radiation-induced hypothyroidism and carotid vascular stenosis, respectively.
- Periodic history and examination focusing on other aerodigestive cancers (e.g., cough, hemoptysis, dysphagia) and chest radiography due to significant risk for second primary malignancies.

PROGNOSIS

- 2-year survival for larynx cancer treated with concurrent chemoradiation is 75%.
- Neck metastases are the most important prognostic factor for HNC.
- Metastatic HNC survival is measured in months (<12 typical).
- Patients with negative postchemoradiation PET/CT have very good prognosis, with low risk of failure.
- HPV-positive HNC 59% reduction in death compared to HPV-negative HNC (HR=0.41).
- Patients treated for HNC (smoking/alcohol related) have 3% to 7% yearly risk of lung or esophagus cancers, which may prove fatal.

REFERENCES

Cancer 2008;113:S1911.
Head Neck 2007;29:986.
Head Neck 2003;25:791.
Lancet Oncology 2009;10:1086.
N Engl J Med 2008;359:1116.
N Engl J Med 2008;359:1143.
N Engl J Med 2007;357:1705.
N Engl J Med 2004;350:1937.
N Engl J Med 2003;349:2091.
Radiology 2005;235:580.
Radiother Oncol 2009;92:4 .

BACKGROUND

- Sarcomas are a group of malignant neoplasms arising from mesenchymal tissues, such as skeletal or smooth muscle, bone, cartilage, adipose tissue, and endothelium; this is a very diverse group of cancers (over 50 subtypes), so only a brief approach to extremity soft-tissue sarcoma (STS) and retroperitoneal sarcoma (RPS) will be presented (GIST covered in separate chapter).
- Sarcomas constitute <1% of all cancers, with soft tissue predominating over bone sarcomas in adults (approximately 9200 and 2400 annual cases, respectively).
- The most common STS subtypes in adults include leiomyosarcoma, liposarcoma, and high-grade undifferentiated pleomorphic sarcoma (formerly malignant fibrous histiocytoma), each accounting for 15% to 20%; other occasionally encountered subtypes include synovial sarcoma, fibrosarcoma, malignant peripheral nerve sheath tumor, and angiosarcoma; osteosarcoma and chondrosarcoma are most common bone-structure sarcomas in adults; Ewing's sarcoma can develop in soft tissue or bone.
  - 60% of adult STS involve the extremities and 15% to 20% constitute RPS or abdominal sarcomas.
- Risk factors: therapeutic radiation incurs small risk, such as angiosarcoma following breast irradiation, lymphangiosarcoma and chronic extremity lymphedema (Stewart-Treves syndrome), STS following prostate irradiation, vinyl chloride and hepatic angiosarcoma, human herpesvirus-8 (HHV-8) infection and Kaposi's sarcoma, Li Fraumeni syndrome (*p53* mutation) and STS, neurofibromatosis (NF1 mutation) and neurofibrosarcoma/malignant nerve sheath tumors, mutation of *Rb1* gene and osteosarcoma, Paget's disease and osteosarcoma.

PATHOBIOLOGY

- Most STS arise from mesodermal tissue and are named according to tissue of origin, for example: rhabdomyosarcoma—skeletal muscle; leiomyosarcoma—smooth muscle; liposarcoma—adipose tissue; angiosarcoma—endothelial/vascular tissue; myofibroblastic tissue—malignant fibrous histiocytoma; and uncertain origin—alveolar soft part sarcoma, synovial sarcoma, clear cell sarcoma; neuroectodermal STS occur on occasion; osteosarcoma in adults has predilection for metaphysis

of long bones, most often femur, tibia, and humerus and quite sensitive to chemotherapy.
- Recurrent chromosomal translocations characterize several sarcomas; examples include:
  - Synovial sarcoma: t(X;18) in >90%.
  - Liposarcoma (myxoid/round cell): t(12;16) in >75%.
  - Ewing sarcoma: t(11;22) in >85%.
- IGF-1 produced by some STS, often large RPS, and may induce autocrine tumor proliferation or cause hypoglycemia.
- Tumor grade is an important prognosticator for sarcoma and is included in the TNM staging system; Ewing's sarcoma is always considered high grade.
- STS of the extremities have metastatic predilection for the lungs; abdominal and RPS often metastasize to the liver; STS and osteosarcoma uncommonly involve lymph nodes (<10%).
- Leiomyosarcoma and liposarcoma are the most common RPS histologic subtypes; may exceed 20 cm in size.

CLINICAL PRESENTATION

- Most STS present as a slow-growing, painless mass lesion, most often involving the extremities or trunk.
- RPS often manifests as abdominal pain, early satiety/fullness, constipation, weight loss; urinary symptoms, or lower extremity edema; neurologic dysfunction can occur in some patients due to local mass effect/tissue invasion.
- Osteosarcoma often presents with a swollen, and often painful, extremity mass.
- Fever, weight loss, anorexia may occur in some patients.
- Symptoms of hypoglycemia (diaphoresis, confusion, dizziness) may complicate large RPS due to production of IGF-1.

PHYSICAL FINDINGS

- A large, fixed (often nontender) mass on an extremity typical for STS; osteosarcoma may have findings of extremity swelling, redness, warmth, and tenderness, especially over metaphyseal areas of long bones.
- Palpable mass common with RPS; lower extremity edema due to venous/lymphatic compression and/or decreased lower extremity sensation/strength if local nerves compressed.

DIAGNOSTIC TESTS AND STAGING

- Extremity STS.
  - MRI optimal imaging study to assess extent of muscle/fat/fascia invasion; superior for extremity sarcomas.

- Chest radiograph or CT to exclude lung metastases.
- Plain radiograph of long limb bones for osteosarcoma.
- PET scan being studied for assessing local involvement, metastatic disease, and response to chemotherapy in high-grade sarcoma.
- Core needle or incisional biopsy (preferred) by experienced radiologist/surgeon to avoid seeding of tissue.
- Bone marrow biopsy for patients with Ewing's sarcoma at any site since considered systemic disease at outset.
- RPS.
  - CT of the abdomen/pelvis accurate to assess RPS extent and involvement of adjacent structures.
  - CT- or MRI-angiogram if suspicion of vascular encasement/occlusion.
  - Radiographic and/or endoscopic assessment of the lower urinary tract or colonoscopy may be useful if involvement of these organ systems is suspected.
  - CT-guided needle core or endoscopically directed biopsy used most often; avoid surgical biopsy—initial surgery of RPS patients should be at definitive resection.
- Osteosarcoma.
  - Plain film radiography classically demonstrates a moth-eaten appearance, periosteal reaction ("sunburst" appearance), or periosteal new bone formation at the margin of soft tissue mass known as Codman's triangle.

Table 22–1 TNM Staging Criteria of STS/RPS

Primary tumor (T)
T1: tumor <5 cm; T1a*: superficial tumor; T1b*: deep tumor; T2: >5 cm; T2a*: superficial tumor; T2b*: deep tumor

Regional lymph nodes (N)
N0: no nodal metastases; N1: nodal metastases present (N1 is considered stage IV)

Distant metastasis (M)
M0: absent; M1: present

Histologic grade (G)
G1: well differentiated; G2: moderately differentiated; G3: poorly differentiated; G4: poorly differentiated or undifferentiated if four-tier grading system used

Stage grouping
Stage I: T1a–2b N0 M0 G1–2 (low-grade tumors) **Stage II:** T1a–2a N0 M0 G3–4 (high-grade tumors) **Stage III:** T2b N0 M0 G3–4 (high-grade tumors) **Stage IV:** Tany N1 M0 Gany; Tany Nany M1 Gany

*Superficial tumor located exclusively above superficial fascia without invasion of fascia; *Deep tumor beneath superficial fascia or superficial to fascia with focal invasion of/through fascia; by definition, RPS, mediastinal, pelvic STS are deep.

- CT demonstrates bone involvement accurately, but MRI superior for assessing soft tissue and intramedullary involvement.
- Chest radiograph or chest CT to assess for lung metastasis.
- Bone scan to exclude bone metastasis, which is common with osteosarcoma.
- Tissue biopsy with large core needle or open surgical biopsy (vital to incorporate biopsy site into future resection site).

TREATMENT

- General treatment principles apply to sarcoma management.
  - Biopsy with core needle or incisional method; biopsy site must be included *en bloc* within future resection site; endoscopic biopsy may be useful for intraabdominal or thoracic sarcoma.
  - Treatment at an institution with experienced surgeons, medical oncologists, radiation oncologists, radiologists, pathologists, and physical therapists is vital for optimal outcome.
  - Adequate surgical margin of 2–3 cm for STS decreases local recurrence; dissection through normal tissue planes; drain sites should exit close to incision edge and must be included in postoperative radiation plan if postoperative radiation is utilized; if specimen reveals positive margins, reresection should be considered if functional outcome not compromised; close margins (<1 cm) may be treated with postoperative radiation.
  - For extremity STS, goal is limb-preservation surgery with or without radiation/chemoradiation; studies reveal similar outcomes compared to amputation; fully trained sarcoma surgeons/orthopedic oncologists should evaluate all patients with extremity sarcoma.
  - Osteosarcoma sensitive to perioperative cisplatin and doxorubicin and is standard of care.
  - Ewing's sarcoma is potentially curable even with metastatic disease and requires immediate multimodality treatment with complex chemotherapy regimen (containing etoposide, ifosfamide, cyclophosphamide, vincristine, and doxorubicin given before and after resection for total of 51 weeks), radiation therapy, and surgical resection.
- Surgical resection is the treatment of choice for sarcoma and is typically the only therapy for low-grade, stage I disease if margin >1 cm; many STS grow along fascial planes, producing a "pseudocapsule"—but wide local excision with negative margins and incorporating the biopsy site is standard; in general, neoadjuvant radiation for STS or chemotherapy for osteosarcoma may increase limb-salvage rates by downsizing the tumor allowing complete resection.
  - Limb-sparing surgery for extremity STS is feasible for many patients except when a negative margin is unachievable or when neurovascular structures are involved that would induce severe functional defects of the limb.

- Randomized trials have shown limb-sparing surgery has low local recurrence rates and not inferior to amputation in most patients.
- Metastatectomy of lung metastasis in patients with osteosarcoma may result in long-term survival.
- Optimal surgery for RPS often necessitates *en bloc* resection of adjacent organs, most often kidney, adrenal, colon, pancreas, or spleen.

- Radiation therapy: adjuvant radiation (in stage II/III disease) increases local control rate in most extremity STS (approximately 85%), obviating the need for disfiguring amputation in most patients; however, radiation does not compensate for suboptimal resection; preoperative and postoperative radiation are options but each have considerations.
  - Preoperative (neoadjuvant) radiation of 50 Gy may allow downstaging and easier resection with less morbidity; smaller radiation fields and doses; higher risk of wound complications due to tissue and vascular fibrosis.
    - Postoperative boost doses are based on resection: close (<1 cm) margin, 10–14 Gy; R1 margin, 16–20 Gy; R2 margin, 20–26 Gy.
    - Intraoperative radiotherapy (IORT) used at select centers.
  - Postoperative radiation improves local control but must involve larger fields to encompass entire operative field (including drain sites) and in higher doses due to surgery-related local tissue hypoxia; some centers utilize intraoperative brachytherapy.
    - 50 Gy typical dose with external beam radiation, with boost based on margin status (see above).
  - Osteosarcoma is radioresistant.
  - Preoperative radiation commonly used for RPS to decrease tumor size, enhance resection, and decrease local recurrence, which is the most common cause of tumor-related demise; less bowel toxicity due to effect of tumor pushing contents out of radiation field.

- Chemotherapy plays little role in small (<5 cm), low-grade, fully resected STS, but anthracyclines and ifosfamide improve survival in patients with high-risk extremity STS (high grade, >5 cm, or locally recurrent); recent meta-analysis on STS adjuvant chemotherapy demonstrated improved local control, disease-free survival, and 4% increase in overall survival for all sites and 7% for extremity STS; other studies show survival benefit of adjuvant ifosfamide/anthracycline for high-grade/recurrent extremity STS in patients with adequate performance status.
  - Metastatic STS is largely incurable in adults but chemotherapy provides palliation and may improve survival; high-dose ifosfamide (an alkylating agent) and doxorubicin (an anthracycline) are the most active agents for metastatic sarcoma—synovial sarcoma is especially sensitive to ifosfamide; gemcitabine and docetaxel active as first-line regimen for leiomyosarcoma; angiosarcoma responsive to taxanes.
  - Single-agent doxorubicin typical agent of choice for metastatic disease; combination regimens (e.g., ifosfamide, MESNA, and doxorubicin [AIM]; doxorubicin and dacarbazine; MESNA, doxorubicin, ifosfamide,

dacarbazine [MAID]) produce higher response rates, but generally, no increased survival compared to doxorubicin alone.

- Neoadjuvant chemotherapy with multiagent regimen followed by limb sparing surgery standard approach to resectable osteosarcoma; active agents included doxorubicin, ifosfamide, cisplatin, and methotrexate
- Trabectedin, an antisarcoma marine-derived agent, has demonstrated objective responses and stable disease of STS refractory to conventional chemotherapy

Table 22–2 Regimens for STS

Selected regimens for metastatic STS
Doxorubicin (single-agent) 50–75 mg/m^2 IV every 21 days
Doxorubicin 20 mg/m^2/day IV continuous infusion days 1–3, ifosfamide 1.5 g/m^2/day IV continuous infusion days 1–4, MESNA 225 mg/m^2 over 1 hour before ifosfamide and at 4 and 8 hours after ifosfamide (can also infuse with ifosfamide at same dose), every 21 days; use G-CSF 480 µg/kg/day for 10 days starting day 5 or pegfilgrastim 6 mg on day 5; other dosing schemes available for ambulatory use, consult comprehensive oncology text for information
MAID regimen: MESNA 2500 mg/m^2/day IV continuous infusion days 1–4, Doxorubicin 20 mg/m^2/day IV continuous infusion days 1–3, ifosfamide 2500 mg/m^2/day IV continuous infusion days 1–3, dacarbazine 300 mg/m^2/day IV continuous infusion days 1–3, every 21 days
Gemcitabine 900 mg/m^2 IV days 1,8 and docetaxel 100 mg/m^2 IV day 8, every 21 days (consider pegfilgrastim 6 mg day 9; full-dose docetaxel may not be tolerated by some patients)

CAV/IE regimen for Ewing's sarcoma
Cyclophosphamide 1200 mg/m^2 IV day 1, doxorubicin 75 mg/m^2 IV day 1, vincristine 2 mg IV day 1 (CAV); when doxorubicin cumulative dose reaches 375 mg/m^2, change to dactinomycin 1.25 mg/m^2 for remainder of CAV cycles
AND
Ifosfamide 1800 mg/m^2 IV days 1–5 and etoposide 100 mg/m^2 IV days 1–5 (IE) Alternate CAV with IE every 21 days for total of 17 cycles; timing of surgery and radiation at discretion of treating team; growth factor support necessary

COMPLICATIONS OF TREATMENT

- Limb radiation may cause slow wound healing/breakdown or infection when given preoperatively; limb edema, skin changes, and joint stiffness not uncommon.
- Surgical resection may result in wound infection, bleeding, need for skin grafting, venous thromboembolism with extremity sarcoma.
- Resection of RPS may result in wound infection, ileus, venous thromboembolism, bleeding, injury to adjacent organs (e.g., bowel, great vessels, ureter, bladder).

- Abdominal radiation for RPS may cause diarrhea/enteritis in 50% of patients; vomiting, infection, ileus, obstruction, and fistula may occur; late second cancer.
- Chemotherapy may cause nausea, vomiting, myelosuppression, febrile neutropenia/sepsis, fatigue, alopecia; certain agents, however, have unique complications.
  - Ifosfamide: electrolyte-wasting nephropathy, encephalopathy, seizures, hemorrhagic cystitis due to acrolein metabolite (must be administered with MESNA, a sulfhydryl compound that binds acrolein in the bladder), hyponatremia.
  - Cyclophosphamide: hemorrhagic cystitis (administer with MESNA), cardiotoxicity/hemorrhagic myocardial necrosis, second malignancy (bladder cancer, leukemia), hyponatremia.

FOLLOW-UP CARE

- Little data available regarding optimal follow-up for STS/RPS; however, higher-grade/stage tumors more likely to recur, most often within 5 years.
- Periodic imaging of primary site with CT or MRI (e.g., extremity, retroperitoneum) should be considered (every 6 to 12 months for 3 years, then as clinically indicated or annually) depending on recurrence risk (highest with large, high-grade sarcomas).
- Stage I sarcomas can be followed with history and physical examination every 3 to 6 months for 2 to 3 years with chest radiography every 6 to 12 months.
- Stage II and III sarcomas require history, examination, and chest imaging every 3 to 6 months for 2 to 3 years and then every 6 months for 2 to 3 more years and then annually because late relapse may occur; other imaging is directed at symptoms and signs.

PROGNOSIS

- Tumor histology and grade are most important variables predicting relapse and overall survival.
- Tumor size affects 5-year survival rate: 2.6–4.9 cm (77%); 5.0–9.9 cm (62%); 10–14.9 cm (51%); 15–20 cm (42%).
- A validated prognostic diagram for individual patients to predict probability of 12-year sarcoma-specific death was developed by Kattan and may assist with patient counseling (*J Clin Oncol* 2002;20:791).
- Response to chemotherapy most important prognostic factor in localized osteosarcoma; long-term survival of 60% to 80% in patients with extremity osteosarcoma treated with neoadjuvant multiagent chemotherapy and limb-sparing surgery.
- For RPS, degree of resection is the most important factor influencing long-term survival, with median survival of 103 months for gross total

resection and 18 months for incomplete resection; overall, poor prognosis with 33% to 35% 5-year survival; may recur in 40% of 5-year disease-free patients by 10 years.

- Patients with metastatic/unresectable RPS have median survival of 10 months.

REFERENCES

Ann Surg Oncol 1999;6:8.
Cancer 2008;112:1585.
Cancer Imaging 2005;5:89.
Curr Probl Surg 2009;46:445.
J Clin Oncol 2007;25:2755.
J Clin Oncol 2005;23:105.
J Clin Oncol 1996;14:1679.
J Clin Oncol 1989;7:1208.
Lancet 1997;350:1647.
N Engl J Med 2005;353:701.
N Engl J Med 2003;348:694.

BACKGROUND

- Small cell lung cancer (SCLC) accounts for approximately 15% of lung cancer cases and is characterized by a rapid doubling time, early dissemination, and nearly universal relapse following primary treatment.
- Approximately 35,000 cases of SCLC occur annually in United States; most patients ultimately die of their disease.
- Over 95% of cases of SCLC result from smoking; hence, the diagnosis of SCLC in a nonsmoker should be suspect.
- Standard-of-care chemotherapy (platinum and etoposide) has not changed in recent years despite active clinical research.

PATHOBIOLOGY

- SCLC is a neuroendocrine neoplasm derived from embryonic neural crest cells that manifests several classic histologic characteristics: round/ovoid or spindle-shaped, small cells with scant cytoplasm and inconspicuous nucleoli, numerous mitoses, nuclear molding, and crush artifact.
- Immunohistochemical staining typically positive for combinations of TTF-1, CK7, CD56, synaptophysin, chromogranin, and neuron-specific enolase.
- SCLC proliferates via autocrine growth loops by secretion of growth-promoting peptides such as gastrin-releasing peptide, stem cell factor, and neuromedin B that bind to specific receptors that stimulate cell proliferation.
- Amplification of MYC oncogenes and dysfunction of tumor-suppressor genes such as p53, Rb1, and RASSF1 are found in >75% of SCLC; loss of chromosome 3p is present in >90% of SCLC, resulting in loss of several tumor-suppressor genes that normally reside at this location.
- SCLC has a predilection for early hematogenous metastasis and is considered a systemic disease at diagnosis; favored sites of metastasis include brain (18% at diagnosis), liver, bone, and adrenal glands, although virtually any organ can be affected with disseminated disease.

CLINICAL PRESENTATION

- Most patients are symptomatic at presentation; only 5% are diagnosed incidentally on chest imaging and have stage I disease (e.g., T1–T2 tumor).

- Because SCLC typically involves central airways, most patients present with thoracic symptoms such as cough, dyspnea, hoarseness, wheezing, hemoptysis, or chest discomfort.
- Compression of the superior vena cava may produce headache, confusion, epistaxis, visual blurring, or pulmonary symptoms.
- Metastatic SCLC may present with weight loss, weakness, anorexia, or fatigue or symptoms based on the location of metastases.
  - Brain: headache, diplopia, paresis, parasthesia, seizure, syncope.
  - Bone: back pain, extremity pain due to pathologic fracture.
  - Liver: abdominal pain, pruritis, dark urine.
  - Adrenal glands: fatigue, anorexia, orthostatic dizziness.
- Paraneoplastic syndromes occur in 15% of patients (not related to tumor stage) and result from tumor cell release of peptide hormones (systemic syndromes) or antibodies that induce damage to the nervous system (neurologic syndromes).
  - Hyponatremia: most common paraneoplastic syndrome (15% of patients); ectopic release of antidiuretic hormone (ADH) reduces renal free water excretion and hyponatremia, which lead to fatigue, nausea, or neurologic symptoms (e.g., confusion, seizures).
  - Cushing syndrome: 2% to 5% of patients; ectopic release of corticotropin (ACTH) leads to hypercortisolism, resulting in symptoms from hyperglycemia (polyuria, polydypsia), hypokalemia (generalized weakness), or adrenal corticosteroids (acne, proximal muscle weakness, generalized, weakness, confusion).
  - Lambert-Eaton syndrome: 3% of patients; antibodies to voltage-gated calcium channels, resulting in proximal muscle weakness, dry mouth, constipation, impotence, or orthostatic dizziness.
  - Neuropathy or encephalomyelitis: <1% of patients; antibodies (anti-Hu) to neurologic tissue resulting in parasthesias, weakness, confusion, or ataxia.
  - Cancer-associated retinopathy: <1% of patients; antirecoverin antibodies to retinal cells result in visual loss.

PHYSICAL FINDINGS

- Limited-stage (LS) SCLC: rales, rhonchi, or ipsilateral supraclavicular adenopathy; if superior vena cava compression present: plethora, dilated chest wall veins, stridor, engorged retinal vessels, jugular vein distension.
- Extensive-stage (ES) SCLC: cachexia, contralateral supraclavicular adenopathy, bone tenderness, dullness to percussion (pleural effusion), hepatomegaly, focal neurologic findings (cranial nerve paresis, limb weakness), hypotension (adrenal metastasis).
- Paraneoplastic syndromes: Cushingoid facies, muscle wasting, proximal muscle weakness, decreased sensation, reflex alterations, ataxia.

DIAGNOSTIC TESTS AND STAGING

- Chest radiograph typically reveals a central/hilar mass; atelectasis or pleural effusion may be present.
- Because treatment of SCLC depends on whether disease is limited to a hemithorax that can be encompassed within a safe radiation portal (LS, 30%) or beyond (ES, 70%), adequate radiographic staging of common metastatic sites is mandatory.
  - CT scan of chest and abdomen to include liver and adrenal glands.
  - MRI is preferred study to exclude brain metastasis; CT of brain with contrast alternative.
  - Bone scan.
  - PET scan sensitive for detecting metastases; may obviate bone scan; typically not necessary if good-quality CT scan, MRI, and bone scan obtained.
- CBC may reveal cytopenia or leukoerythroblastic changes indicative of bone marrow metastases; increased alkaline phosphatase may indicate bone or liver metastasis; increased LDH typically from rapid cell turnover, but may signify liver involvement; bone marrow biopsy generally does not change management but may be useful if unexplained anemia or elevated alkaline phosphatase present without obvious ES disease (<5% of patients).

Table 23–1 Veterans Administration Lung Study Group Staging for SCLC

Limited stage
Disease limited to one hemithorax that can be safely encompassed within tolerable radiation portal; with or without ipsilateral/contralateral mediastinal lymphadenopathy or ipsilateral supraclavicular lymphadenopathy

Extensive stage
Disease beyond ipsilateral hemithorax including contralateral hilar/supraclavicular lymphadenopathy; malignant pleural/pericardial effusion; distant metastasis

TREATMENT

- Chemotherapy plays a central role in the management of LS and ES SCLC, because micrometastases are assumed at diagnosis; platinum-based doublet chemotherapy is standard with overall and complete response rates of 75% to 90% and 50%, respectively, for LS disease, and 50% and 25%, respectively, for ES disease.
  - Response is often dramatic, occurring within several days to 3 weeks, and may result in improvement in performance status; tumor lysis syndrome may occur in patients with significant disease burden.
  - Cisplatin and etoposide for four cycles administered concurrently with thoracic radiation is the preferred regimen for patients with LS disease; carboplatin may be preferable in elderly/infirm patients with ES disease.
  - Use of G-CSF or pegfilgastrim is generally given because myelosuppression common, especially with carboplatin.

- Concurrent chemoradiotherapy with a platinum doublet for four cycles is standard-of-care for LS SCLC and results in improved outcome (5% absolute survival benefit at 3 years) compared to sequential therapy.
  - Commencing radiation with the first cycle is superior compared to later administration.
  - Twice-daily (hyperfractionated) radiation to 45 Gy has been shown to improve median survival (23 vs. 19 months) and 5-year survival (26% vs. 16%) compared to daily radiation to same dose, but with more esophageal and hematologic toxicity.
  - Daily radiation to 60–70 Gy is most widely used regimen combined with chemotherapy; less toxic and more convenient than hyperfractionated regimen.
- The rare patient with an isolated lesion found to be stage I SCLC at surgery should receive adjuvant chemotherapy if node-negative and chemoradiation if node-positive.
- Prophylactic cranial irradiation (PCI) is standard of care for LS patients with complete response and is suggested for ES patients with a favorable response to first-line platinum-based chemotherapy; several principles regarding PCI are outlined below.
  - Brain metastasis are present in approximately 20% of patients at diagnosis and up to 80% of patients at 2 years; at relapse, one-third of patients will have brain-only disease and another one-third have systemic and brain disease.
  - Multiple parenchymal metastases most common, but leptomeningeal disease may occur.
  - Administration of PCI improved 3-year survival by 5.4% when administered following systemic therapy to complete responders with LS disease and is now standard of care.
  - Recently, an EORTC randomized trial demonstrated that ES SCLC patients administered 20–30 Gy of PCI following any response to initial therapy experienced a decrease in symptomatic brain metastasis by 77% (HR=0.23, $p<0.001$) and at 1 year (14.6% vs. 40.4%); median overall survival was 6.7 months vs. 5.4 months ($p=0.003$) and survival at 1 year was 27.1% vs. 13.3%. Based on this data, PCI should be administered to ES SCLC patients within 4 to 6 weeks following a favorable response to initial chemotherapy.
- Relapsed chemoresistant-disease is virtually inevitable; patients who relapse <3 months following standard platinum chemotherapy are considered refractory and have <10% chance of meaningful response to second-line treatment; patients relapsing >3 months are considered sensitive and have response rates of approximately 20%; single-agent topotecan is the only FDA-approved agent in this setting, although paclitaxel or the CAV (cyclophosphamide, doxorubicin, vincristine) can be considered, although these regimens do not confer survival benefit compared to topotecan but may improve symptoms; if relapse occurs >6 months following initial treatment, readministration of the original regimen can be considered.

Table 23–2 Chemotherapy Regimens for SCLC

Limited-stage disease (administered concurrently with radiation)
Cisplatin 60 mg/m² IV day 1 and etoposide 120 mg/m² IV days 1–3 × 4 cycles
Cisplatin 80 mg/m² IV day 1 and etoposide 100 mg/m² IV days 1–3 × 4 cycles
Carboplatin AUC 5–6 IV day 1 and etoposide 100 mg/m² IV days 1–3 × 4 cycles
Note: cisplatin recommended platinum in LS disease

Extensive-stage disease (maximum of four–six cycles)
Cisplatin 75–80 mg/m² IV day 1 and etoposide 80–100 mg/m² IV days 1–3
Cisplatin 25 mg/m² IV days 1–3 and etoposide 100 mg/m² IV days 1–3
Carboplatin AUC 5–6 IV day 1 and etoposide 100 mg/m² IV days 1–3

Relapsed disease
Topotecan 1.5 mg/m² IV days 1–5, every 21 days
Paclitaxel 80–100 mg/m² IV days 1,8,15 every 28 days
CAV regimen: cyclophosphamide 1000 mg/m² IV day 1, doxorubicin 40 mg/m² IV day 1, vincristine 2 mg IV day 1, every 21 days

COMPLICATIONS OF TREATMENT

- Chemoradiation: esophagitis (grade III common), dysphagia, oral/pharyngeal/esophageal candidiasis, pneumonitis, fatigue, nausea, vomiting, cytopenia; cisplatin-related: vomiting, ototoxicity, neurotoxicity, electrolyte-wasting, anemia, thrombotic microangiopathy, thrombosis; carboplatin more myelosuppressive than cisplatin.
- PCI: headache, nausea, vomiting, fatigue, dermatitis, alopecia, anorexia.

FOLLOW-UP CARE

- Because relapse usually occurs within several months after initial therapy, history, physical examination, and chest imaging should be performed every 2 to 3 months; monitoring of blood counts and LDH reasonable.

PROGNOSIS

- Without treatment, the median survival for LS SCLC is <6 months, and only 2 to 4 months if ES disease present; 95% of patients with SCLC die from their disease.
- Median survival for LS SCLC is 14 to 23 months, with 5-year survival of 12% to 17%.
- Median survival for ES SCLC is 7 to 12 months; 2-year survival approximately 5%, but 5-year survival only 2%.
- Risk of second primary lung cancer is 2% to 10% per patient per year.

REFERENCES

J Clin Oncol 1994;12:2022.
J Clin Oncol 1992;10:282.
J Clin Oncol 1992;10:890.
Lancet 2005;366:1385.
N Engl J Med 2007;357:664.
N Engl J Med 1999;340:265.
N Engl J Med 1999;341:476.

- Non-small cell lung cancer (NSCLC) is the leading cause of cancer death (29% of all cancer deaths in the United States), accounting for 85% of total lung cancer cases, and is divided into three major types: adenocarcinoma (AC), squamous cell carcinoma (SCC), large cell carcinoma (LCC).
- Approximately 215,000 cases and 162,000 deaths in the United States annually; NSCLC is the leading cause of cancer death in both men and women.
- Most patients present with unresectable, advanced-stage disease; 85% of patients with NSCLC ultimately die from their disease within 5 years of diagnosis.
- Approximately 10% to 15% of NSCLC cases arise in nonsmokers, with AC the predominant histology; many nonsmokers with adenocarcinoma are females, which may reflect gender differences in carcinogen metabolism or the presence of estrogen receptors in neoplastic cells.
- Risk factors: cigarette smoking is responsible for 85% to 90% of NSCLC cases; radon exposure is second leading cause of NSCLC; less common risks include environmental exposure to arsenic, chromium, nickel, or asbestos, radiation therapy for prior malignancy (especially Hodgkin's lymphoma), and secondhand tobacco smoke (increases risk 20% to 30%), which may account for up to one-fourth of cancers in never-smokers.
- Risk of NSCLC increases with duration of smoking and number of cigarettes smoked daily; duration imparts a larger risk; although risk of developing cancer after smoking cessation decreases significantly, it likely does not return to that of never-smokers, as evidenced by the fact that 50% of cases occur in former smokers.
- Cigar smoking increases risk of NSCLC but not to the degree as cigarette smoking.

PATHOBIOLOGY

- Significant progress in defining biology and host susceptibility to NSCLC; polymorphisms in cytochrome P-450 (which metabolizes carcinogens, such as polycyclic aromatic hydrocarbons), glutathione-S-transferase (an enzyme that detoxifies carcinogens, such as polycyclic aromatic hydrocarbons), and various DNA-repair enzymes, may account for differing risks among individual smokers.

- Smoking-induced NSCLC induces genetic/epigenetic changes within cells that eventually result in "clonal patches" of premalignant tissue capable of abnormal cell proliferation, invasive capacity, and invasive cancer with metastatic phenotype.
- Smoking-related cancers often harbor mutations of p53, KRAS, and EGFR, all of which result in disordered cell growth, invasive potential, enhanced survival, and proliferation.
  - Mutations of EGFR are more common in AC, especially in Asian patients (up to 50% vs. 10% in U.S.) and are more common in females; EGFR mutations are associated with unusual sensitivity to EGFR inhibitors (e.g., erlotonib); EGFR mutations in exon 19 and L858R mutant within exon 21 are associated with improved prognosis.
  - Although erlotonib improves survival in all types of NSCLC, females, nonsmokers, and Asians are especially likely to respond, often in dramatic fashion.
  - KRAS mutations are mutually exclusive of EGFR mutations and confer resistance to EGFR inhibitors and cytotoxic chemotherapy.
- Increased serum levels of VEGF correlate with tumor growth and prognosis; bevacizumab, a monoclonal antibody directed at VEGF, improves survival in nonsquamous NSCLC.
- Lung cancer cells may produce growth factors (e.g., IGF-1) and receptors that induce autocrine cell growth; ongoing research to target IGF-1 and other autocrine factors.
- Until recently, patients with advanced NSCLC were treated the same; however, subtypes of NSCLC have been shown to respond differently to specific chemotherapy agents, due to histology-specific biologic characteristics.
  - AC: >50% of NSCLC; typically peripheral location with tendency to metastasize early, often to the brain; histologic glandular pattern that may produce mucin; typically CK7+, often TTF-1+; most common subtype in nonsmokers, often in association with EGFR mutations; recent data suggest that AC has higher response rate to multifolate inhibitor, pemetrexed; EGFR is expressed in approximately 85% of NSCLC cases; presence of EGFR exon 19 deletion or exon 21 L858 mutation (found in 10% to 15% of whites and 30% to 40% of Asians) predicts response to EGFR tyrosine kinase inhibitors; the AC subtype bronchioloalveolar carcinoma (BAC) typically grows in "lepidic" fashion along alveoli and is associated with diffuse infiltrates and responsiveness to EGFR inhibitors.
  - SCC: 25% of NSCLC; often central location arising from lobar/mainstem bronchi; tumor cavitation common (SCC precludes treatment with VEGF inhibitor, bevacizumab, due to hemorrhagic risk); tendency to metastasize late; histologic features of intercellular bridging, pearl formation, and keratinization; typically CK5/6+ and CK7+; may be associated with hypercalcemia due to production of parathyroid hormone related peptide (PTHrP); recent data suggest SCC has higher response rate to gemcitabine-based chemotherapy.

- LCC: 10% of NSCLC; often display neuroendocrine features; poorly differentiated cells with large nucleoli; often associated with paraneoplastic syndromes.

CLINICAL PRESENTATION

- Most patients with NSCLC present with advanced disease and symptoms; some patients may be diagnosed with chest imaging in the absence of symptoms and are more likely to have resectable stage I/II disease.
- Symptoms of locally advanced NSCLC result from tumor involvement of major airways (cough, hemoptysis, stridor, wheezing, dyspnea), superior vena cava (headache, epistaxis, visual blurring, dyspnea), brachial plexus (neck pain or parasthesia involving ulnar nerve distribution in cases of superior sulcus [Pancoast] tumors), esophagus (dysphagia), recurrent laryngeal nerve (hoarseness), pleura (dyspnea, pleuritic pain from pleural effusion), or systemic symptoms (fatigue, weight loss, anorexia).
- Symptoms of metastatic NSCLC are protean because any organ can be affected; most common areas of involvement include the brain (headache, seizures, diplopia, nausea, extremity weakness), bones (pain, sudden fracture), liver (abdominal pain or fullness), adrenal glands (orthostatic dizziness, fatigue, anorexia), lungs (progressive cough, dyspnea, hemoptysis), and spine (back pain, leg weakness/incontinence if spinal cord compression present).
- Paraneoplastic syndromes may be the initial manifestation of NSCLC or recurrent disease; hypercalcemia (from release of PTHrP from SCC) may cause confusion, fatigue, polyuria, weakness, constipation; hypertrophic pulmonary osteoarthropathy (HPOA) may complicate AC and cause long bone pain and limb swelling; Trosseau's syndrome may present with limb swelling and pain from venous thrombosis.

PHYSICAL FINDINGS

- Locally advanced disease: rhonchi, wheezing, rales common; decreased breath sounds if endobronchial lesion present; elevated neck veins, engorged retinal vessels, plethora, dilated chest wall veins with superior vena cava compression; Horner's syndrome (miosis, ptosis, anhidrosis of face) with superior sulcus (Pancoast) tumor.
- Metastatic/inoperable disease: supraclavicular adenopathy; dullness to percussion with pleural effusion; neck vein distention, hypotension, pulsus paradoxus with pericardial effusion; bone tenderness with metastatic involvement; cranial nerve palsies or extremity weakness with brain metastasis; bilateral leg weakness, areflexia, decreased anal tone with spinal cord compression.
- Miscellaneous: finger clubbing; long bone tenderness/swelling with HPOA.

DIAGNOSTIC TESTS AND STAGING

- Chest radiography: may reveal isolated lung lesion in stage I/II disease; advanced-stage NSCLC often associated with large mass, cavitation (especially SCC), hilar fullness due to adenopathy, pleural effusion (stage IIIB), or bone destruction.
- CT of chest thru liver and adrenal glands: initial diagnostic test of choice if lung cancer suspected; may reveal hilar/mediastinal adenopathy but sensitivity/specificity limited (65% to 75%) and cannot exclude node metastasis; although lymphadenopathy may represent benign hyperplasia, nodes >1 cm on CT require mediastinoscopy with biopsy for definitive staging; adrenal fullness or mass may indicate metastasis.
- PET/CT: very useful for staging to delineate extent of primary tumor, involvement of mediastinal nodes (sensitivity/specificity of approximately 90%), and distant metastasis; nodes <1 cm on CT that are negative on PET have high negative predictive value for metastasis and may not require preoperative mediastinoscopy (although nodes need to be assessed at surgery); PET adequate to exclude bone metastasis in most patients.
- Bone scan: obtained if bone/back pain, increased alkaline phosphatase, or hypercalcemia; may be omitted if staging PET/CT performed.
- Brain imaging: MRI with gadolinium preferred; not necessary in stage I/II patients but consider in stage III disease or in patients with neurologic symptoms or headache; isolated brain metastasis does not preclude resection (of primary and metastatic lesion) if systemic metastasis are absent.
- Tissue diagnosis: bronchoscopy with forceps biopsy of endobronchial lesion; transbronchial needle biopsy of adjacent lymph node(s); CT-guided percutaneous needle biopsy (for peripheral lung lesions); endoscopic bronchial ultrasound (EBUS)-guided needle aspiration cytology of lymph node(s); thoracentesis with cytology; CT-guided percutaneous needle biopsy of metastatic site (liver, bone, adrenal).
- Mediastinoscopy: because clinical staging often differs from pathologic staging, accurate assessment of mediastinal lymph nodes (N2/N3) is vital, because mediastinal involvement (especially bulky N2 and N3) almost always precludes curative surgery; mediastinoscopy may be deferred if CT reveals mediastinal nodes <1 cm and PET is negative.
- EBUS with trans-airway biopsy: emerging technology to assess enlarged nodes preoperatively; not yet standard of care for mediastinal staging.
- Preoperative evaluation: careful assessment of performance status/exercise tolerance, forced vital capacity (FVC), fractional expiration volume at 1 second (FEV1), and diffusing capacity (DLCO) to determine risk for postoperative complications and ability to tolerate lobectomy or pneumonectomy; referral to a pulmonologist should be considered.

Table 24-1 TNM7 Staging Criteria (Revised in 2009)

Primary tumor (T)
T1: tumor ≤3 cm, surrounded by lung or visceral pleura, without bronchoscopic evidence of invasion more proximal than lobar bronchus; **T1a:** tumor ≤2 cm; **T1b:** tumor >2 cm but ≤3 cm; **T2:** tumor >3 cm but ≤7 cm with any of the following: involves main bronchus ≥2 cm distal to carina, invades visceral pleura, associated with atelectasis/obstructive pneumonitis extending to hilum but not involving entire lung; **T2a:** tumor >3 cm but ≤5 cm; **T2b:** tumor >5 cm but ≤7 cm; **T3:** tumor >7 cm or invading any of following: chest wall, diaphragm, mediastinal pleura, parietal pericardium, or main bronchus <2 cm distal to carina but without involving carina, associated atelectasis/obstructive pneumonitis of entire lung, or separate tumor nodules within same lobe; **T4:** tumor of any size invading any of the following: heart, great vessels, trachea, esophagus, recurrent laryngeal nerve, vertebral body, carina; or, separate tumor nodules in a different ipsilateral lobe

Regional lymph nodes (N)
N0: nodal metastasis absent; **N1:** metastasis involving ipsilateral peribronchial and/or hilar nodes and/or intrapulmonary nodes including involvement by direct extension of primary tumor; **N2:** metastasis involving ipsilateral mediastinal and/or subcarinal nodes; **N3:** metastasis involving contralateral mediastinal/hilar, ipsilateral or contralateral scalene, or supraclavicular nodes

Distant metastasis (M)
M0: absent; **M1a:** separate tumor nodules in contralateral lung; pleural tumor nodules; malignant pleural effusion; **M1b:** distant/systemic metastasis

Stage grouping
Stage IA: T1a,b N0 M0
Stage IB: T2a N0 M0
Stage IIA: T1a,b N1 M0; T2a N1 M0; T2b N0 M0
Stage IIB: T2b N1 M0; T3 N0 M0
Stage IIIA: T1–3 N2 M0; T3 N1 M0; T4 N0–1 M0
Stage IIIB: Tany N3 M0; T4 N2 M0
Stage IV: Tany Nany M1a,b

TREATMENT

- Surgical resection (lobectomy or pneumonectomy) is the best chance for cure of NSCLC, but only one-third of patients at presentation are potential candidates (stage I/II disease); one-third present with locally advanced (stage IIIA/B) disease, which is typically treated with combined chemoradiation; and one-third present with metastatic (stage IV) disease, which is treated with chemotherapy and palliative radiation directed at symptomatic areas.
- Surgery for resectable disease (stage I/II, some stage IIIA).
  - Lobectomy superior to wedge resection in regards to recurrence and survival; pneumonectomy may be required if tumor involves major

fissure or mainstem bronchus; wedge resection can be considered for smaller, peripheral lesions in patients with limited reserve.

- Video-assisted thoracoscopic surgery (VATS) should be considered, providing standard oncologic surgical principles are not compromised, due to lower postoperative morbidity and mortality compared to thoracotomy.
- Patients with superior sulcus (Pancoast) tumors are treated with combined preoperative chemoradiation (cisplatin and etoposide) followed by surgery, which may require chest wall resection; 2-year survival rates range from 50% to 70%.
- Neoadjuvant chemotherapy may be considered in younger patients with nonbulky stage IIIA NSCLC; mediastinoscopy following two cycles of chemotherapy is necessary, because patients with residual mediastinal node involvement do not benefit from surgery and should complete treatment with radiation or chemoradiation.
- Routine postoperative radiation for stage II/III resected SCC reduces local recurrence but does not increase survival; postoperative radiation is detrimental for stage I patients.

- Adjuvant chemotherapy for resected disease (stage II/IIIA).
  - Several large phase III trials and meta-analyses show statistically significant survival benefit for four cycles of adjuvant platinum-based doublet chemotherapy for pathologic stage II/IIIA NSCLC; stage IB patients with tumor >4 cm may derive some benefit from chemotherapy, but this remains a controversial area.
    - The NCIC and ANITA studies utilized adjuvant cisplatin and vinorelbine postresection and demonstrated increases in 5-year survival of 54% vs. 69% ($p=0.03$) and 43% vs. 51% ($p=0.017$), respectively, compared to surgery alone.
    - Recent meta-analyses have shown 11% relative and 4% to 5% absolute risk reduction in mortality following platinum-based chemotherapy.
    - Radiation following chemotherapy should be considered in pathologic N2 nodes; positive resection margins should receive postoperative concurrent chemoradiation.
  - Cisplatin is superior to carboplatin in the adjuvant setting and data suggests combination with vinorelbine or etoposide; docetaxel reasonable option as is pemetrexed if AC histology, although trials are lacking.
- Definitive radiation for resectable (stage I/II, some stage IIIA) but medically inoperable disease.
  - High-dose radiation (up to 77.4 Gy) to tumor and nodal areas may result in long-term survival in 15% to 30% of patients who have medical contraindications for surgery, although adequate lung function is necessary; studies ongoing regarding stereotactic radiation to small tumors with encouraging results.
- Definitive chemoradiation up to 74 Gy for locally advanced disease (bulky stage IIIA, IIIB without pleural effusion).

- Some patients with IIIA disease may experience long-term survival with multimodal treatment, but IIIB is generally incurable with survival similar to stage IV patients.
- The uncommon patient with satellite lung metastasis in the same lobe as primary tumor (T3) may be potentially cured with surgery; surgical referral is indicated in these settings.
- RTOG study demonstrated increased survival with concomitant chemoradiation compared to sequential therapy, although increased risk of toxicity (esophagitis, pneumonitis).
- Chemotherapy can be administered with full-dose cisplatin/etoposide for optimal treatment of micrometastatic disease or in lower weekly radiosensitizing doses of carboplatin and paclitaxel; a concern with weekly dosing is that micrometastases are not adequately treated; a CALGB study showed a trend toward increased survival with induction full-dose carboplatin/paclitaxel prior to chemoradiation (11.4 vs. 14 months, $p=0.154$) with 1-year survival of 48% vs. 54%; another option is to administer two to three cycles of full-dose chemotherapy following chemoradiation, if the patient can tolerate this.

- Chemotherapy for stage IV NSCLC.
  - Several randomized studies show a survival benefit for doublet chemotherapy in patients with stage IV NSCLC, provided adequate performance status (≤ 2): 1-year survival rate of 10% vs. 35% to 40% for untreated vs. treated patients; chemotherapy also improves quality of life and decreases tumor-related symptoms.
  - In general, platinum-based doublet regimens with newer generation drugs (taxanes, vinorelbine, gemcitabine, pemetrexed) are preferred; elderly patients with limited performance status may benefit from single-agent vinorelbine as demonstrated in ELVIS trial; patients with severe comorbidity and/or performance status of 3/4 do not benefit from chemotherapy.
  - Carboplatin may be preferable to cisplatin for patients with stage IV disease due to palliative intent and improved tolerability with ease of administration compared to cisplatin; myelosuppression, however, may be significant.
  - Until recently, choice of doublet (paclitaxel/platinum, gemcitabine/platinum, docetaxel/platinum, vinorelbine/platinum) has not significantly influenced median overall survival, and regimens are often utilized based on physician preference and convenience; however, recent studies revealing improved histology-specific response rates to gemcitabine (for SCC) and the multifolate antagonist, pemetrexed (for AC) and improved survival with the anti-VEGF agent, bevacizumab, in non-SCC NSCLC, have altered treatment of these patients and are changing standard of care.
    - Pemetrexed for AC: pemetrexed is a novel, multitargeted antifolate that has been demonstrated in phase III trials, in combination with cisplatin for first-line treatment, to increase median survival in patients with advanced/metastatic AC by approximately 2 months

compared to gemcitabine and cisplatin; pemetrexed is well tolerated if folate/B12 and steroids are administered to prevent hematologic and skin toxicity, respectively; also indicated as monotherapy for second-line treatment with better efficacy against AC compared to docetaxel, but with improved toxicity profile; "maintenance" pemetrexed administered immediately to non-SCC patients with at least stable disease following non-pemetrexed-based platinum doublet therapy improved overall survival compared to best supportive care (13.4 vs. 10.6 months, HR=0.50, p=0.012)—this benefit was especially evident for the subgroup of AC histology (16.8 vs. 11.5 months, HR=0.73, p<0.0001).

- Gemcitabine for SCC: gemcitabine and cisplatin improves median survival by 1 month compared to pemetrexed and cisplatin, leading many physicians to recommend this drug for initial treatment in patients with advanced SCC.
- Bevacizumab for nonsquamous NSCLC: ECOG phase III trial compared carboplatin/paclitaxel to carboplatin/paclitaxel/bevacizumab showed improved median overall survival for triplet regimen: 12.3 vs. 10.3 months (HR=0.79, p=0.003), with 50% 1-year survival; use of bevacizumab contraindicated in patients with untreated brain metastasis and SCC due to higher risk of brain hemorrhage and fatal hemoptysis, respectively.
- Cetuximab, a monoclonal antibody directed at the EGFR receptor, recently shown to increase survival in phase III FLEX trial when administered with cisplatin and vinorelbine, but only by 1 month.
- More than four to six cycles of doublet chemotherapy do NOT confer survival benefit leads to increased toxicity.
- Second-line chemotherapy: inevitably, the majority of patients with advanced/metastatic NSCLC will progress within 3 to 6 months after initial therapy; docetaxel and pemetrexed are approved in this setting and impart similar 1-year median survival (29.7% for both), but pemetrexed is better tolerated; as noted, pemetrexed is superior in AC histology and should be considered if not used first-line.
- Erlotinib: an oral EGFR tyrosine kinase inhibitor indicated for second-line and beyond treatment in patients who may not tolerate cytoxics; NCIC BR21 trial demonstrated improved overall survival in all histologies compared to placebo in patients with IIIB/IV NSCLC previously treated with chemotherapy (6.7 vs. 4.7 months, HR=0.70, p<0.001); patients with EGFR-positive tumors who received erlotinib had improved survival compared to placebo patients and patients whose tumors did not express EGFR—other studies have demonstrated similar findings; presence of EGFR mutations exon 19 deletion or exon L858R, nonsmoking status, female gender, and Asian ethnicity predict responsiveness to erlotinib, which may be dramatic.
- Brain metastasis: patients with solitary brain lesion and control of systemic disease should be considered for surgical resection followed

- by whole brain radiation (WBRT); stereotactic radiosurgery (SRS) followed by WBRT is another option in this setting.
- Malignant pleural effusion: if thoracentesis and chemotherapy do not control symptomatic pleural effusion, options include talc pleurodesis following tube thoracostomy drainage or video-assisted thoracoscopy (VATS); a tuneled pleural catheter is an option for patients to self-drain as fluid reaccumulates.
- Superior vena cava syndrome: radiation or chemoradiation should be considered if symptoms are present; stent placement can be considered, although data are limited.

Table 24–2 Chemotherapy Regimens for NSCLC

Adjuvant regimens*
Cisplatin 50 mg/m^2 IV days 1,8 and vinorelbine 25 mg/m^2 IV days 1,8,15,22 every 28 days × 4 cycles
Cisplatin 100 mg/m^2 IV day 1 and vinorelbine 30 mg/m^2 IV days 1,8,15,22 every 28 days × 4 cycles
Cisplatin 75–80 mg/m^2 IV day 1 and vinorelbine 25–30 mg/m^2 IV days 1,8 every 21 days × 4 cycles
Cisplatin 100 mg/m^2 IV day 1 and etoposide 100 mg/m^2 IV days 1–3 every 21 days × 4 cycles
Cisplatin 75 mg/m^2 IV day 1 and docetaxel 75 mg/m^2 IV day 1 every 21 days × 4 cycles
Carboplatin AUC 6 day 1 and paclitaxel 200 mg/m^2 IV day 1 every 21 days × 4 cycles (for patients with contraindication to cisplatin)

Regimens used with radiation
Carboplatin AUC 2 IV and paclitaxel 45–50 mg/m^2 IV weekly with concurrent radiation to 63 Gy (consider 2 cycles of carboplatin AUC 6 IV and paclitaxel 200 mg/m^2 IV every 21 days following chemoradiation in fit patients, although phase III data are not available)
Cisplatin 50 mg/m^2 IV days 1,8,29,36 and etoposide 50 mg/m^2 IV days 1–5 and 29–33 with concurrent radiation to 61 Gy (preferred regimen based on randomized trial data); (consider 3 cycles of docetaxel 75 mg/m^2 IV every 21 days following chemoradiation in fit patients, although not all studies show definitive benefit)
Carboplatin AUC 6 IV day 1 and paclitaxel 200 mg/m^2 IV day 1 every 21 days × 2 cycles followed by radiation to 63 Gy beginning day 42

Advanced/metastatic (stage IV) disease*
Carboplatin AUC 6 IV day 1, paclitaxel 200 mg/m^2 IV day 1, and bevacizumab 15 mg/kg IV day 1 every 21 days; do not administer > 6 cycles of chemotherapy but bevacizumab can be continued until progression as tolerated
Carboplatin AUC 6 IV day 1 and paclitaxel 200 mg/m^2 IV day 1 every 21 days × 4–6 cycles

*Based on randomized phase III trials, cisplatin is recommended platinum agent for adjuvant therapy.

(continued)

Table 24–2 (*Continued*)

Carboplatin AUC 6 IV day 1 and docetaxel 75 mg/m^2 IV day 1 every 21 days × 4–6 cycles
Carboplatin AUC 5 IV day 1 and gemcitabine 1000 mg/m^2 IV day 1,8 every 21 days × 4–6 cycles
Carboplatin AUC 6 IV day 1 and vinorelbine 25 mg/m^2 IV days 1,8 every 28 days × 4–6 cycles
Carboplatin AUC 5 IV day 1 and pemetrexed 500 mg/m^2 IV day 1 every 21 days × 4–6 cycles; folate 400 mcg by mouth daily and vitamin B12 1000 mcg IM every 9 weeks during regimen to prevent toxicity/cytopenia; dexamethasone 4 mg by mouth twice a day the day prior to, day of, day after pemetrexed to prevent rash
Cisplatin 80 mg/m^2 IV day 1, vinorelbine 25 mg/m^2 IV days 1,8, and cetuximab 400 mg/m^2 IV loading dose then 250 mg/m^2 IV weekly every 21 days × 4–6 cycles
Cisplatin 80 mg/m^2 IV day 1 and paclitaxel 175 mg/m^2 IV day 1 every 21 days × 4–6 cycles
Cisplatin 75 mg/m^2 IV day 1 and docetaxel 75 mg/m^2 IV day 1 every 21 days × 4–6 cycles
Cisplatin 100–120 mg/m^2 IV day 1 and vinorelbine 25–30 mg/m^2 IV days 1,8,15 every 28 days × 4–6 cycles
Cisplatin 75 mg/m^2 IV day 1 and pemetrexed 500 mg/m^2 IV day 1 every 21 days × 4–6 cycles; folate 400 mcg by mouth daily and vitamin B12 1000 mcg IM every 9 weeks during regimen to prevent toxicity/cytopenia; dexamethasone 4 mg by mouth twice a day the day prior to, day of, day after pemetrexed to prevent rash
Cisplatin 60–75 mg/m^2 IV day 1 and etoposide 100–120 mg/m^2 IV days 1–3 every 21–28 days × 4–6 cycles
Second-line/salvage therapy
Docetaxel 75 mg/m^2 IV every 21 days
Pemetrexed 500 mg/m^2 IV every 21 days; folate 400 mcg by mouth daily and vitamin B12 1000 mcg IM every 9 weeks during treatment regimen to prevent toxicity/cytopenia; dexamethasone 4 mg by mouth twice a day the day prior to, day of, day after pemetrexed to prevent rash
Erlotinib 150 mg by mouth daily

*Because treatment is palliative in advanced/metastatic setting, carboplatin often utilized due to favorable toxicity profile and ease of administration, but consider cisplatin in younger, fit patients as data from adjuvant setting suggest slightly improved efficacy; consider neurokinin antagonist, aprepitant (125 mg by mouth 1 hour prior and 80 mg by mouth daily days 2,3), for cisplatin containing regimens; consider granulocyte growth factors in heavily pretreated patients or those who develop severe neutropenia with first cycle.

COMPLICATIONS OF TREATMENT

- Surgical resection: perioperative cardiac complications, venous thromboembolism, infection; impaired pulmonary function.
- Chemoradiation: esophagitis (may be severe), oropharyngeal candidiasis, pneumonitis, skin erythema/desquamation, fatigue, nausea, vomiting, cytopenia.

- Chemotherapy (limited list of adverse effects, please refer to pharmacology text for specific agents): cytopenias, infection, hemorrhage, neuropathy, pneumonitis, nausea, vomiting, diarrhea, rash, alopecia (taxanes), fatigue, neuropathy (cisplatin, vinorelbine), electrolyte wasting (cisplatin), hypersensitivity reactions (taxanes, carboplatin, etoposide), increased liver enzymes, arterial thrombosis (cisplatin), thrombotic microangiopathy (cisplatin, gemcitabine).
- Bevacizumab: hypertension, headache, proteinuria, epistaxis, hemorrhage, impaired wound healing, bowel perforation, venous/arterial thrombosis, reversible posterior leukoencephalopathy.
- Erlotonib: acneiform/pustular rash, dry skin, diarrhea, nausea, fatigue, mucositis, interstitial lung disease (rare, more common in Japan).
- Cetuximab: infusional-hypersensitivity (hypotension, rash, chills, fever, bronchospasm—more common in North Carolina/Rocky Mountain states), acneiform/pustular rash, dry skin, diarrhea, fatigue, paronychia, interstitial lung disease (rare), hypomagnesemia.

FOLLOW-UP CARE

- Following resection or definitive chemoradiation: history, physical examination, and chest CT every 4 to 6 months for 2 years and then annually.

PROGNOSIS

- Overall, the long-term prognosis of NSCLC is poor, with only a 15% 5-year survival.
- Favorable prognostic factors at diagnosis include early-stage disease, performance status ≤2, absence of weight loss, and female gender.
- 5-year survival is correlated with stage at diagnosis: stage I/II, 38% to 67% (pathologic staging) and 22% to 61% (clinical staging); stage IIIA, (23% to 25%, pathologic staging) and 9% to 13% (clinical staging); stage IIIB <5%; and stage IV ≤1%.
- Patients with metastatic NSCLC have median survival of 7.9 months with 12-month overall survival of 33%; survival times may be increasing with more efficacious chemotherapy directed at histology. For instance:
  - Adenocarcinoma patients treated with pemetrexed and cisplatin had higher median overall survival compared to gemcitabine and cisplatin (12.6 months vs. 10.9 months) in phase III trial.
  - Pemetrexed "maintenance" after four cycles of a platinum doublet increased median overall survival to 13.4 months compared to 10.4 months for placebo in nonsquamous NSCLC patients in phase III study.

REFERENCES

Cancer 1982;50:2751.
J Clin Oncol 2008;21:3543.
J Clin Oncol 2008;26:3543.
J Clin Oncol 2004;22:1589.
J Clin Oncol 2004;22:3852.
J Clin Oncol 2000;18:2529.
J Clin Oncol 1998;16:3316.
J Clin Oncol 1995;13:2166.
J Natl Cancer Inst 1999;91:66.
Lancet 2009;374:1432.
Lancet Oncol 2006;7:719.
N Engl J Med 2008;359:1367.
N Engl J Med 2006;355:2542.
N Engl J Med 2005;353:123.
N Engl J Med 2004;350:351.
N Engl J Med 2002;346:92.
N Engl J Med 2000;343:1217.
Proc Am Soc Clin Oncol 2008;26:abstract 3.

25 ■ MALIGNANT PLEURAL MESOTHELIOMA

- Malignant pleural mesothelioma (MPM) is an aggressive and typically incurable neoplasm that is increasing in frequency worldwide that results from exposure to asbestos; the association between asbestos and MPM is stronger than cigarette smoking and bronchogenic carcinoma.
  - Peritoneal mesothelioma accounts for approximately 20% to 30% of mesothelioma cases; other rarely involved structures include the pericardium and the tunica vaginalis; none of these nonpleural subtypes will be discussed.
- Approximately 2500 cases occur annually in the United States; it is estimated that there will be 72,000 deaths in the United States from MPM over the next 40 years.
- The characteristic feature of MPM is a prolonged latency between exposure and disease—often 20 to 50 years; as such, cases will increase for another 2 or 3 decades.
- Most cases of MPM occur during the fifth through seventh decades, with a significant male predominance, primarily due to occupational exposure; although most patients report prolonged exposure, exposure of only 1 to 2 years can cause MPM, which reinforces the importance of a detailed occupational/environmental history.
- Risk factors: there are three principle epidemiologic exposure patterns to asbestos-related MPM:
  - Direct occupational exposure through mining, milling, or processing.
  - Occupational exposure during chain of manufacture and utilization of asbestos-containing products such as carpenters, plumbers, boilermakers, defense personnel, shipbuilding, brake manufacturing, or insulation installers.
  - Incidental or unknowing exposure, such as wives who washed clothing of spouses who worked in asbestos mines and people exposed to asbestos tailings used as landfill, playground materials, or road surfaces.
- In contrast to lung cancer, MPM is not caused by smoking.

PATHOBIOLOGY

- Asbestos is a general term for a group of various mineral silicates that includes chrysotile, amosite, and crocidolite.
  - The most carcinogenic fibers are the long, slender fibers known as amphiboles; serpentine fibers known as chrysotiles may also cause MPM, but at rates lower than that of amphiboles.

151

- The pathogenesis of MPM is complex, but the carcinogenic effects result primarily from the physical properties of asbestos rather than chemical structure; the long, rod-like amphiboles are able to reach terminal air units.
- Mesothelial cells envelop the visceral and pleural surfaces and facilitate a gliding movement by production of lubricating glycoproteins; malignant transformation may result from several processes.
  - Mesothelial cells proliferate in response to injury from asbestos fibers puncturing the lung surface, which causes them to "stick out" and repeatedly scratch the parietal mesothelium, leading to inflammation, repair/proliferation, and eventual malignant transformation.
  - Asbestos fibers may pierce and damage the mitotic spindle apparatus, thereby disrupting mitosis; aneuploidy and chromosomal damage may occur, such as deletion of chromosome 22.
  - Asbestos may induce generation of reactive oxygen species (ROS) that damage DNA.
  - Asbestos induces phosphorylation of MAP and ERK kinases involved in cell proliferation.
- Transformed mesothelial cells possess several biologic features: response to growth factors such as epidermal growth factor (EGF), platelet-derived growth factors (PDGF), and transforming growth factor β (TGFβ) in an autocrine or paracrine fashion; over 90% of MPM cells produce telomerase, an enzyme that prevents telomere shortening, which allows cells to continue indefinite cell division (to become immortal, a hallmark of malignancy); loss of tumor-suppressor genes such as p16, p14, NF2; up-regulation of the antiapoptosis protein Bcl-x$_L$; and increased angiogenesis.
- The oncogenic DNA virus simian virus 40 (SV40) is frequently isolated from MPM tissue and may play a role in pathogenesis by inhibiting tumor-suppressor genes; contamination of poliovirus vaccines decades ago by SV40 has been postulated in the pathogenesis of MPM, although this remains controversial.
- Three histologic variants of MPM include epithelioid (most common, favorable prognosis), sarcomatoid (least common, poor prognosis), and mixed histology.
- Tumor cell release of interleukin (IL)-6 may induce a systemic inflammatory response known as "cancer cachexia" syndrome, which is characterized by anorexia, sarcopenia, weight loss, fevers, and increases in serum inflammatory markers.

CLINICAL PRESENTATION

- Most patients with MPM are symptomatic at presentation, with dyspnea occurring in most patients; ipsilateral chest wall pain is common and, when accompanied by a pleural effusion, is suggestive of MPM.
- Symptoms of superior vena cava syndrome (dyspnea, headache, visual blurring, epistaxis) may occur due to encasement of the superior vena cava.

- Invasion of thoracic vertebrae may cause back pain or, rarely, paraparesis from cord compression.
- Advanced MPM often produces systemic symptoms such as fever, night sweats, anorexia, fatigue, and weight loss.

PHYSICAL FINDINGS

- Most patients have evidence of pleural effusion: dullness to percussion and diminished breath sounds; decreased inspiratory chest wall excursion may result from encasement/fixation of the chest wall musculature.
- Evidence of cancer cachexia syndrome may complicate advanced MPM: cachexia, sarcopenia, pallor, symmetric muscle weakness.
- Superior vena cava compression may cause plethora, conjuctival injection, retinal engorgement, dilated chest wall veins, stridor, and neck vein distention.
- Patients who have undergone thoracentesis, tube thoracostomy, or thoracoscopy often develop visible/palpable tumor nodules at the insertion site due to tumor cell migration into the tissue tracts formed by these procedures.

DIAGNOSTIC TESTS AND STAGING

- Chest radiography typically reveals a pleural effusion and/or a pleural mass(es) with a right-sided predominance (60%); a characteristic finding is a pleural effusion with lack of contralateral shift due to fixation of the chest wall; calcified pleural plaques are a sign of asbestos exposure, but are not precursors to MPM.
- CT is the most useful initial imaging study for MPM and may reveal pleural-based masses in isolation or as an encircling rind (90%), pleural effusion (70% to 75%), interlobular tissue thickening (85%), or compression of vascular and/or mediastinal structures.
- MRI may be useful in potential surgical candidates to determine if tumor invades ribs, vertebrae, or diaphragm.
- PET is useful for distinguishing benign versus malignant pleural masses and for detecting mediastinal node involvement and metastatic disease during preoperative staging; metastasis may involve the skeleton, adrenal glands, liver, and kidneys.
- Serum levels of mesothelin-related protein (SMRP) are elevated in approximately 80% of cases of MPM and <5% of cases of benign pleural disease; the test is currently available in research centers.
- Routine blood testing often reveals thrombocytosis, anemia, hypoalbuminemia, elevated sedimentation rate, and hyperglobulinemia—manifestations of cancer cachexia syndrome from circulating IL-6.
- Pulmonary function tests typically reveal a restrictive ventilatory pattern.

- Assessment of mediastinal nodes (nodal stages similar to bronchogenic carcinoma) with mediastinoscopy should be considered in potential candidates for aggressive surgery.
- Definitive diagnosis of MPM relies on cytologic or histologic analysis of pleural fluid or pleural tissue, respectively; throacentesis or FNA of pleural masses are the initial studies of choice; cytologic evidence of MPM in the pleural fluid may be found in 33% to 84% of patients, but often more than one thoracentesis is necessary; thoracoscopic pleural biopsy is indicated if pleural fluid is not diagnostic and leads to diagnosis in over 90% to 95% of cases.
- The typical immunohistochemical findings of MPM include:
  - Positive staining for Wilms' tumor 1 antigen (WT-1, a mesothelial marker), epithelial membrane antigen (EMA), caltretinin, cytokeratin 5/6, and mesothelin; typical adenocarcinoma markers are negative.

Table 25–1 International Mesothelioma Interest Group (IMIG) staging system for MPM

Primary tumor (T)
T1: tumor limited to ipsilateral parietal pleura including mediastinal and/or diaphragmatic pleura; small foci may involve visceral pleura; **T2:** tumor limited to ipsilateral pleural surface with at least one of the following: involvement of diaphragm, confluent visceral pleural tumor, or invasion of lung parenchyma; **T3:** locally advanced, but potentially resectable with at least one of the following: involvement of endothoracic fascia, mediastinal fat, a solitary focus extending into chest wall soft tissue, or nontransmural pericardial invasion; **T4:** unresectable with at least one of the following: diffuse tumor extension or multiple foci involving chest wall, transdiaphragmatic invasion of peritoneal cavity, direct extension to contralateral pleura, invasion of mediastinal organs or spine, or extension to internal surface of pericardium with or without effusion or myocardial invasion

Regional lymph nodes (N)
N0: nodal metastasis absent; **N1:** metastasis involving ipsilateral peribronchial/intrapulmonary or hilar nodes; **N2:** metastasis involving subcarinal or ipsilateral mediastinal nodes; **N3:** metastasis involving contralateral mediastinal and/or ipsilateral or contralateral supraclavicular nodes

Distant metastasis (M)
M0: absent; **M1:** present

Stage groupings
Stage I: T1 N0 M0
Stage II: T2 N0 M0
Stage III: Any T3 Any N1 or N2 M0
Stage IV: Any T4 Any N3 Any M1

TREATMENT

- Surgery is most often utilized for diagnostic (thoracoscopy with biopsy) or palliative purposes (thoracoscopic pleurodesis for pleural effusion); a minority of patients may be considered for aggressive therapeutic surgical procedures.
  - Pleurectomy/decortication is a cytoreductive procedure with removal of grossly involved visceral and parietal pleura; this procedure is rarely curative, and R0 resection is unusual; relatively low-mortality procedure and can be performed by many thoracic surgeons; postoperative radiation is problematic because the lung remains in place, which increases risk for radiation pneumonitis and fibrosis.
  - Extrapleural pneumonectomy (EPP) is an aggressive procedure that should only be performed by experienced surgeons in fit/younger patients due to significant operative morbidity and mortality; involves *en bloc* resection of entire parietal and visceral pleura enveloping the lung, pericardium, and mediastinal nodes; because pneumonectomy is performed, higher doses adjuvant radiation can be delivered; for optimal outcome, adjuvant radiation and chemotherapy are suggested, with survival times of 2 years reported by some authors.
- Radiation therapy utilized alone has little effect on survival, because MPM is generally radioresistant; when utilized postoperatively, intensity-modulated radiotherapy (IMRT) is the most effective method.
  - The primary role of radiation is in the adjuvant setting following EPP or PD, although the remaining lung tissue in the latter surgery is at significant risk for radiation damage, which limits the amount that may be safely delivered, because MPM is a diffuse neoplasm requiring large treatment fields.
  - Radiation delivered to sites of thoracentesis puncture, tube thoracostomy, or thoracoscopy decreases risk of seeding of tissue tracts and subsequent tumor growth.
- Chemotherapy, until recently, has had minimal impact on advanced MPM due to relative chemoresistance; recent trials have demonstrated improved survival with novel agents.
  - Pemetrexed is a multitargeted antifolate that inhibits three key enzymes involved in tumor cell purine and pyrimidine synthesis: dihydrofolate reductase, thymidylate synthase, and glycinamide ribonucleotide formyltransferase; enters cell via reduced folate carrier and undergoes intracellular polyglutamation, trapping the drug within the cell.
    - Pemetrexed with cisplatin administered every 3 weeks is the standard of care for MPM based on a phase III trial demonstrating a response rate (RR) of 41% versus 17% ($p<0.001$) and a median overall survival (OS) of 12.1 months versus 9.3 months for cisplatin alone ($p=0.02$); most patients are treated with four to eight cycles depending on response and toxicity, although studies regarding maintenance single-agent pemetrexed following doublet therapy are ongoing.

- Phase II trials have shown that substitution of carboplatin for cisplatin resulted in a RR of 25% and median OS of 14 months; although no phase III data exist, this regimen should only be considered in patients unable to tolerate cisplatin.
- Co-administration of folate 400 μg orally daily (beginning 7 to 10 days prior) and vitamin B12 1000 μg IM (beginning 7 to 10 days prior and every 9 weeks) are required during pemetrexed therapy to prevent drug-induced toxicity; dexamethasone 4 mg orally twice daily the day prior, of, and after pemetrexed is required to prevent rash.

  - Gemcitabine is a nucleoside analogue that inhibits DNA synthesis and is reasonably well tolerated, even in the elderly.
    - Byrne et al. reported a 48% RR and a median OS of 9.4 months with a combination of gemcitabine and cisplatin; symptom improvement occurred in 90% of patients; gemcitabine has also been combined with carboplatin or oxaliplatin with similar efficacy, but, because phase III data are not available, pemetrexed and cisplatin remains standard first-line care.
  - Other drugs that have shown activity against MPM include vinorelbine and vinflunine, although available data is limited.
- Palliation of MPM is frequently required as disease progresses and may involve various modalities.
  - Dyspnea due to recurrent pleural effusion may be treated with repeat thoracentesis but is best controlled with definitive talc pleurodesis via tube thoracostomy or thoracoscopy; oral or sublingual morphine may provide subjective relief from dyspnea.
  - Pain is very common in advanced MPM and results via one or more of three mechanisms: chest wall invasion causes somatic pain that may be relieved with anti-inflammatory or opiate drugs; intercostal nerve or vertebral invasion can cause neuropathic pain that may respond to anticonvulsant drugs (gabapentin, carbamazepine, or valproic acid) or intercostal nerve block; organ invasion results in visceral pain, which typically requires opiates.

Table 25–2 Regimens for MPM

Cisplatin and pemetrexed*: cisplatin 75 mg/m² IV day 1 and pemetrexed 500 mg/m² IV day 1 every 21 days × 4–8 cycles (standard-of-care first-line regimen)
Carboplatin and pemetrexed: carboplatin AUC 5 IV day 1 and pemetrexed 500 mg/m² IV day 1 every 21 days × 4–8 cycles
Cisplatin and gemcitabine: cisplatin 100 mg/m² IV day 1 and gemcitabine 1000 mg/m² IV day 1,8,15 every 28 days
Carboplatin and gemcitabine: carboplatin AUC 5 IV day 1 and gemcitabine 1000 mg/m² IV day 1,8,15 every 28 days

*Patients treated with pemetrexed should receive folate 400 μg by mouth daily and vitamin B12 1000 μg IM every 9 weeks beginning 7–10 days prior to commencing treatment and continued during treatment; dexamethasone 4 mg by mouth twice daily the day prior, of, and after pemetrexed as rash prophylaxis.

COMPLICATIONS OF TREATMENT

- Extrapleural pneumonectomy/PD: bronchial fistula, empyema, chylothorax, vocal cord paralysis, atrial fibrillation, venous thromboembolism, wound infection, sepsis, death.
- Radiation: pneumonitis, lung fibrosis, dermatitis, fatigue, nausea, vomiting
- Pemetrexed: pancytopenia (decreased with folate/B12 supplementation), fatigue, nausea/vomiting, rash (prevented with prophylactic dexamethasone), fever, and diarrhea.
- Gemcitabine: cytopenia (especially thrombocytopenia), edema, capillary-leak syndrome (hypotension, edema, body cavity effusions), nausea, vomiting, diarrhea, flulike syndrome, pneumonitis, thrombotic microangiopathy (rare).
- Cisplatin: nausea, vomiting, fatigue, ototoxicity, nephrotoxicity, electrolyte-wasting (magnesium, potassium), peripheral neuropathy, cytopenia.
- Carboplatin: nausea, vomiting, fatigue, diarrhea, cytopenia (especially thrombocytopenia).

FOLLOW-UP CARE

- There is no standard follow-up regimen, but in patients who have undergone surgical resection follow-up every 3 months with history, physical examination, and chest imaging (chest radiography and/or CT) is reasonable; patients with advanced disease may undergo CT or PET to assess for disease response, but this is often of short duration.

PROGNOSIS

- Prognosis for the vast majority of patients is dismal, with most deaths occurring from local extension within the mediastinum or chest cavity.
- The median survival of MPM from time of diagnosis is 12 months; chemotherapy may improve upon this by several weeks to a few months; a few patients may survive >2 years following EPP and adjuvant chemotherapy and radiation.
- Poor prognostic factors include poor performance status, male gender, leukocytosis, anemia, thrombocytosis, chest wall pain, and sarcomatoid histology.

REFERENCES

Am J Med Sci 2005;329:29.
Ann Oncol 2008;19:370.
Br J Cancer 2008;99:44.
Clin Lung Cancer 2003;4:294.
J Thorac Oncol 2006;1:25.
J Clin Oncol 1999;17:25.
Lancet 2008;371:1685.
N Engl J Med 2005;353:1591.
Oncologist 2007;12:850.

BACKGROUND

- The myelodysplastic syndromes (MDS) are a heterogeneous group of clonal hematologic diseases characterized by peripheral blood cytopenia(s) and hypercellular bone marrow.
- MDS is typically a disease of the elderly with a mean age of 68 years at diagnosis, although MDS can uncommonly occur in patients <50 years; there is a male predominance.
- Most cases arise *de novo*, although treatment-related MDS (tMDS) may follow administration of alkylating agents (typically within 5 to 7 years of therapy) or topoisomerase inhibitors (typically within 2 to 3 years of therapy); tMDS often transforms into therapy-resistant acute myeloid leukemia (AML).
- Risk factors: advanced age, radiation exposure, benzene, chemotherapy, smoking, agricultural chemicals, genetic syndromes (e.g., Diamond-Blackfan syndrome, Fanconi anemia, Shwachman-Diamond syndrome, and dyskeratosis congenita).

PATHOBIOLOGY

- Despite a hypercellular marrow in most cases of MDS, peripheral blood cytopenia(s) is present due to ineffective erythropoiesis, apoptosis of marrow precursors, and hyporesponsiveness to endogenous growth factors; abnormal cell proliferation and differentiation also contribute to cytopenia.
- Transforming genetic mutations of the hematopoietic stem cell are central to development of MDS; mutations of NRAS and TET2 are common.
- Recent research has shown that epigenetic changes, abnormal cytokine production, immune dysregulation, and an abnormal bone marrow stroma all contribute to the development of MDS.
  - Epigenetic changes, such as abnormal DNA methylation of transcription promoter regions, leads to gene silencing of tumor-suppressor genes and emergence of a neoplastic clone (targeted by hypomethylating agents).
  - Increased marrow production of VEGF, tumor necrosis factor (TNF), and other inflammatory cytokines, such as IL-6 contribute to pathobiology.

- Common hematologic and bone marrow findings of MDS:
  - Peripheral blood smear: thrombocytopenia, anisocytosis, macroovalocytosis, dimorphic red cell population, hypogranular neutrophils, unilobed or bilobed neutrophils ("pseudo-Pelger Huet" cells), circulating blasts in advanced stage disease.
  - Bone marrow aspirate/biopsy: hallmark is dyspoiesis of erythroid and myeloid precursors characterized by bizarre nucleus, hypogranular cytoplasm, abnormal hemoglobinization, and nuclear-cytoplasmic dyssynchrony; dyspoietic megakaryocytes, ringed sideroblasts, and myeloblasts may be noted; reticulin fibrosis; the 5q- variant associated with hypolobulated micromegakaryocytes.
- Clonal chromosomal derangements are present in 40% to 70% of patients and include trisomy 8, deletions of entire or portions of chromosome 5 or 7 (often present following alkylating chemotherapy; associated with shorter survival), 11q23 (following therapy with topoisomerase inhibitors, such as anthracyclines and epipodophyllotoxins), deletion of portions of chromosome 13 and 20; the presence of specific chromosomal derangements is an important prognosticator (see below); interstitial deletion of 5q31is associated with an MDS variant known as 5q- syndrome, which has unique hematologic findings (macrocytosis, elevated platelet count, erythroid hypoplasia, and hypolobulated megakaryocytes), presentation (middle-aged females with severe anemia), treatment, and favorable prognosis; loss of chromosome Y is common but does not confer an adverse outcome.
- Hypoplastic MDS, similar to aplastic anemia, is often associated with expression of HLADR15 and/or trisomy 8 and abnormal T-lymphocyte damage to marrow cells and is important to recognize due to dramatic response to immune suppression therapy (IST) in select patients.
  - Hypocellular marrow reminiscent of aplastic anemia and often paroxysmal nocturnal hemoglobinuria (PNH) clone detected.
- Over time, acquisition of new genetic mutations leads to further cellular instability and evolution to acute leukemia, most often acute myeloid leukemia (AML).

CLINICAL PRESENTATION

- Many patients with MDS are asymptomatic, with anemia discovered during evaluation for other reasons.
- Symptomatic MDS patients typically present with manifestations of anemia: fatigue, dyspnea, angina, palpitations, headache, syncope; neutropenia may manifest as recurrent fever or symptoms of infection, typically of the skin or respiratory tract; thrombocytopenia may manifest as mucosal bleeding (epistaxis, hematuria, melena) or bruising.
- Ophthalmic symptoms such as visual loss, eye tearing, or pain may complicate MDS-related corneal ulcers, iritis, vitreous/retinal hemorrhage, or optic neuritis.

- Some patients may note rashes, which may be autoimmune or due to acute neutrophilic dermatosis (e.g., Sweet's syndrome).
- Evolution to AML is often associated with the above symptoms as well as fever, night sweats, bone pain, anorexia, weight loss, and rapid decline in performance status.

PHYSICAL FINDINGS

- Pallor of skin, mucous membranes, conjunctiva, and nail beds if anemia is severe.
- Mucosal bleeding (e.g., nose, gingiva), petechia, purpura if thrombocytopenia is severe.
- Erythematous nodular plaques may indicate Sweet's syndrome.

DIAGNOSTIC TESTS AND STAGING

- Initial diagnostic test is a CBC, which most often shows normocytic or macrocytic anemia; thrombocytopenia and/or leukopenia not uncommon; bilobed pseudo-Pelger cells may be noted; circulating blasts may be present with advanced-stage MDS; isolated neutropenia or thrombocytopenia (associated with loss of 20q).
- Reticulocyte count is typically low due to ineffective erythropoiesis.
- Exclusion of other disorders that cause marrow dyspoiesis: B12/folate levels, human immunodeficiency virus (HIV) testing in at-risk patients, copper level (malnourished patients), lead or arsenic levels if suspicion high.
- Bone marrow aspiration, biopsy, cytogenetic study for classification and prognosis.
  - >80% of bone marrow biopsies are hypercellular; dyspoiesis in ≥10% of cells in any erythroid or myeloid lineage necessary for diagnosis of MDS.
  - Cytogenetic analysis necessary for determining prognosis (see Table 26–1).
- Serum erythropoietin: predictive of response to erythropoietic stimulating agents (ESAs), such as recombinant erythropoietin, if level <500 mU/mL.
- The WHO classification system is based on marrow morphology, presence of unilineage or multilineage dysplasia, and percentage of circulating and bone marrow blasts.
  - Refractory cytopenia with unilineage dysplasia (RCUD): refractory anemia (Hb <10 gm/dl); refractory neutropenia (ANC <1.8 × 10⁹ cells/L); refractory thrombocytopenia (platelets <100,000 cells/L); all with <5% marrow blasts.
  - Refractory anemia with ringed sideroblasts (RARS): isolated anemia (Hb<10 gm/dL) with marrow dysplasia limited to erythroid line, ≥15% ringed sideroblasts, and <5% blasts.

- Refractory anemia with multilineage dysplasia (RCMD), with or without ringed sideroblasts: ≥2 peripheral cytopenias; marrow dysplasia involving ≥2 cell lineages, <5% blasts, > or <15% ringed sideroblasts, no Auer rods.
- Refractory anemia with excess blasts-1 (RAEB-1): ≤2% to 4% circulating blasts; 5% to 9% marrow blasts and absence of Auer rods.
- Refractory anemia with excess blasts-2 (RAEB-2): 5% to 19% circulating blasts; 10% to 19% marrow blasts, and/or presence of Auer rods.
- MDS variant del5(q), "5q- syndrome": anemia and normal or elevated platelet count; isolated erythroid dysplasia, <5% blasts, isolated del 5q on metaphase spread.
- MDS, unclassified (MDS-U): peripheral cytopenia(s); marrow unilineage dysplasia or no dysplasia in presence of typical MDS cytogenetic changes with <5% blasts.

- The International Prognostic Scoring System (IPSS) is based on a multivariate analysis of data from several studies of untreated patients with *de novo* MDS; the IPSS combines clinical, morphologic, and cytogenetic data to predict survival duration and risk of leukemic transformation.

Table 26–1 International Prognostic Scoring System (IPSS)*

Prognostic variable	Value	Score
Marrow blasts	<5%	0
	5% to 10%	0.5
	11% to 20%	1.5
	21% to 30%	2.0
Karyotype**	Good	0
	Intermediate	0.5
	Poor	1.0
Number of cytopenias	0–1	0
	2–3	0.5

Risk category (% of IPSS pts.)	Sum of scores	Median survival without therapy
Low (33%)	0	5.7 years
INT-1 (38%)	0.5–1.0	3.5 years
INT-2 (22%)	1.5–2.0	1.1 years
High (7%)	≥2.5	0.4 years

Blood 1997;89:2079

**Cytogenetics: Good=normal, isolated -Y, isolated del(5q), isolated del(20q); Poor= ≥3 (complex) abnormalities or abnormal chromosome 7; intermediate=all others

TREATMENT

- The only curative therapy for MDS is allogenic stem cell transplantation, but, due to increased age and comorbidities of most MDS patients, is an option for relatively few patients (advanced-stage disease, young age, good performance status); ongoing research with reduced intensity conditioning regimens may expand the population eligible for transplant in the future.
- Supportive care is the mainstay for low-risk disease and elderly/infirm patients and includes transfusion of leukoreduced (irradiated and cyto-megalovirus [CMV]-matched if stem cell transplant planned) red cells and platelets and administration of ESAs and granulocyte-stimulating growth factors (G-CSF).
  - Recombinant erythropoietin 40,000–60,000 U subcutaneously one to three times per week or darbopoietin 150–300 mcg subcutaneously weekly or 500 mcg subcutaneously monthly.
  - Filgrastim (G-CSF) 300–480 mcg one to three per week may be added to ESAs if erythroid response suboptimal; not indicated for neutropenia in absence of repeated bacterial infection.
- Hypomethylating agents (azacytadine, decitabine) remove methyl groups from promoter sequences of transcription genes, which reverses hyper-methylation-induced gene silencing of tumor-suppressor genes, allowing for restoration of normal gene functions critical for cell proliferation and differentiation.
  - These agents delay time to leukemic transformation, improve cytopenias and symptoms, and, in the case of azacytidine, improve survival for patients with advanced-stage (INT-2 and high-risk) disease compared to supportive care alone (24.5 months vs. 15 months); complete remissions may occur in 10% to 17% of patients treated with azacytidine.
  - Recent meta-analysis showed azacytidine and decitabine prolonged survival (HR=0.66) and time to leukemic transformation or death (HR=0.69); azacytidine, but not decitabine, improved survival (HR=0.56) on subgroup analysis.
  - Several cycles, often four to six, may be necessary before hematologic responses are noted.
- Lenolidamide is an immunomodulating agent related to thalidomide; in a pivotal trial of 148 patients with 5q- variant of MDS, it demonstrated impressive activity at rapidly reducing transfusion requirements.
  - Median time to response was 4.6 weeks, with median rise in hemoglobin of 5.4 g/dL; cytogenetic improvement (including complete cytogenetic remission) was common, and transfusion independence was maintained for >1 year in 62% of lenalidomide responders; based on these data, lenalidomide is standard treatment for 5q- syndrome with symptomatic/severe anemia.
- Induction-type chemotherapy for RAEB-2 or AML may be attempted, but complications are common and disease is often refractory.

- Antithymocyte globulin (ATG) and/or cyclosporine should be considered in pancytopenic patients with hypoplastic MDS, especially those with detectable paroxysmal nocturnal hemoglobinuria (PNH) clone and/or expression of HLADR15.
- Chelation therapy for patients transfused with >20–30 units of red cells or serum ferritin >1000 mg/dL; can use infusional deferoxamine or oral desfirasirox.

Table 26–2 Regimens for MDS

Azacytidine 75 mg/m^2 SQ or IV daily for 5–7 days every 28 days
Decitabine 15 mg/m^2 IV every 8 hours for 3 days
Lenalidomide 10 mg by mouth daily or 10 mg by mouth daily for 21 days every 28 days
Antithymocyte globulin (equine) 40 mg/kg IV daily for 4 days

COMPLICATIONS OF TREATMENT

- Transfusion therapy: acute transfusion reactions, infection, alloimmunization, delayed hemolysis, iron overload.
- ESAs: diarrhea, hypertension, seizures, venous thromboembolism (especially if hemoglobin >12 gm/dL).
- Filgrastim: bone pain, myalgias, splenic rupture (rare).
- Hypomethylating agents: fatigue, nausea, vomiting, edema, neutropenia, thrombocytopenia, infection.

FOLLOW-UP CARE

- Patients with low-risk disease should be monitored every few months with a CBC to detect worsening cytopenias or transformation to leukemia; serum ferritin should be monitored after 15–20 units of red cells are administered.
- High-risk patients should be examined and have CBC every several weeks for evidence of bleeding, infection, or symptoms/signs of AML.

PROGNOSIS

- The IPSS, recently refined, is useful to counsel patients with regards to prognosis, with median survivals as follows: low risk, 97 months; intermediate-1 risk, 63 months; intermediate-2 risk, 26 months; and high risk, 11 months.
- Overall, best prognosis for RARS and worst for RAEB-2.

REFERENCES

Ann Intern Med 2002;137:156.
Curr Oncol Rep 2008;10:372.
Haematologica 2009;epub, ahead of print.
J Clin Oncol 2002;20:2429.
Lancet Oncol 2009;10:223.
Leukemia 2005;19:2223.
N Engl J Med 2009;361:1872.
N Engl J Med 2006;355:1456.

27 ■ ACUTE MYELOID LEUKEMIA

BACKGROUND

- Acute myeloid leukemia (AML) is a group of neoplasms arising from a clonal hematopoietic stem cell in which failure of differentiation and overproliferation of the malignant progeny results in accumulation of nonfunctional cells known as myeloblasts.
  - It is the abnormal function of myeloblasts and decreased production of normal hematopoietic cells that give rise to the cardinal manifestations of AML: anemia (red cells), infection (neutrophils), and bleeding (platelets).
- There are approximately 13,000 cases and 9000 deaths attributed to AML annually in the United States; the incidence may rise as the age of the population increases and, with that, the rate of myelodysplastic syndromes (MDS); the increased number of cancer survivors (e.g., breast/testicular cancer and Hodgkin's disease patients) who have received myelotoxic chemotherapy and/or therapeutic radiation may further increase the risk of AML due to marrow stem cell damage and treatment-related MDS (tMDS).
- The median age at diagnosis is 68 years, with an age-adjusted population-incidence of 17.6 cases per 100,000 population for those >65 years and 1.8 cases per 100,000 population for those <65 years.
- AML therapy is highly age dependent, with patients >60 years considered elderly and possessing different disease biology and markedly inferior prognosis to those <60 years—treatment paradigms generally differ in these populations: less intense/supportive therapy versus aggressive chemotherapy/stem cell transplantation, respectively.
- Risk factors: although most cases in patients <60 years arise *de novo*, several established risk factors for AML exist: ionizing radiation (therapeutic, atomic bomb survivors); occupational benzene, petrochemical, paint, or pesticide exposure; cigarette smoking; chemotherapy (most commonly alkylating agents); and the antipsoriasis agent, bimolane, which has been linked to acute promyelocytic leukemia (APL).

PATHOBIOLOGY

- Abnormal proliferation and failure of differentiation underscore the pathogenesis of AML; the subtype APL has a unique biology and will be discussed separately.

- AML cells infiltrate the marrow, blood, and other tissues, such as the skin, bone, gingiva (monocytic AML), and meninges (monocytic AML); a mass lesion of leukemic blasts known as a granulocytic sarcoma can involve virtually any organ.
- Failure of erythroid, megakaryocyte, and neutrophil precursor generation by the infiltrating blast population results in severe anemia, hemorrhage, and infections, respectively.
- Any type of AML, especially APL, can induce a consumptive coagulopathy and a disseminated intravascular coagulation (DIC) picture.

- APL is important to recognize due to its unique pathogenesis and disease-specific therapy and complications.
  - Translocation of the promyelocytic (PML) gene on chromosome 15 and the retinoic acid receptor-α (RAR-α) gene on chromosome 17 [t(15;17)] results in a fusion-gene that produces the PML-RARα protein, which blocks normal myeloid gene transcription and differentiation, leading to growth arrest at the promyelocyte stage.
  - Accumulation of promyelocytes with their abundant coagulophilic granules, leads to consumptive coagulopathy/DIC characterized by hypofibrinogenemia and thrombocytopenia, which accounts for hemorrhagic death before or during induction therapy.
  - Modern therapy of APL hinges upon the differentiating agent, all-*trans* retinoic acid (ATRA), which induces rapid (within hours to days) differentiation of promyelocytes into maturing neutrophils; maturing cells adhere to the pulmonary vasculature *via* surface adhesion molecules and release cellular contents into the circulation, frequently leading to "differentiation syndrome," which is characterized by cytokine-induced fever, tachycardia, and a vascular-leak syndrome, resulting in life-threatening pulmonary edema, pleural/pericardial effusions, peripheral edema, and hemoconcentration with shock.

- Morphologic, immunohistochemical, and cell-surface markers are useful in characterization of different AML subtypes.
  - AML blasts are 12–20 μm in diameter, contain multiple nucleoli, and often contain azurophilic granules within the cytoplasm; a pathognomonic feature is the presence of plasmic Auer rods; undifferentiated AML (M0) may not contain granules.
  - Most cases of AML (especially M1–M4) stain positive for myeloperoxidase (MPO), whereas monocytic leukemias (M4, M5) stain for nonspecific esterase (NSE); periodic acid Schiff (PAS)-positive staining may be noted in some cases, especially acute erythroleukemia (M6).
  - APL cells contain prominent cytoplasmic granules and Auer rods; the hypogranular variant of APL, however, typically possesses a bilobed or folded nucleus and absence of cytoplasmic granules.
  - Cell surface markers (often in abnormal combinations) typically detected by flow cytometry are helpful in determining subtype.
    - Most AML blasts express antigens found on normal immature myeloid cells: CD13, CD33, and CD34; APL blasts are typically HLA-DR4 negative.

- Monocytic blasts typically express CD14.
- Erythroid leukemia (M6) and megakaryocytic leukemia (M7) express CD36/71 and CD41a/61, respectively.
- Cytogenetic and molecular biology profiles are of key importance in disease biology and providing prognostic information that determines treatment strategy.
  - Beside age, cytogenetics are the most important factor predicting survival and response to chemotherapy and are divided into three categories: favorable [t(8;21) and inv16 or t(16;16)]—the so-called core-binding-factor leukemias; intermediate (normal karyotype); and high-risk (abnormalities of chromosome 5 and/or 7, trisomy 8, 11q23 translocation, or complex abnormalities); the intermediate-risk group comprises the largest group and is heterogeneous with regards to prognosis.
    - Nonrandom molecular mutations in cytogenetically normal AML have recently been shown to provide prognostic information: internal tandem duplication (ITD) of the FLT3 (FLT3-ITD) gene that encodes a growth factor receptor (20% to 40% of cases) and mutation of the NPM1 gene (20% to 30% of cases) that encodes a nucleolar-cytoplasmic shuttling protein; both may occur in isolation or as double mutations.
    - A single NPM1 mutation confers a favorable outlook—similar to the favorable cytogenetic-risk group and presence of FLT3-ITD is associated with inferior survival; patients who express both mutations have a prognosis between those with isolated mutations.
    - Recent data suggest that cKIT or BAALC mutations predict inferior survival, whereas mutation of CEBPA predicts improved survival.
  - APL is considered separately due to different biology and therapy and is characterized by the t(15;17) translocation; the gene product, the APL-RARα fusion-protein, can be detected in marrow or peripheral blood via reverse transcriptase polymerase chain reaction (RT-PCR).
  - Karyotyping of bone marrow by metaphase cytogenetics is mandatory in all patients at presentation to categorize an individual patient into one of the above risk groups.
- Secondary AML arises in the setting of an antecedent blood disorder, most commonly in elderly patients with MDS (24% to 56% in patients >60 years compared to 8% for those <60) either de novo or following a myeloproliferative disorder or chemotherapy (see below).
- Patients >60 have higher incidence of antecedent MDS, unfavorable cytogenetic profiles (chromosome 5 and/or 7 abnormalities, trisomy 8, or complex aberrations), and lower incidence of favorable cytogenetic profiles (t(8;21), t(16;16), inv16, and t(15;17)) compared to their younger counterparts—all factors that contribute to more aggressive disease biology and inferior outcomes.
  - AML cells in the elderly have a higher incidence (71% vs. 35% in those <60 years) of harboring the multidrug resistance gene MDR1

and its product, the P-glycoprotein drug-efflux pump, which confers less chemosensitivity and lower rates of complete remission.
- Underlying comorbidity, as well as altered drug-metabolism, particularly for cytarabine, contributes to inferior outcome and greater treatment morbidity/mortality in the elderly.
- The pathogenesis of chemotherapy-related AML generally depends on the type of agent and duration since therapy.
  - Characteristics of alkylating agent-related AML (melphalan, cyclophosphamide, nitrosureas): prolonged latency (5 to 7 years), development of MDS prior to AML, frequent derangements of chromosomes 5 and/or 7, and poor response to therapy.
  - Characteristics of topoisomerase II inhibitor-related AML (anthracyclines, etoposide): short latency (1 to 2 years), monocytic morphology, derangements of chromosome 11q23, and lack of preceding MDS.

CLINICAL PRESENTATION

- Most patients are symptomatic for a relatively short period (<12 weeks) before diagnosis and often present with nonspecific symptoms such as fatigue, weakness, and anorexia; weight loss is common, and fever may be the only manifestation in 10% of patients.
- Bruising and mucosal bleeding may complicate coagulopathy or thrombocytopenia.
- Sudden, severe headache or seizure may occur with cerebral hemorrhage, especially in patients with APL-related coagulopathy or monocytic leukemia.
- Severe neutropenia may present with oral ulcers or evidence of infection of oral or soft tissues (fluctuance, erythema, and warmth may be absent).
- Patients with significant leukocytosis (>100,000 cells/mm^3) may present with symptoms of leukostasis: visual changes, headache, confusion, dyspnea, cough.

PHYSICAL FINDINGS

- Low-grade fever is not uncommon; tachycardia may result from fever or anemia.
- Pallor of the skin, conjunctiva, nail beds, and mucosal surfaces results from anemia.
- Gingival enlargement is characteristic of monocytic leukemia.
- Blood in the nares/oral cavity or petechiae suggest thrombocytopenia, whereas large ecchymoses are suggestive of coagulopathy/DIC.
- Papular skin lesions may result from leukemic infiltration (*leukemia cutis*).
- Hepatomegaly, splenomegaly, and lymphadenopathy may occur but are uncommon in AML.

DIAGNOSTIC TESTS AND STAGING

- Uric acid, creatinine, potassium, phosphorus, calcium, and LDH should be obtained at diagnosis and during therapy to monitor for tumor lysis and renal dysfunction.
- Exclusion of coagulopathy with PT, PTT, and fibrinogen is indicated in all patients, especially those with APL due to the very high occurrence in this subtype.
- Evaluation of left ventricular function with nuclear gated scan or echocardiography prior to anthracycline therapy.
- Assessment of CMV serostatus, especially for allogenic transplant candidates.
- Bone marrow aspiration and biopsy with morphologic, immunohistochemical, flow cytometric, and cytogenetic examinations; molecular studies to assess for NPM1 mutation or presence of FLT3-ITD suggested.
- HLA antigen testing on initial marrow evaluation if transplant anticipated; also useful for platelet matching if refractoriness develops during treatment; HLA typing of family members should be performed quickly in patients found to have high-risk disease.
- Routine lumbar puncture with cytology is not routinely indicated in most AML patients; however, it should be considered for patients with WBC >100,000 cells/mm^3 and/or monocytic differentiation (M4/M5).

TREATMENT

- Placement of a subcutaneously tunneled multilumen catheter is necessary for frequent blood draws and administration of blood products and cytotoxic chemotherapy.
- Urine alkalinization with intravenous sodium bicarbonate (1 to 2 ampules added to a liter of 5% dextrose in water or half-normal saline) and allopurinol (300 mg orally daily).
  - Rasburicase (recombinant urate oxidase) should be considered for patients at high-risk of or with end-organ dysfunction from tumor lysis (renal failure, hyperkalemia, acidosis, arrhythmia).
- Posaconazole antifungal prophylaxis (200 mg orally three times daily) significantly decreases incidence of fungal infections during induction therapy compared to fluconazole.
- Acyclovir or a derivative can be considered to prevent latent oral herpes infection.
- Principles of blood product transfusion support include use of leukoreduced and irradiated products to decrease risk of alloimmunization and transfusion-associated graft-versus-host disease, respectively; red cell transfusion for Hb <8 grams; single-donor aphereis platelets for platelet count <10,000 cells/mm^3 (<20,000 cells/mm^3 in presence of fever or active infection) or with evidence of bleeding; CMV-negative blood should be administered for potential transplant candidates, although leukoreduction affords protection against CMV transmission as well.

- Patients with APL-coagulopathy should receive cryoprecipitate to maintain serum fibrinogen >150 mg/dL and platelet transfusion to maintain count >50,000 cells/mm^3.

- Use of myeloid growth factors such as filgrastim following induction therapy decreases duration of neutropenia by 5 to 7 days (but not mortality) and may be considered after day-14 bone marrow aspiration.

- Febrile neutropenia episodes should be treated with broad-spectrum antimicrobials (after cultures of blood from catheter and peripheral site) to cover Gram-negative and Gram-positive organisms (e.g., antipseudomonal penicillin in combination with aminoglycoside, aztreonam, or quinolone; monotherapy with cefepime or carbapenem; vancomycin should be considered if the likelihood of a line infection is significant or if severe oral mucositis is present, which can result in fatal toxic-shock syndrome from oral viridians streptococci); fever persisting beyond 7 days should be empirically treated with an antifungal agent different from the prophylactic agent (e.g., voriconazole, caspofungin, amphotericin).

- Oral, perineal, eye, and skin care should be instituted in all patients; women of menstruating age should receive ovarian suppression.

- The goal of induction chemotherapy is to significantly decrease the myeloblast count to allow normal hematopoiesis to occur and to provide a complete hematologic remission (CHR); the day-14 marrow aspirate is to ensure that chemotherapy has induced adequate cytoreduction/marrow aplasia, with <5% marrow blasts signifying successful induction); a CHR is defined as an absolute neutrophil count (ANC) >1000 cells/mm^3, platelets >100,000 cells/mm^3, and no evidence of extramedullary disease, however, it is important to realize that CHR does not equate to cure or eradication of the leukemic clone; induction regimens are identical for non-APL subtypes and will be discussed separately.

  - AML (non-APL): the standard induction regimen has remained unchanged for many years and consists of infusional cytarbine for 7 days and an anthracycline (daunorubicin, idarubicin, or mitoxantrone) daily for the first 3 days of therapy ("7 + 3" regimen); idarubicin may be slightly superior to daunorubicin due to prolonged intracellular retention times; mitoxantrone (an anthracenedione) may be considered if concern of cardiotoxicity exists; a recent study, however, demonstrated that daunorubicin 90 mg/m^2 IV for three doses during induction significantly improved CR rates and survival in patients <50 years with favorable- or intermediate-risk cytogenetics; 65% to 75% of patients <60 years achieve CR following induction (two-thirds after one cycle and one-third after two cycles); fit elderly patients can be treated with 7 + 3, but treatment-related morbidity/mortality are significant and remission rates are much lower; frail patients can be treated with cytarbine 20 mg subcutaneously twice daily for 10 days monthly or daily hydroxyurea, although CR rate of 18% and a survival benefit have been shown for subcutaneous cytarabine compared to hydroxyurea (1% CR rate and no survival benefit).

- 7 to 10 days following completion of induction, a bone marrow aspirate is performed to document aplasia and <5% blasts; patients with residual leukemia are typically treated with the same regimen as induction (may be shortened to 5 + 2 if toxicity a concern).
- Patients who fail to achieve CR following two induction cycles are high-risk and should be transferred to a transplant center for an allogeneic hematopoietic stem cell transplantation (HSCT; if a suitable donor can be indentified in timely fashion) or a clinical trial.
- APL: the discovery that retinoic acid is able to induce remission in most patients with APL is a milestone in modern medicine; ATRA acts as a differentiating agent upon promyelocytes, inducing release of maturation arrest and formation of neutrophils; ATRA should be administered orally if APL is suspected, before results of testing for t(15;17) are available; administration of idarubicin for 3 days remains standard of care; the role of cytarabine is controversial, but should be considered in patients with "high-risk" APL (WBC >10,000 cells/mm^3 and/or platelet count <40,000 cells/mm^3); data are emerging for a "chemotherapy-free" regimen of arsenic trioxide (ATO, an agent that causes apoptosis of APL cells) and ATRA—a regimen that may be considered in patients who may not tolerate cytotoxic chemotherapy; addition of the gemtuzumab-ozagomicin (an anti-CD33 monoclonal antibody attached to a calicheamicin, a cytotoxic agent) to ATO-ATRA can be considered in high-risk patients receiving this induction regimen.
  - As noted above, careful monitoring for coagulopathy with as-needed correction with platelets, cryoprecipitate, and/or frozen plasma is vital to keep platelets >50,000 cells/mm^3 and fibrinogen >150 mg/dL, respectively; the ATRA-differentiation syndrome should be treated with dexamethasone 10 mg IV twice daily for 3 to 5 days, followed by a 14-day taper, with supportive care as necessary; prophylactic dexamethasone should be administered to patients with WBC >30,000 cells/mm^3 at the time of induction; patients receiving ATO should have periodic electrocardiography to monitor the QT interval and daily monitoring of potassium and magnesium levels to maintain above 4.0 meq/dL and 1.8 mg/dL, respectively.
- Following induction, virtually all patients with AML will relapse within several months if not administered consolidation chemotherapy, with the goal of further cytoreduction to the point of cure or in anticipation of HSCT.
  - AML (non-APL): consolidation therapy in younger patients is based primarily on cytogenetic profile; favorable-risk patients should receive three to four cycles of high-dose cytarabine (HiDAC; 3 grams/m^2 IV every 12 hours on days 1, 3, 5), which is associated with cure rates similar to allogeneic HSCT, but with a significantly lower morbidity and mortality (5% mortality and 12% neurologic/cerebellar toxicity for HiDAC); patients with intermediate-risk AML should typically receive (HiDAC) as well, with HSCT reserved for relapse, unless a matched sibling is available for a young patient in first remission; patients

with high-risk cytogenetics, normal karyotype but with poor molecular features (such as presence of FLT-ITD and absence of NPM1 mutation), should be referred to a transplant center for preparation for HSCT; patients who require two induction cycles to achieve remission or those who are refractory should be transferred to a transplant center for consideration of HSCT; older fit patients may receive lower dose (1–2 grams/m^2) cytarabine or the 5 + 2 regimen for consolidation, but most will relapse, and a clinical trial should always be considered; data are emerging to support consideration for reduced-intensity conditioning allogeneic HSCT in select elderly patients.

- APL: goal of consolidation is to achieve molecular remission, with absence of PML-RARα in blood and marrow; typically, three cycles of consolidation anthracycline with 15 days of ATRA (45 mg/m^2 orally); consolidation cytarabine does not appear to benefit low- and intermediate-risk patients, but should be considered in high-risk patients; ATO consolidation following anthracycline/ATRA induction is being studied and may emerge as a standard of care; consolidation with ATO (or cytarabine) should be considered in high-risk patients; APL patients should receive 1 to 2 years of oral maintenance ATRA with or without methotrexate and 6-mercaptopurine (6-MP), because trials have shown decreased relapse rates: 35% for no maintenance; 21% for ATRA; and 8% for ATRA, methotrexate, and 6-MP; however, patients with low-risk disease and postconsolidation molecular remission may not receive a significant absolute benefit from maintenance therapy.

- Relapse of AML after initially successful therapy is not uncommon and is approached differently based upon AML versus APL and patient age.
  - AML (non-APL): younger patients who relapse <12 months following induction chemotherapy should be assessed at a transplant center for possible clinical trial or HSCT; patients with late relapse may receive the same induction regimen followed by preparation for a HSCT from a sibling, unrelated donor, or cord blood; patients >60 years with AML relapse may be considered for reinduction with the initial regimen if they are fit and have a long remission, gemtuzumab ozogamicin, or best supportive care (transfusions, antibiotics); gemtuzumab ozogamicin is approved for treatment of relapsed AML in older patients; hypomethylating agents such as azacytidine may be considered in some patients.
  - APL: patients who have not achieved molecular remission at the end of consolidation or who develop molecular relapse should receive ATO, which can induce molecular remission in 70% to 80% of patients as monotherapy; patients with relapsed APL may have central nervous system involvement, and intrathecal chemotherapy is recommended; patients who achieve molecular remission following relapse therapy benefit from autologous HSCT; gemtuzumab ozogamicin is an effective salvage regimen for relapsed APL and may be considered in nontransplant candidates; allogenic HSCT should be considered for salvage.

Table 27–1 Regimens for AML/APL

Induction
AML (non-APL)
"7 + 3" regimen: cytarabine 100 mg/m^2/day IV continuous infusion × 7 days, combined with any one:
Idarubicin 12 mg/m^2 IV days 1,2,3; daunorubicin 60–90 mg/m^2 IV days 1,2,3; Mitoxantrone 12 mg/m^2 IV days 1,2,3
APL
AIDA: ATRA 45 mg/m^2 by mouth daily and idarubicin 12 mg/m^2 IV days 2,4,6,8 (consider continuous infusion cytarabine in high-risk patients)

Consolidation
AML (non-APL)
HiDAC: cytarabine 3000 mg/m^2 IV every 12 hours days 1,3,5
"5 + 2" regimen: same induction regimen but with 5 days of cytarabine and 2 days of anthracycline
APL
"5 + 2" regimen or single agent anthracycline for 2–3 cycles with ATRA 45 mg/m^2 by mouth followed by 2 years of ATRA (consider daily 6-mercaptopurine and weekly methotrexate in high-risk patients)

Salvage
Cytarabine 20 mg/m^2 SQ daily for 10 days every 28 days (for elderly, infirm patients)
Gemtuzumab ozogamicin 9 mg/m^2 IV, repeat in 14 days; premedication with acetaminophen 650–1000 mg by mouth and diphenhydramine 50 mg by mouth

COMPLICATIONS OF TREATMENT

- Anthracyclines (daunorubicin, idarubicin, mitoxantrone [actually, an anthracenedione]): myelosuppression, nausea, vomiting, alopecia, cardiotoxicity (arrhythmia, heart failure), rash, mucositis, diarrhea, reddish urine discoloration (except for mitoxantrone, which may cause blue urine), rash.
- High-dose cytarabine: myelosuppression, vomiting, diarrhea, oral mucositis, enteritis, pancreatitis, alopecia, eccrine hidradenitis, cerebellar toxicity/neurotoxicity (especially in patients >60 years and/or patients with renal dysfunction), conjunctivitis (prophylaxis with steroid eye drops mandatory for HiDAC therapy), hand-foot syndrome, pneumonitis, noncardiogenic pulmonary edema, viridans streptococcal sepsis.
- Gemtuzumab ozogamicin: infusion reaction, nausea, vomiting, protracted thrombocytopenia, hepatitis, veno-occlusive disease of liver (typically in patients receiving HSCT after treatment).
- ATRA: differentiation syndrome, vitamin A toxicity (headache, fever, dry skin, rash, pruritis, conjunctivitis), flushing, hypotension, cardiotoxicity, hyperlipidemia, neurologic toxicity, constipation, diarrhea, earache/aural fullness, *pseudotumor cerebri.*

- Arsenic trioxide: differentiation syndrome, leukocytosis, headache, nausea, vomiting, diarrhea, myalgias, hyperglycemia, prolongation of QT interval, *Torsades de pointes*, ventricular tachycardia/fibrillation.

FOLLOW-UP CARE

- Bone marrow aspiration with or without biopsy on day 10–14 of induction to assess for marrow aplasia and presence of <5% blasts; if >5% blasts or if the presence of residual leukemia is equivocal, repeat marrow 7 days later (growth factors should NOT be administered prior to marrow aspirate because they may induce morphologic changes resembling leukemia); patients with APL should NOT undergo marrow aspiration until 4 to 6 weeks posttreatment, after blood counts have recovered, because differentiation of APL cells may take weeks and lead to overtreatment; criteria to document morphologic remission include:
  - Absolute neutrophil count >1000 cells/mm^3, platelets ≥100,000 cells/mm^3, and no evidence of extramedullary involvement.
  - Relapse is defined as reappearance of blasts in the blood, >5% marrow blasts, or evidence of extramedullary relapse.
- Patients in CR following consolidation therapy should undergo a CBC every 1 to 2 months for 2 years and then every 3 to 6 months for a total of 5 years; routine surveillance bone marrow aspiration/biopsy is not recommended and is performed only if abnormal blood counts are discovered.
- Detection of minimal residual disease with metaphase cytogenetics, flow cytometry, fluorescence *in situ* hybridization to detect chromosomal aberrations, and PCR to detect molecular abnormalities (most sensitive method) are important to assess for early disease relapse.
  - Monitoring peripheral blood every 3 months for 2 years after successful consolidation therapy for APL for appearance of the PML-RARα protein with RT-PCR allows early institution of salvage therapy before overt disease is evident.

PROGNOSIS

- Overall, AML has a poor prognosis—only one-third of patients diagnosed between ages 18–60 years will be cured; long-term survival rates in the elderly are approximately 5%.
- Age and cytogenetic category are the dominant predictors of long-term survival, although it is being recognized that various molecular alterations in cytogenetically normal AML patients have powerful prognostic ability.
  - Retrospective reviews have shown 5-year survivals based on cytogenetic categories: 55% to 60% for favorable, 25% to 35% for intermediate, and 5% to 12% with poor risk.

- The intermediate-risk group is heterogeneous; recent data indicate that patients harboring a mutant NPM1 gene and absence of an IDT duplication of the FLT3 gene have a prognosis similar to favorable-risk cytogenetics.
- Retrospective data suggest that a delay of >5 days from diagnosis to commencement of therapy may adversely impact outcome.
- Patients who achieve a hematologic CR after one cycle have longer disease-free intervals than patients who require >1 induction cycle to achieve CR.

REFERENCES

Blood 2010;115:453.
Blood 2009;113:28.
Clin Lymphoma Myeloma 2009;9:s281.
Haematologica 2008;93:1767.
J Clin Oncol 1990;8:272.
N Engl J Med 2009;361:1249.
N Engl J Med 2007;356:348.
N Engl J Med 2001;344:175.
N Engl J Med 1994;331:896.
N Engl J Med 1991;324:1385.
Oncologist 2008;13:1097.

BACKGROUND

- Multiple myeloma (MM) is the most common of the plasma cell disorders—diseases characterized by neoplastic monoclonal cells derived from common progenitors cells within the B-lymphocyte lineage.
- The protean clinical features of these disorders result from expansion of the neoplastic cells within various organ systems, secretion of diverse biologically active molecules, and host-response.
- MM is characterized by the accumulation of monoclonal plasma cells within the bone marrow that typically secrete intact immunoglobulins or light chains; the most common end-organs affected include the kidneys and bone, but widespread organ dysfunction can occur due to tumor-released humoral factors.
- There are approximately 21,000 cases and 11,000 deaths annually in the United States; MM accounts for approximately 1% of all cancers.
- Monoclonal gammopathy of uncertain significance (MGUS, see below for criteria) is usually diagnosed incidentally during evaluation of another problem; MGUS affects up to 10% of patients >75 years.
- There is a slight male predominance with a mean age at diagnosis of 62 years.
- Blacks have twice the incidence of MM compared to whites; MM causes 33% of hematologic malignancies compared to 13%, respectively.
- Risk factors: black race, age, farming, woodworking, leather industry, petroleum exposure.

PATHOBIOLOGY

- Normally, maturation of B-lymphocytes to mature, Ig-secreting plasma cells is stimulated by antigen to which the surface Ig is specific; however, in MM this regulation is lost via complex gene changes and cells produce monoclonal Ig (usually intact Ig or light chains).
- Various gene and chromosomal derangements are common in MM.
  - The most common chromosomal abnormalities include 13q and 17p deletions and 11q derangements; common translocations include t(11;14), t(4;14); hyperploidy is common; 13q deletion, 17p deletion, and t(4;14) are poor prognosticators and associated with a more aggressive phenotype.
  - Overexpression of *ras* or *myc* genes and mutations involving tumor-suppressor genes p53 and Rb1 occur in some cases.

- There is a complex interaction between the malignant plasma cell and the surrounding marrow stroma and vasculature, which results in tumor growth via autocrine and paracrine mechanisms.
  - The MM cell binds to bone marrow stromal cells via adhesion molecules, triggering a cascade of events increasing cell proliferation, survival, and drug-resistance, in part via production of IL-6 and VEGF.
  - This MM cell/stromal cell interaction also up-regulates growth pathways such as Ras/Raf/MAPK, JAK/STAT, and PI3K/Akt.
- Bone lesions in MM result from tumor cell growth, osteoclast activation, and osteoblast suppression; osteoclast activation is a complex but factors such as IL-1, VEGF, macrophage inhibitory factor (MIP), TNF, and receptor activator of nuclear factor kappa-β ligand (RANK-L) play a dominant role.
  - Bone lesions are lytic due to enhanced osteoclast activity and hence are not detected on isotope bone scans; large bone lesions may become expansile (plasmacytoma).
  - Bone resorption commonly causes diffuse osteopenia and/or hypercalcemia, which can lead to neurologic and cardiac dysfunction.
- Renal failure is a hallmark of MM with a variety of pathologic mechanisms.
  - Hypercalcemia is most common cause and results in calcium phosphate precipitation and volume depletion with tubular necrosis; hyperuricemia may contribute.
  - Light-chain excretion damages renal tubular epithelium and may form obstructing deposits within the nephron ("cast nephropathy") and proteinuria; light chains may induce Fanconi's tubulopathy, which is characterized by glucosuria, phosphaturia, and amino aciduria.
  - Amyloid production may cause renal failure and nephrotic syndrome.
  - Other causes of renal failure in MM include hyperuricemia, recurrent infections, use of nonsteroidal agents for bone pain, intravenous contrast, and bisphosphonates; myelomatous infiltration of the kidneys is uncommon.
- Immune dysfunction may result in recurrent bacterial infections, typically involving the respiratory and urinary tracts.
  - Infections due to *Streptococcus pneumoniae*, *Staphylococcus aureus*, *Klebsiella pneumoniae*, and *Escherichia coli* predominate.
  - Increased infection susceptibility results from hypogammaglobulinemia from suppression and destruction of normal immunoglobulins, impaired antibody responses, impaired neutrophil and complement function, and various drugs (dexamethasone and chemotherapy/immune-modulating agents).
- Hematologic abnormalities are common and have several mechanisms.
  - Anemia results from plasma cell infiltration of the marrow, inhibition of erythropoiesis by tumor products, mild hemolysis, and B12 deficiency; renal failure with blunted erythropoietin production and gastrointestinal ulcerations from nonsteroidal use may contribute.

- Neutropenia and thrombocytopenia are uncommon but may occur with large tumor burden.
- Coagulopathy and bleeding may result from platelet dysfunction from Ig-coated platelets or interaction of the M-protein with clotting factors such as I, II, V, VII, and VIII; amyloid may bind factor X.
- Venous thromboembolism may occur from impairment of the clotting cascade or administration of thalidomide or lenalidomide, especially in conjunction with dexamethasone.
- Serum hyperviscosity is uncommon but may result from significant elevation of IgM, IgA or, less commonly, IgG (especially subclass 3); hyperviscosity may result in neurologic or respiratory dysfunction from stasis within the microvasculature.
- Nervous system involvement has several pathologic mechanisms.
  - Hypercalcemia and hyperviscosity may result in cerebral dysfunction.
  - Anatomic etiologies include spinal cord compression from vertebral collapse or plasmacytoma and carpal tunnel syndrome from amyloid infiltration.
  - Peripheral neuropathy often results from neuronal damage from antimyeloma agents, most commonly thalidomide, bortezomib, and vincristine.

CLINICAL PRESENTATION

- Bone pain is the most common symptom, affecting 70% of patients, and most often affects the back and/or ribs, although any bone may be affected; sudden, severe pain or the inability to bear weight should suggest pathologic fracture; skeletal pain from MM is typically related to activity.
- Anemia often presents with weakness, fatigue, dyspnea, or angina.
- Immune dysfunction and hypogammaglobulinemia may result in symptoms of repeated infection (e.g., fever, cough, dysuria, skin redness).
- Hypercalcemia may cause delirium, somnolence, fatigue, polyuria, and constipation.
- Hyperviscosity may cause headache, visual changes, epistaxis, and dyspnea.
- Spinal cord/nerve root compression from vertebral fracture or plasmacytoma may cause back pain, radicular pain, extremity weakness/parasthesia, and bowel/bladder dysfunction; median nerve distribution parasthesia due to amyloid in carpal tunnel.

PHYSICAL FINDINGS

- Physical examination may be normal, but often reveals pallor due to anemia.
- Bone tenderness over the spine is common; an expansile palpable skeletal or soft tissue mass may occur with plasmacytoma; spinal cord

compression causes leg weakness, hyporeflexia, clonus, and decreased anal tone.

- Confusion, somnolence, dry oral mucosa, and reflex changes occur with hypercalcemia.
- Common signs of infection include rales (pneumonia), sinus tenderness (sinusitis), flank tenderness (pyelonephritis), and skin erythema/warmth (cellulitis).
- Hyperviscosity syndrome may produce retinal vessel engorgement/hemorrhage, neurologic deficits, or tachypnea from pulmonary involvement.

DIAGNOSTIC TESTS AND STAGING

- Patients with suspected MM require an array of diagnostic blood, urine, bone marrow, and radiographic tests.
- CBC most often reveals normocytic anemia; thrombocytopenia and leucopenia are uncommon but may occur with increased tumor load; rare patients manifest plasma cell leukemia with >2000 plasma cells/μl; the peripheral smear often reveals rouleaux formation.
- Bone marrow aspiration and biopsy findings of MM include: ≥10% plasma cells, often with binucleate or multinucleate cells; flow cytometry reveals a CD138-positive phenotype; metaphase cytogenetics and fluorescence *in situ* hybridization (FISH) panel to at least assess for del 13, del 17, t(4;14), t(11;14), and t(14;16) translocations or hyperploidy.
- β-2-microglobulin is a marker of disease burden and, with serum albumin, is required for adequate staging.
- Serum protein electrophoresis (SPEP) typically shows a sharp peak ("M-spike") within the gamma-region and provides a quantitative measure (g/dL) of the protein; hypogammaglobulinemia is common; confirmation of a monoclonal protein in this region requires immunoelectrophoresis, which demonstrates light and heavy chain type.
  - Quantitative (SPEP) and qualitative assessment of proteins provides the most useful way of monitoring disease progression and/or response to therapy.
  - 60% to 80% of MM involves IgG and 20% involves IgA; 1% of cases do not secrete any Ig (nonsecretory MM).
- Urine protein electrophoresis (UPEP) and immunoelectrophoresis provide similar information as the serum counterpart with regards to urinary excretion of the monoclonal protein and serve as a useful tool for monitoring response to therapy; 24-hour urine protein collection.
  - 20% of cases of MM produce only light chains, which are excreted into the urine as "Bence-Jones" proteins; these proteins are especially toxic to the renal tubules and can induce renal failure (light chain nephropathy); most patients with a serum M-spike also excrete urine light chains.
- A thorough discussion of response criteria is beyond the scope of this chapter (see *J Natl Cancer Inst* 2009;7:916); complete response (CR)

requires absence of serum and urine monoclonal protein by immunofixation for at least 6 weeks, <5% marrow plasma cells, and no increase is size of lytic bone lesions; patients not fulfilling CR criteria are categorized as partial response (PR) or minimal response (MR); patients with CR or deep PR have improved outcomes compared to patients with MR; relapsed MM is characterized by reappearance (if prior CR) or increase in serum/urine paraprotein, increased lytic lesions, hypercalemia, and/or ≥5% marrow plasma cells.

- Serum-free light chain assay may be useful for low or undetectable M-protein levels.
- Levels of serum and ionized calcium and creatinine are necessary to exclude hypercalemia and renal failure, respectively.
- Skeletal survey includes plain radiographs of the skull, axial, and appendicular skeletons to screen for lytic bone lesions or diffuse osteopenia; sclerotic bone lesions should suggest a myeloma variant known as POEMS syndrome (Polyneuropathy, Organomegaly, Endocrinopathy, Multiple myeloma, Skin changes).
- MRI of the spine is very sensitive at detecting vertebral involvement that is not detected on skeletal survey.
- In summary, essential criteria for the diagnosis of MM includes: serum M-spike ≥3 g/dL (except if nonsecretory MM), ≥10% marrow plasma cells, and evidence of end-organ disease—anemia, renal failure, hypercalcemia, and/or lytic bone lesions; in contrast, MGUS is characterized by an M-spike <3 g/dL, <10% marrow plasma cells, and absence of end-organ dysfunction; a variant known as "smoldering" MM is characterized by an M-spike of ≥3 g/dL, ≥10% marrow plasma cells, but no end-organ damage.

Table 28–1 International Staging System (ISS)

Stage	Criteria	Median survival
I	Serum β-2-microglobulin <3.5 mg/L and serum albumin ≥3.5 g/dL	62 months
II	Not stage I or III	44 months
III	Serum β-2-microglobulin ≥5.5 mg/L	29 months

TREATMENT

- The treatment of MM has progressed rapidly in recent years with introduction of several novel agents that have dramatically impacted the outlook for patients with this disease; only a brief treatment overview will be offered.
- Urgency of systemic therapy is based on degree and rapidity of end-organ damage, most importantly acute renal failure and hypercalemia; asymptomatic secretory MM patients can be monitored every 3 months

until symptoms or end-organ dysfunction develops; MGUS requires no active therapy.

- General indications for treatment include increasing M-protein in blood and/or urine, bone lesions with fractures or pain, increasing anemia and/or other cytopenias, hypercalcemia, recurrent infections, plasmacytoma.

- The typical patient should be approached with regards to whether autologous peripheral blood stem cell (PBSCT) is an option—a procedure shown in randomized trials to increase overall survival by approximately 1 year with complete response rates of 25% to 40%.
  - Generally, criteria for PBSCT include age <70 years, good performance status, and preserved cardiac and pulmonary function; renal failure is not a contraindication if due to MM.

- Several active agents are available for MM.
  - Dexamethasone: single-agent activity of approximately 40%; provides 80% of antimyeloma activity of the VAD regimen (infusional vincristine, infusional doxorubicin, oral dexamethasone), a regimen used infrequently due to more effective therapies.
  - Thalidomide: a pleiotropic immune-modulating drug (iMID) with antiproliferative, antiangiogenic, and anticytokine properties; typically administered with oral dexamethasone (TD regimen), which in phase III trials resulted in response rates of 63% compared to dexamethasone monotherapy; significant toxicity (including fatal thromboembolism) may limit this regimen in many patients; TD is an acceptable induction regimen in PBSCT-eligible patients and does not seem to impair stem cell collection; posttransplant maintenance thalidomide improved 5-year event-free survival in a phase III trial; thrombotic prophylaxis with aspirin, warfarin, or low-molecular-weight heparin is suggested with TD.
  - Lenalidomide: iMID related to thalidomide but different side-effect profile; demonstrated significant activity in relapsed MM but currently used by many oncologists as first-line therapy with dexamethasone (RevDex), with response rates of 90% noted in trials, or in combination with bortezomib (RVD); although excellent responses have been shown in phase I/II trials, phase III data are not available for the RVD regimen; RevDex is a commonly used induction regimen prior to PBSCT, because damage to stem cells is nil based on the literature; thrombotic prophylaxis with aspirin, warfarin, or low-molecular-weight heparin is suggested with RevDex.
  - Bortezomib: a unique boron-containing molecule that inhibits the 26S proteosome, an organelle that degrades ubiquinated intracellular proteins; proteosome paralysis results in inhibition of ubiquinated protein lysis, which disrupts cell-signaling pathways leading to cell death (apoptosis); also down-regulates NF-kappaβ pathway, with inhibited release of cell growth factors and increased chemosensitivity; initially shown to have a 30% response rate in relapsed and refractory MM patients; shown to be active in relapsed disease

with liposomal doxorubicin for relapsed/refractory disease; now often used first-line in combination with dexamethasone (VD regimen) or dexamethasone and lenolidamide (RVD) in transplant-eligible and ineligible patients.

- Liposomal doxorubicin: liposome-encapsulated form of doxorubicin with decreased uptake into normal tissues with less cardiotoxicity; active regimen when combined with bortezomib for patients with relapsed MM showed improved median time to progression and response duration in phase III trial.
- Melphalan and prednisone: the MP regimen has been utilized for decades and is useful for disease control but uncommonly results in complete or near-complete responses; because melphalan is an alkylating agent, stem cell damage is expected, making this drug contraindicated in PBSCT candidates; MP is a reasonable initial therapy in elderly non-transplant-eligible patients; recent phase III data demonstrate improved response rates and overall survival when MP is combined with thalidomide (MPT regimen) or bortezomib (MPV regimen).
- High-dose melphalan: used for PBSCT after induction therapy with non-stem-cell damaging regimen (e.g., TD, RevDex); typical dose is 200 mg/m^2 (or 140 mg/m^2 for reduced renal function) after adequate stem cell mobilization and collection following several days of filgrastim (with or without cyclophosphamide); patients who do not achieve a CR or near CR should be considered for a second PBSCT ("tandem" transplant).
- Bisphosphonates (zoledronic acid and pamidronate): both drugs inhibit osteoclast activity and are indicated to treat hypercalcemia and bone disease in MM; both agents have been shown to delay the time to a skeletal-related event (SRE) and improve quality of life; zolendronic acid is easier to administer than pamidronate (15-minute vs. 90-minute infusion), but it must be adjusted for decreased renal function due to renal toxic effects; all patients should undergo pretreatment dental/oral examination due to the risk of osteoneurosis of the jaw (ONJ).

- Painful vertebral collapse or fracture may be treated with balloon kyphoplasty or vertebroplasty and injection of methylmethacrylate cement; pain relief may be almost immediate.
- Local radiation is indicated for symptomatic medullary or extramedullary plasmacytoma (which typically involves nasopharyngeal area), painful bone lesions, or areas of impending pathologic fracture.
- Treatment of hypercalcemia includes volume repletion, steroids, bisphosphonates, and, if a rapid response is required, calcitonin.
- Plasmapheresis should be considered with severe acute renal failure due to light chain nephropathy or symptomatic hyperviscosity syndrome.
- Erythropoietin or darbopoietin should be considered for disease- or treatment-related symptomatic anemia (avoid hemoglobin >11–12 and use with TD or RevDex due to risk of venous thrombosis).

- Intravenous immune globulin (IVIG) should be considered in patients with documented hypogammaglobulinemia and recurrent bacterial infection.
- Prophylactic oral acyclovir, valacyclovir, or famcyclovir should be administered to patients receiving bortezomib due to increased incidence of varicella reactivation.

Table 28–2 Regimens for MM

Induction regimens for transplant-eligible patients
VD: bortezomib 1.3 mg/m^2 IV days 1,4,8,11 and dexamethasone 20 mg by mouth day of and after bortezomib
RevDex: lenalidomide 25 mg by mouth days 1–21 and dexamethasone 40 mg by mouth days 1–4, 9–12, and 17–20 for first 4 cycles every 28 days
VTD: Bortezomib 1.3 mg/m^2 IV days 1,4,8,11, thalidomide 100–200 mg by mouth daily, dexamethasone 40 mg by mouth days 1–4, 9–12, and 17–20 or 40 mg by mouth weekly
RVD: lenalidomide 15–25 mg by mouth days 1–14, bortezomib 1.3 mg/m^2 IV days 1,4,8,11 and dexamethasone 20 mg on day of and after bortezomib every 21 days

Induction regimens for nontransplant-eligible patients
MP: melphalan 8–10 mg/m^2 by mouth days 1–4 and prednisone 60 mg/m^2 by mouth days 1–4 every 6 weeks
MPT: melphalan 0.25 mg/kg by mouth days 1–4, prednisone 1.5 mg/kg by mouth days 1–4, thalidomide 100 mg by mouth daily every 28 days
MPV: melphalan 9 mg/m^2 by mouth days 1–4, prednisone 60 mg/m^2 by mouth days 1–4, bortezomib 1.3 mg/m^2 IV days 1,4,8,11,22,25,29,32 every 6 weeks × 4 cycles; then, melphalan 9 mg/m^2 by mouth days 1–4, prednisone 60 mg/m^2 by mouth days 1–4, bortezomib 1.3 mg/m^2 IV days 1,8,22,29 every 6 weeks × 5 cycles
TD: thalidomide 200 mg by mouth daily and dexamethasone 40 mg by mouth days 1–4 every 28 days
Rev/dex: lenalidomide 25 mg by mouth days 1–21 and dexamethasone 40 mg by mouth days 1,8,15,22 every 28 days
VAD: vincristine 0.4 mg/day IV continuous infusion days 1–4, doxorubicin 9 mg/m^2 IV continuous infusion days 1–4, dexamethasone 40 mg by mouth days 1–4, 9–12, 17–20 every 28 days
Dexamethasone: 40 mg IV or by mouth days 1–4, 9–12, and 17–20 every 21 days

Regimens for relapsed disease
Bortezomib 1.3 mg/m^2 IV days 1,4,8,11 every 21 days
TD: thalidomide 200 mg by mouth daily and dexamethasone 40 mg by mouth days 1–4 every 28 days
Rev/dex: lenalidomide 25 mg by mouth days 1–21 and dexamethasone 40 mg by mouth days 1,8,15,22 every 28 days
Bortezomib 1.3 mg/m^2 IV days 1,4,8,11 and liposomal doxorubicin 30 mg/m^2 IV day 4 every 21 days

COMPLICATIONS OF TREATMENT

- Dexamethasone: anxiety, mood changes, psychosis, insomnia, dyspepsia, gastrointestinal ulceration/perforation, edema, hypertension, skin break-down, infection, hyperglycemia, hypokalemia, leukocytosis.
- Thalidomide: venous thromboembolism (especially when combined with dexamethasone), sedation, orthostatic hypotension, neuropathy, consti-pation, bradycardia, rash (Steven-Johnson syndrome reported), infection, teratogenicity (pregnancy test MUST be performed in all females of child-bearing age; two forms of birth control are necessary).
- Lenalidomide: nausea, vomiting, diarrhea, constipation, venous thrombo-embolism (especially when combined with dexamethasone), neutropenia, thrombocytopenia, teratogenicity (pregnancy test MUST be performed in all females of child-bearing age; two forms of birth control are necessary).
- Bortezomib: fatigue, nausea/vomiting, diarrhea, fever, peripheral neu-ropathy, orthostatic hypotension, constipation, herpes-zoster reactiva-tion in 10% to 15% of patients, thrombocytopenia, neutropenia.
- Liposomal doxorubicin: infusion reaction, nausea, vomiting, diarrhea, mucositis, alopecia, skin hyperpigmentation, hand-foot syndrome, myelosuppression, hepatotoxicity, cardiotoxicity (uncommon).
- High-dose melphalan: oral mucositis (may be severe, necessitating intra-venous narcotic analgesia and parenteral nutrition; may result in virid-ians *Streptococcus* septic shock with respiratory failure; may be effectively prevented with oral cryotherapy—sucking ice cubes before, during, and after melphalan infusion), infusional hypersensitivity, nausea, vomiting, diarrhea, pneumonitis, myelosuppression, late malignancies (especially hematologic).
- Melphalan and prednisone: nausea, vomiting, fatigue, diarrhea, hyperg-lycemia, infection, myelosuppression.
- Bisphosphonates: flulike symptoms, renal insufficiency, ONJ (more common with zoledronic acid; risk factors include periodontal disease, history of tooth extraction, and denture use), hypocalcemia, hypophosphatemia, hypomagnesemia.

FOLLOW-UP CARE

- Periodic history, physical examination, and serum and urine studies should be monitored every several weeks during active therapy and every 3 to 4 months following drug therapy or PBSCT; the following are most commonly utilized:
  - CBC, creatinine, calcium, LDH, β-2-microglobulin.
  - SPEP and UPEP with immunofixation and serum-free light chains.
  - Skeletal imaging and bone marrow biopsy as indicated by symptoms or suspicion of relapse.
- Careful oral hygiene and dental examinations are important to monitor for ONJ.
- Administration of pneumococcal and influenza vaccines as necessary.

PROGNOSIS

- MGUS has a favorable prognosis, with a 1% incidence of progression to MM annually; the survival of MGUS patients is 2 years shorter compared to age-matched controls.
- The median overall survival of MM is 5 to 6 years; a few patients may survive a decade, but cure rarely, if ever, occurs.
- The ISS staging system (see above) is useful for assessing 5-year survival and should be obtained in all patients.

REFERENCES

Blood 2008;111:2962.
Blood 2005;106:4050.
Clin Lymphoma Myeloma 2009;9:375.
Clin Lymphoma Myeloma 2005;6:181.
J Clin Oncol 2009;27:5015.
J Clin Oncol 2007;24:abstract 8002.
J Clin Oncol 2006;24:431.
J Clin Oncol 2005;23:3412.
N Engl J Med 2003;348:1875.

29 ■ CHRONIC MYELOGENOUS LEUKEMIA

BACKGROUND

- Chronic myelogenous leukemia (CML) is the prototype disorder representing successful treatment of a neoplastic disease with a therapy targeted (imatinib mesylate) at a specific protein product (*bcr-abl* protein) which results from a recurrent genetic translocation ([t(9;22)(q34;q11)]) within hematopoietic cells; the protein product of *bcr-abl* contains a constitutively active tyrosine kinase that results in uncontrolled cellular proliferation resulting in the characteristic phenotype of CML—it is this tyrosine kinase that is inhibited by imatinib mesylate, a drug that has revolutionized the concept of "targeted" cancer care.
- The annual incidence of CML is 1.6 cases per 100,000, with a slight male-to-female predominance; median age at diagnosis is 55 years.
- There are approximately 5100 cases and 470 deaths annually in the United States.
- Many patients are diagnosed in chronic phase (CP), a typically asymptomatic phase of the disease characterized by leukocytosis, that is often detected on a routine blood count.
- There are no common risk factors for CML; atomic bomb survivors from Japan are at increased risk.

PATHOBIOLOGY

- As noted, CML results from a recurrent translocation between chromosomes 9 and 22 which results in juxtaposition of the ABL protooncogene on 9q34 to the BCR gene on 22q11.
- The breakpoint of the ABL gene on chromosome 9 is variable and may occur over an area of over 200 kilobases; the breakpoint on chromosome 22 occurs in one of three small regions in a 5.8-kb sequence known as the "breakpoint cluster region," which is present in the majority of Philadelphia (Ph)-positive CML and one-half of cases of Ph-positive acute lymphoblastic leukemia (ALL).
    - The protein product of the *bcr-abl* fusion gene is a 210- kilodalton hybrid protein that contains a constitutively active tyrosine kinase that induces a continuous proliferative signal via various transduction pathways (e.g., STAT, RAS, MYC, JUN), resulting in myeloproliferation, cytokine independence, and resistance to apoptosis.
- Bone marrow morphology of CML reveals exuberant myelopoiesis, with cellularity often exceeding 90%.

186

- Continuous cell division during CP results in secondary genetic defects, most commonly trisomy 8; others include additional t(9;22) or 17p-, a phenomenon known as "clonal evolution," which usually results in disease progression known as accelerated-phase (AP) CML or a pre-terminal condition known as "blast crisis"; time from CP to AP CML is usually 3 to 4 years, with AP lasting several months before terminating in blast crisis.

CLINICAL PRESENTATION

- Common symptoms of CP CML include fatigue, weight loss, or symptoms of splenomegaly, such as early satiety or a "dragging" sensation in the left upper quadrant.
- Increased cell breakdown with release of urate can precipitate acute gouty arthritis with severe joint pain (e.g., first metatarsophalangeal joint, knee).
- Elevated serum histamine from increased circulating basophils may cause pruritis, flushing, and/or diarrhea.
- Extreme leukocytosis (>100,000–200,000 cells/mm^3) may induce stasis within the microvasculature (leukostasis), causing cerebral ischemia/hemorrhage (headache, visual changes, paralysis, confusion, seizures), pulmonary insufficiency (dyspnea, cough, hemoptysis), cardiac ischemia (angina pectoris), priapism, or venous thromboembolism (leg swelling, dyspnea, hemoptysis).
- Progression to AP or blast crisis typically presents with increased fatigue, weight loss, anorexia, fever, night sweats, bone pain or mucosal bleeding (epistaxis, gingival bleeding, hematuria, menorrhagia).

PHYSICAL FINDINGS

- Splenomegaly (which may be massive) is the most common physical finding associated with CP CML.
- Acute urate arthropathy manifests as joint effusion, erythema, and warmth.
- Lymphadenopathy is uncommon but may occur with AP disease.

DIAGNOSTIC TESTS AND STAGING

- Leukocytosis is the *sinequonon* of CP CML, with many asymptomatic patients having leukocyte counts exceeding 50,000 cells/mm^3; thrombocytosis is common; anemia may occur in some patients, but is more common in AP and blast crisis; thrombocytopenia may occur later in the course.
  - The peripheral smear during CP reveals leukocytosis with a leftward shift; promyelocytes, myelocytes, metamyelocytes, and band forms are common; basophilia is an important clue; abundant circulating

platelets are evident; <5% myeloblasts are typical of CP CML but are markedly increased during AP and blast crisis.

- Leukocyte alkaline phosphatase (LAP) score is low in CML cells; serum B12 often elevated.
- Bone marrow aspirate and biopsy findings include hypercellularity (may approach 100%) with a marked increase of the myeloid:erythroid ratio; all stages of myeloid maturation are present, with abundant basophilic and eosinophilic precursors; reticulin may be noted.
- Bone marrow metaphase cytogenetic analysis reveals the Philadelphia chromosome, which results from a reciprocal translocation between chromosomes 9 and 22 [t(9;22)]; FISH is more sensitive at detecting the translocation and is also useful for monitoring disease response and/or recurrence.
- Polymerase chain reaction (PCR) of marrow or blood for the bcr-abl protein or, more accurately, mRNA, is the most sensitive (may detect 1 CML cell out of 10^4–10^6 hematopoietic cells) method for diagnosis and is a mainstay for monitoring disease course and response to therapy.
- Disease evolution to AP manifests as worsening anemia, thrombocytopenia, and increased circulating blasts; blast crisis synonymous with acute leukemia (≥20% peripheral blasts); blast crisis is usually myeloid (acute myelogenous leukemia), although some patients may develop acute lymphoid leukemia.
- Although there is no TNM staging system for CML per se, a widely utilized prognostic staging system known as the Sokal score is a mathematical equation determined by multivariate analysis of prognostic features in CML patients that includes the percentage of circulating blasts, spleen size, platelet count, age, and cytogenetic clonal evolution; this system was devised in the pre-imatinib era, but some authors have demonstrated utility in imatinib-treated patients.

TREATMENT

- Although the only curative treatment for CML is allogeneic stem cell transplantation, which should be considered in young patients with a matched sibling donor, the vast majority of patients are initially commenced on imatinib mesylate given the impressive phase III data with regards to durable survival; importantly, there is no evidence that imatinib therapy adversely affects outcome of subsequent transplantation.
  - Imatinib mesylate is an oral inhibitor of the ATP binding site on the ABL kinase that results in inhibition of phosphorylation of proteins involved with signal transduction and, consequently, cell proliferation; imatinib also induces apoptosis in bcr/abl expressing cells.
  - The phase III IRIS trial was a comparative trial between interferon-alpha and cytarabine versus imatinib 400 mg orally daily in 1106 treatment-naïve CML patients that established this drug as standard-of-care initial therapy.

- Rates of complete cytogenetic response (CCR, absence of Ph-positive cells in the marrow) were 76% at 18 months and 85% at 5 years; additional 5-year follow-up data revealed progression-free survival of 83% and overall survival of 89%.
- All patients who achieved a major molecular remission (MMR, ≥3-log reduction in bcr-abl transcripts by PCR of peripheral blood) by 18 months were free of disease progression at 5-year follow-up.
- No patient who achieved CCR during year 1 of treatment progressed to advanced stage at 5-year follow-up.
  - Imatinib displays modest activity in AP disease, with a 40% 4-year survival; however, survival for blast crisis is <10% in imatinib-treated patients; suggested dose in AP and blast crisis is 600 mg orally daily and may be used as a "bridge" to allogeneic transplantation in appropriate patients.
  - Despite impressive responses, some patients develop resistance to imatinib by one of several mechanisms: mutations at kinase site, gene amplification, up-regulation of drug-efflux proteins, and alternative growth-signaling mechanisms.
    - Mutations in kinase domain are most common mechanism and may be treated with higher doses (800 mg daily) or one of two novel agents: dasatanib or nilotinib; however, a specific mutation T315I is resistant to all three drugs and remains a treatment challenge.
- Dasatanib is an oral bcr-abl and Src kinase inhibitor that is over 300 times more potent than imatinib against the bcr-abl kinase, but is not active against T315I mutation.
  - Studies show ability of dasatanib administered at 100 mg daily to induce hematologic, cytogenetic, and molecular remission in various degrees in imatinib-resistant/intolerant patients; also some activity demonstrated in AP and blast crisis patients; symptomatic pleural effusions occurred in 22% of patients and required drainage in 7% of patients in a recent trial.
- Nilotinib is an oral bcr-abl kinase inhibitor 30 times more potent than imatinib that has also demonstrated activity in imatinib-resistant/intolerant patients at a dose of 400 mg orally twice daily; the drug is inactive against the T315I mutation; sudden death occurred in several patients during clinical trials, possibly related to QT interval prolongation.
- Hydroxyurea (1–4 grams daily orally in divided doses) may be considered if rapid cytoreduction is necessary.
- Leukapheresis should be considered for patients with cerebral and/or pulmonary symptoms of leukostasis.
- Induction chemotherapy for blast crisis may be employed but response rates are low.
- Evaluation at a transplant center is indicated in the following situations: absence of hematologic remission at 3 months; no cytogenetic response at 6 months; minor or nil cytogenetic response at 12 months; cytogenetic relapse at 12 months; partial, minor, or no cytogenetic response or

cytogenetic relapse at 18 months; T315I kinase mutation; or presentation of CML in AP or blast crisis.
- Donor leukocyte infusions (DLI) may induce durable remission, often at the expense of severe graft-versus-host disease, in many patients with relapse following allogeneic transplant.

Table 29–1 Regimens for CML

Imatinib mesylate 400 mg by mouth daily for CP and 600 mg by mouth daily for AP/blast crisis
Dasatinib 100 mg by mouth daily
Nilotinib 400 mg by mouth twice daily
Hydroxyurea 1–4 gm by mouth daily in divided doses
Interferon-α 5 million IU/m^2 SQ daily and cytarabine 20 mg/m^2 SQ daily for 10 days every month

COMPLICATIONS OF TREATMENT

- Imatinib: myelosuppression (especially early in therapy), nausea and vomiting (improved if taken with food), diarrhea, edema (periorbital and peripheral), myalgias, fluid retention and body cavity effusions, weight gain, cytopenias, rash (Stevens-Johnson syndrome reported).
- Dasatinib: fluid retention in 50% (edema and pleural effusions which may require thoracentesis), nausea, vomiting, diarrhea, anorexia, fatigue, bleeding complications from platelet dysfunction, prolonged QT interval, hypocalcemia, hypophosphatemia, myelosuppression.
- Nilotinib: anorexia, nausea, fatigue, myelosuppression, hyperlipasemia, hypocalcemia, hypophosphatemia, hypomagnesemia, hyponatremia, hyperbilirubinemia, prolonged QT interval, sudden death (rare).
- Interferon: fever, chills, myalgia, headache, fatigue, arthalgia, anorexia, confusion, delirium, rash, alopecia, depression (suicide reported), myelosuppression, hepatitis, proteinuria, hypocalcemia, nephrotic syndrome, cardiotoxicity, autoimmune syndromes (thyroiditis, vasculitis, lupus).

FOLLOW-UP CARE

- Complete hematologic remission (CHR)—normalization of blood counts and resolution of splenomegaly—occurs in the majority of patients within the first several weeks of imatinib therapy and should be monitored with every 2-week blood counts after the first several weeks of initiation of therapy and then decreased in frequency.
- Every 3 month measurement of *bcr-abl* transcripts by PCR and/or FISH from peripheral blood should be performed to monitor depth of response; once FISH is negative or there is a ≥3-log reduction in *bcr-abl,* bone marrow aspiration for cytogenetic analysis should be obtained.

- Thereafter, every 3- to 4-month follow-up with history, examination, blood counts, and peripheral blood PCR analysis (sent to the same lab to avoid interlaboratory variation) is suggested.
  - PCR revealing rise in *bcr-abl* transcripts should be repeated and, if confirmed, switching to dastanib or nilotinib considered; mutational analysis should be considered, and patients with T315I mutation should be referred to a transplant center for possible allogenic transplantation or clinical trial.

PROGNOSIS

- Imatinib has revolutionized CML management, with overall survival rates of approximately 90% in patients experiencing a CCR or MMR within the first year of therapy.
- Prognosis for most patients with blast crisis is dismal, with median survival of 6 months or less, with most patients dying from infection or bleeding.
- Allogenic transplantation imparts long-term survival (cure) in 65% to 80% of patients with a matched-related donor, but chronic graft-versus-host disease is commonly associated with significant morbidity and, occasionally, mortality; optimal results occur when transplant is performed within the first 2 years of CP.

REFERENCES

Blood 2007;109:2303.
Br J Haematol 2004;125:613.
Curr Oncol Rep 2008;10:365.
N Engl J Med 2006;354:2531.
N Engl J Med 2006;354:2542.
N Engl J Med 2006;355:2408.
N Engl J Med 2003;348:994.
N Engl J Med 2007;357:258.

BACKGROUND

- Chronic lymphocytic leukemia (CLL) is the most common leukemia in the United States; although often associated with a prolonged smoldering course in elderly patients, some cases occur in younger individuals, which may follow an aggressive and often fatal course.
- There are approximately 15,000 cases diagnosed annually in the United States, but due to prolonged survival the total prevalence of CLL is much higher; there are over 5000 deaths annually in the United States due to CLL.
- CLL is typically a disease of the elderly (mean age 65–70 years); it is more common in men and blacks but is uncommon in Asians; approximately 20% of patients are younger than 55 years.
- The tissue counterpart of CLL is small lymphocytic lymphoma (SLL) and is so-named when nodal disease predominates the clinical picture with minimal or no leukemic counterpart.
- Risk factors: none firmly established.

PATHOBIOLOGY

- Although there is some degree of increased cell proliferation, CLL primarily results from prolonged cell survival due to impaired apoptotic mechanisms from overexpression of the antiapoptotic protein, BCL2, which is present in the majority of cases; conversely, underexpression of the proapoptotic protein BCL_x is decreased.
- Complex interactions between neoplastic lymphocytes and bone marrow stromal cells via various chemokines leads to accumulation of leukemic cells.
- The biologic behavior of CLL in large part relates to the mutation status of the V_H gene: lymphocytes from one-half of patients harbor an unmutated and lymphocytes from the other half of patients harbor V_H genes that are mutated from postgerminal center B cells.
  - Unmutated V_H CLL is an aggressive disease with shorter survival and commonly expresses the ZAP-70 protein, which increases signal transduction.
  - Unmutated V_H CLL is more frequently associated with unfavorable cytogenetic abnormalities (e.g., 17p- and 11q-), and mutated V_H CLL is more frequently associated with favorable cytogenetic abnormalities (e.g., 13q-).

- Cytogenetic abnormalities, most commonly deletions or trisomies, are common in CLL and impact disease biology; for instance, deletion of chromosome 17p results in dysfunction of the tumor suppressor gene, p53, and imparts an aggressive course and relative refractoriness to nucleoside analogues.
- Autoimmune phenomena are not uncommon, with 20% to 30% of cases having a positive Coomb's test with clinical hemolysis developing in many of these; autoimmune thrombocytopenia and neutropenia (rare) may also occur; pure red cell aplasia is a rare complication and likely has an autoimmune pathobiology.
  ◦ The etiology of autoimmune complications is not firmly established, but abnormalities in T-regulatory cells (Tregs) may play a role.
- Increased susceptibility to infection is a pathologic hallmark of CLL and is reflective of hypogammaglobulinemia, abnormal complement activation, impaired lymphocyte function, and neutropenia if marrow infiltration is severe.
  ◦ Defective opsonization of microorganisms especially increases risk for infection due to *Streptococcus pneumoniae, Staphylococcus aureus,* and *Haemophilus influenzae.*
- CLL is known for its propensity to biologically transform into more aggressive disease variants.
  ◦ Approximately 3% to 15% of cases of CLL (especially those with 17p deletion) eventually transform into diffuse large B cell lymphoma (DLBCL)—a phenomenon known as Richter's transformation, which is characterized by an aggressive and often fatal course.
  ◦ Uncommonly, CLL transforms into an aggressive leukemia known as prolymphocytic leukemia (PLL), which is typically fatal.

CLINICAL PRESENTATION

- Most cases of CLL are discovered when a CBC is obtained for unrelated reasons in an otherwise asymptomatic patient.
- Symptomatic patients often note fatigue, night sweats, weight loss, and fever; some patients may notice node enlargement in the neck or axillae.
- Dark-colored urine occurs with hemolysis.
- Symptoms of recurrent infection (especially of the skin or respiratory tract) may be the presenting manifestations of CLL and is suggestive of hypogammaglobulinemia.
- Symptoms of Richter's transformation include rapidly progressive lymphadenopathy, fevers, night sweats, weight loss, and fatigue.
- Symptoms of PLL transformation include increasing fatigue, cachexia, fevers, abdominal discomfort due to splenic enlargement, and progressive lymphadenopathy.

PHYSICAL FINDINGS

- Patients with asymptomatic CLL often have a normal examination or the presence of diffuse, painless, rubbery adenopathy.
- Patients with advanced-stage CLL often exhibit significant splenomegaly and hepatomegaly; bulky lymphadenopathy suggests presence of the 11q deletion.
- Icterus may be noted if hemolysis supervenes.
- Patients with Richter's transformation often manifest rapidly growing widespread lymphadenopathy, pallor, and cachexia; those with PLL transformation are often cachectic with rapidly growing lymphadenopathy and splenomegaly.

DIAGNOSTIC TESTS AND STAGING

- CBC: clonal lymphocytosis exceeding 5000 cells/mm^3 is required for diagnosis of CLL; a count less than this value has been termed MLUS (monoclonal lymphocytosis of uncertain significance); thorough evaluation and exclusion of other etiologies of anemia and thrombocytopenia are essential, because the presence of one or both determines disease stage if due to marrow infiltration and poor marrow function; nonmalignant causes of anemia and thrombocytopenia in the CLL patient include:
  - Coomb's positive autoimmune hemolytic anemia (AHIA) should be excluded in anemic patients with direct Coomb's test, haptoglobin, LDH, and reticulocyte count; the presence of AIHA (auto immune hemolytic anemia) as a cause for anemia does not affect disease stage or prognosis.
  - Immune thrombocytopenia alone or in conjunction with AIHA (Evan's syndrome) may occur and, if suspected, bone marrow biopsy should be considered, which typically reveals megakaryocytic hyperplasia as opposed to megakaryocytopenia in cases of malignant thrombocytopenia; autoimmune thrombocytopenia does not affect disease stage or prognosis.
  - Pure red cell aplasia manifests as severe anemia and reticulocytopenia; bone marrow biopsy reveals absence of erythroid elements.
  - Anemia and/or thrombocytopenia may complicate hypersplenism from splenic involvement; consumptive cytopenia does not affect staging or adversely affect prognosis.
- Peripheral blood smear typically reveals a monomorphous population of small, mature-appearing lymphoid cells with scant cytoplasm; "smudge" cells are common and represent leukemic cells damaged during slide preparation; the presence of spherocytes and reticulocytes is suggestive of AIHA, and decreased platelets may indicate marrow infiltration with CLL, splenic sequestration, or immune thrombocytopenia.
- Flow cytometry of peripheral blood is adequate for diagnosis with CLL cells displaying a characteristic immunophenotype: CD5+ (aberrant

T-cell marker), CD10-, CD19+, CD20+, CD23+, dim surface immunoglobulin (dim sIg) expression, and cyclin D1-.

- CLL may be confused with mantle cell lymphoma (MCL), because both are CD5+; however, MCL is characteristically CD23- and cyclin D1+.

• Bone marrow aspiration and biopsy, although not necessary for diagnosis, is useful to exclude other etiologies of anemia and thrombocytopenia and for assessing pattern of lymphoid infiltration (e.g., nodular vs. diffuse).

• Cytogenetics of blood and/or marrow are abnormal in approximately one-half of CLL patients at diagnosis and should be obtained in most patients.

  - Deletion of 13q is most common abnormality, present in approximately 50% of patients, and confers a favorable prognosis with a near-normal life span.
  - Deletion of 11q occurs in 15% to 20% of cases and is often associated with bulky lymphadenopathy.
  - Trisomy 12 occurs in 15% to 20% of cases and is generally associated with a poor prognosis.
  - Deletion of 17p , associated with disruption of tumor-suppressor gene p53, occurs in <15% of cases but is associated with aggressive disease characterized by resistance to purine analogues (e.g., fludarabine) and a short survival without allogeneic stem cell transplant.

• FISH panel for prognostic stratification is more accurate than metaphase cytogenetics for determining each of the above chromosomal abnormalities, but routine use of this technology is still being studied; however, FISH panel should be obtained in younger patients with CLL.

• Determination of immunoglobulin heavy chain gene sequences via PCR reveal unmutated sequences (poor prognosis) or mutated sequences (favorable prognosis).

  - Unmutated V_H is more commonly positive for ZAP-70, which may serve as a disease prognosticator if mutation testing is unavailable; unmutated cases are also commonly CD38+, but the association is not as robust; as stated, unmutated V_H CLL is more commonly associated with unfavorable cytogenetics.

• Lymph node biopsy is typically unnecessary if other criteria for CLL are met, but, if performed, reveals nodal replacement with small malignant lymphocytes.

• Metabolic profile including electrolytes, creatinine, lactate dehydrogenase, and uric acid; SPEP often reveals hypogammaglobulinemia, which may increase risk of infection.

• CT of chest, abdomen, and pelvis may be helpful to identify nonpalpable visceral adenopathy, splenomegaly, or hepatomegaly, which are common with advancing disease.

• Patients with Richter's transformation usually have progressive anemia, thrombocytopenia, and rising LDH; PET is useful for staging in this situation; lymph node biopsy should be obtained, which reveals DLBCL; PLL transformation is characterized by >55% circulating large prolymphocytes with a conspicuous nucleolus and an immunophenotype expressing CD19, CD20, CD22, CD24, and FMC7.

Table 30–1 Rai staging system for CLL

Stage	Clinical features	Median survival
0	Lymphocytosis only	>10 years
I	Lymphocytosis + lymphadenopathy	8.5 years
II	Lymphocytosis + lymphadenopathy + splenomegaly +/– hepatomegaly	6 years
III*	Lymphocytosis + anemia	1.5 years
IV*	Lymphocytosis + thrombocytopenia	1.5 years

*Anemia and thrombocytopenia must not be immune-mediated.

TREATMENT

- Treatment of CLL has changed significantly over the last several years; however, asymptomatic patients with low-risk Rai stage (0/I) disease generally do not require therapy unless in the context of a clinical trial; patients with high-risk cytogenetic derangements, such as deletion of 17p, should be enrolled into trials to determine whether therapy instituted prior to symptomatic or cytopenic disease is beneficial.
- A rapid lymphocyte doubling time (<6 months) and autoimmune cytopenia not responsive to steroids are general indications to consider therapy.
- Patients with Rai stage II may or may not require therapy at presentation depending on age, comorbidities, and symptomatology of nodal and hepatosplenic bulk; patients with marrow failure (Rai stage III/IV) almost always require systemic therapy due to the poor outlook without treatment (<1.5 year survival).
  - The subgroup of patients with SLL and a low International Prognostic Index (IPI) score can typically be observed, but symptomatic patients and those with a high IPI score have an inferior survival and should generally be treated in similar fashion to CLL.
- The historic reference drug for CLL is the oral alkylating agent chlorambucil; this agent rarely, if ever, induces complete remission but may be useful for cytoreduction and palliation of symptoms in elderly patients who may not tolerate aggressive treatment.
- The purine analogue, fludarabine, is the most active agent used alone or in combination with cyclophosphamide (FC) or cyclophosphamide and rituximab (FCR); regimens containing fludarabine are the preferred initial therapy for younger patients requiring treatment.
  - Fludarabine monotherapy may be appropriate for elderly patients, and is associated with an overall response of up to 70% and a complete response rate of approximately 15% to 25%.
  - Fludarabine markedly suppresses production of CD4 lymphocytes for up to a year after completion of treatment, which increases the risk of opportunistic infections such as *Pneumocystis* and herpesviruses; prophylactic trimethoprim-sulfamethoxazole orally twice daily three

times per week and acyclovir 400 mg orally twice daily (or a related agent) are suggested until several weeks following treatment.

- Rituximab, a monoclonal antibody directed at the CD20 antigen, has minimal activity for CLL when used alone, but is synergistic when combined with fludarabine.
  - A CALGB study demonstrated the efficacy of concurrent fludarabine and rituximab (FR regimen) with an overall response rate of 95%; other trials suggest that this combination may also improve survival, which has been difficult to achieve even with novel agents.
  - The FCR regimen devised by M. D. Anderson is a very active regimen with a complete remission rate of approximately 70%, half of which are molecular remissions that may last several years; this regimen is typically well tolerated in fit patients and is used first-line by most U.S. oncologists in patients not enrolled in clinical trials.
- Pentostatin is a purine analogue that may be better tolerated in elderly patients but is not as active as fludarabine; this agent is commonly combined with cyclophosphamide and rituximab (PCR regimen).
- Alemtuzumab is a monoclonal antibody that targets the CD52 antigen present on both B- and T-lymphocytes and is indicated for treatment of CLL that relapses following fludarbine-containing regimens; alemtuzumab is more active than nucleoside analogues in patients with the 17p deletion; alemtuzumab is associated with rapid peripheral blood clearance of malignant lymphocytes (often within days); bulky nodal disease (especially associated with deletion of 11q) is less responsive to alemtuzumab.
  - Alemtuzumab is frequently associated with cytomegalovirus (CMV) reactivation, which can lead to pneumonitis, colitis, marrow failure, or hepatitis; monitoring for CMV viremia by PCR is suggested with ganciclovir initiated if viremia ensues.
- Bendamustine is a bifunctional alkylating agent recently approved in the United States for the treatment of CLL, although the drug has been utilized in Germany for many years.
  - Bendamustine may be used as monotherapy for relapsed CLL or combined with rituximab (BR regimen), which has resulted in overall response rates of 77% and CR rates of 15%; this regimen produces less neutropenia than FCR.
- Relapsed CLL is defined as progression of disease >12 months following completion of therapy that attained a partial or CR; refractory CLL is defined as disease progression <12 months after completion of therapy or disease that does not respond to purine-analogue-based treatment.
  - The choice of second-line therapy depends on patient age, presence of comorbidities, remission duration, and most recent prior therapy.
  - Patients with a remission duration >12 months following fludarabine-based treatment may be treated with the initial regimen; patients initially treated with an oral alkylating agent should be treated with a fludarabine-based regimen if tolerated.

- Alemtuzumab monotherapy should be considered if patients received prior fludarabine or harbor the 17p deletion; alemtuzumab can be added to fludarabine, but toxicity is significant.
- Allogeneic HSCT is an option for younger, fit patients with adverse features, especially fludarabine-refractory disease and 17p deletion; although treatment-related complications are significant, patients may experience long-term survival and even cure, so early referral to a transplant center is encouraged in appropriate patients.

Table 30–2 Regimens for CLL

First-line regimen*
FCR: fludarabine 25 mg/m^2 IV days 1–3, cyclophosphamide 250 mg/m^2 IV days 1–3, rituximab 375 mg/m^2 IV day 1 first cycle and 500 mg/m^2 IV day 1 subsequent cycles every 28 days × 6 cycles (preferred regimen for fit patients); consider pegfilgrastim 6 mg SQ day 4 of each cycle; consider prophylactic trimethoprim–sulfamethoxazole DS by mouth twice daily 3× weekly and acyclovir 400 mg by mouth twice daily (or equivalent) during and until 2 months after treatment completion
FR: fludarabine 25 mg/m^2 IV days 1–5 and rituximab 375 mg/m^2 IV day 1 every 28 days × 6 cycles
PCR: pentostatin 2 mg/m^2 IV day 1, cyclophosphamide 600 mg/m^2 IV day 1, rituximab 375 mg/m^2 IV day 1 every 21 days
Bendamustine 70–100 mg/m^2 IV days 1,2 every 28 days
Alemtuzumab (especially for 17p deletion): 30 mg IV daily 3× weekly for maximum of 23 weeks; start with 3 mg IV test dose and escalate to 10 mg IV dose then to 30 mg dose; premedicate with diphenhydramine 50 mg by mouth and acetaminophen 650 mg by mouth prior to infusion; prophylactic trimethoprim–sulfamethoxazole DS by mouth twice daily 3× weekly and acyclovir 400 mg by mouth twice daily (or equivalent) during and until 2 months after treatment completion; monitor for CMV reactivation and institute valganciclovir 900 mg by mouth twice daily if viremia occurs

Regimens for elderly patients
Chlorambucil : several oral regimens available
Bendamustine 50 mg/m^2 IV day 1,2 every 28 days
Pulse corticosteroids
Rituximab 375 mg/m^2 IV weekly × 4 weeks every 6 months × 4 cycles

Second-line regimen†
FCR (if remission >1 year following FCR or first-line alkylator only therapy and fit patient): see above
PCR (if remission >1 year following PCR or first line alkylator only therapy and fit patient): see above
BR: bendamustine 70 mg/m^2 IV day 1,2 and rituximab 375 mg/m^2 IV day 1 first cycle and 500 mg/m^2 IV day 1 subsequent cycles every 28 days × 6 cycles
Alemtuzuab (especially if 17p deletion): see above

* Premedicate with acetaminophen 650–1000 mg by mouth and diphenhydramine 50 mg by mouth/IV, 30 minutes prior to rituximab
†Clinical trial or evaluation for allogeneic HSCT should be strongly considered in younger patients, those with unfavorable cytogenetics, or short first remission duration.

- AIHA or autoimmune thrombocytopenia is treated with corticosteroids (e.g., prednisone 1 mg/kg orally for several days followed by a taper); intravenous immune globulin (IVIG) or rituximab can be considered for recurrent hemolysis despite corticosteroids; although AIHA does not preclude the use of fludarabine, these patients require careful management; autoimmune pure red cell aplasia may be treated with cyclosporine (5–10 mg/kg orally daily with attention to serum levels and renal function), prednisone, or antithymocyte globulin (ATG).
- Hypogammaglobulinemia associated with recurrent infections is an indication for IVIG, 0.3–0.5 g/kg monthly to maintain IgG nadir level of >500 mg/dL.
- Treatment of Richter's transformation is difficult and associated with a high mortality rate; some patients may achieve remission with DLBCL regimens (e.g., R-CHOP—rituximab, cyclophosphamide, doxorubicin, vincristine, prednisone), although relapse is frequent; assessment at a transplant center should be considered in younger patients.
- Transfusion therapy in patients with CLL should be with irradiated blood products to avoid transfusion-associated graft-versus-host disease.

COMPLICATIONS OF TREATMENT

- Chlorambucil: nausea, vomiting, fatigue, rash (rare cases of Stevens-Johnson syndrome), gonadal toxicity, seizures (rare), myelosuppression (may be prolonged), hyperuricemia, pneumonitis, secondary malignancy (myelodysplastic syndrome/acute myeloid leukemia).
- Fludarabine: nausea, vomiting, fever, fatigue, rash, myelosuppression, immunosuppression due to decreases in CD4 and CD8 T-lymphocytes (risk of infection with opportunistic fungi, herpesviruses, and *Pneumocystic jirovecii*), autoimmune hemolytic anemia, hepatitis, tumor lysis syndrome (in setting of significant disease burden and if combined with rituximab), pneumonitis, transfusion-associated graft-versus-host disease (all blood products should be irradiated).
- Pentostatin: nausea, vomiting, headache, fatigue, fever, chills, myalgias, conjunctivitis, otalgia, visual changes, myelosuppression, hepatitis, immunosuppression due to decreases in B- and T-lymphocytes (risk of infection with opportunistic fungi, herpesviruses, and *Pneumocystis jirovecii*), neurotoxicity (rare).
- Cyclophosphamide: nausea, vomiting, diarrhea, fatigue, rhinitis, hemorrhagic cystitis, alopecia, skin/nail hyperpigmentation, infusional headache, myelosuppression, hyponatremia/syndrome of inappropriate antidiuretic hormone hypersecretion (SIADH), gonadal toxicity, secondary malignancies (myelodysplasia, acute myeloid leukemia, bladder cancer).
- Bendamustine: nausea, vomiting, fatigue, diarrhea, fever, headache, stomatitis, constipation, anorexia, rash, myelosuppression, infection.

- Rituximab: infusion reaction (fever, chills, bronchospasm, urticaria, flushing, angioedema, hypotension), tumor lysis syndrome, rash (including Stevens-Johnson syndrome), nausea, cough, rhinitis, sinusitis, lymphopenia, reactivation of hepatitis B virus (HBV) or hepatitis C virus (HCV) infection with fulminant viremia and hepatitis, progressive multifocal leukoencephalopathy (PML) from reactivation of JC virus (may manifest as confusion/delirium, ataxia, dysarthria, visual changes; diagnosed with polymerase chain reaction (PCR) for JC virus on cerebrospinal fluid but no effective therapy available with high fatality rate).
- Alemtuzumab: infusion reaction (fever, chills, bronchospasm, urticaria, flushing, angioedema, hypotension), myelosuppression (rare marrow hypoplasia/aplasia), immunosuppression (risk of infection with opportunistic fungi, herpesviruses, CMV, *Pneumocystis jirovecii*, meningitis due to *Listeria monocytogenes*, *Cryptococcus neoformans*, *Candida* species).

FOLLOW-UP CARE

- Patients achieving remission, either partial or complete, after a complete regimen are typically monitored; additional consolidation-like treatment is not standard of care and should not be administered outside of a clinical trial.
- Periodic history, physical examination, and CBC should be considered every 3 to 6 months for 3 to 5 years after therapy; patients who develop symptoms concerning for cytopenia at any time should have a CBC.
- Patients with rapidly progressive adenopathy, night sweats, and weight loss should have an LDH level, CBC, peripheral blood flow cytometry, and excisional lymph node biopsy to exclude Richter's transformation.

PROGNOSIS

- As demonstrated in the Rai staging system, overall survival is highly stage-dependant, with many stage 0 patients surviving for a decade or more and patients with marrow failure (stage III/IV) having a very poor survival (<2 years generally).
  - Recent advances in molecular biology demonstrate, however, that outcome is poor in patients with unmutated V_H and CD38+ CLL, regardless of stage at diagnosis; as such, young patients with these characteristics should be referred to a transplant center for evaluation.
  - Patients with mutated V_H CLL (especially if CD38-) typically display indolent disease behavior and prolonged survival.
- Because infection is a major cause of death in CLL, appropriate use of vaccines, antibiotics, and immune globulin may improve prognosis.
- Patients with CLL have a higher incidence of second cancers, often solid malignancies such as Kaposi sarcoma, melanoma, lung cancer, gastrointestinal cancers, and bladder cancer.

REFERENCES

Ann Oncol 2008;19:S320.
Blood 2004;104:abstract 339.
Blood 2003;101:6.
Blood 1975;46:219.
J Cancer Res Clin Oncol 2001;127:48.
J Clin Oncol 2005;22:4079.
J Clin Oncol 2003;21:1746.
N Engl J Med 2005;352:804.
N Engl J Med 2004;351:893.

31 ■ FOLLICULAR LYMPHOMA

- Follicular lymphoma (FL) is a malignancy of B-lymphocytes that comprises 22% of adult non-Hodgkin lymphoma (NHL) and is the most common indolent lymphoma in the United States.
- Overall, there are approximately 24,000 cases of FL annually in the United States, with a median age at diagnosis of 59 years.
- The clinical course of FL is typically indolent, with many patients surviving for years without treatment; other patients may suffer an aggressive course from the outset or develop aggressive disease from transformation into a high-grade NHL.
- The majority (85% to 90%) of patients exhibit advanced-staged disease (stages III/IV) at diagnosis and are considered incurable, even with modern therapies; patients with stage I/II (10% to 15%), however, may be cured with radiation.
- Risk factors: not well-established for FL but may include immunosuppressive therapy, organ transplantation, inherited immune disease, and rheumatoid arthritis.

PATHOBIOLOGY

- The pathogenesis of FL relates to the translocation of chromosomes 14 and 18 [t(14;18)], resulting in constitutive activation of the BCL2 oncogene, which inhibits apoptosis, leading to the accumulation of transformed, malignant cells.
- Histologically, FL replaces normal nodal architecture with nodular expansions of small lymphocytes with cleaved nuclei (centrocytes) and larger cells (centroblasts).
- Histologic transformation to a high-grade NHL, typically diffuse large B-cell lymphoma (DLBCL), occurs at a rate of 3% per year; transformed FL represents an aggressive phenotype that is often resistant to treatment and ultimately fatal, although some patients may experience remission with aggressive chemotherapy.
- A hallmark of all NHL, including FL, is noncontiguous lymph node spread and frequent extralymphatic involvement—unlike Hodgkin's lymphoma, which is characterized by orderly, contiguous spread.

CLINICAL PRESENTATION

- Although patients with FL may be diagnosed incidentally while under-going imaging for other reasons, many patients note the presence of painless lymphadenopathy.
- Patients with advanced-stage (III/IV) disease may note fever, drenching night sweats, or weight loss ("B" symptoms); anorexia and fatigue are not uncommon, especially in patients with anemia related to bone marrow involvement, which is present in up to one-half of patients.
- Symptoms of transformation to DLBCL include sudden-onset of night sweats, fever, weight loss, and nodal enlargement.

PHYSICAL FINDINGS

- Patients with localized disease (stage I/II) typically manifest palpable nodes that are mobile with a rubbery consistency, in distinction to firm, fixed nodes characteristic of metastatic carcinoma.
- Patients with advanced disease (stage III/IV) may exhibit pallor, diffuse adenopathy, and cachexia.
- Increasing node size over an short interval is suggestive of histologic transformation to DLBCL.

DIAGNOSTIC TESTS AND STAGING

- An excisional node biopsy evaluated by a hematopathologist is essential for accurate diagnosis, because this allows evaluation of nodal architecture; FNA is inadequate, but core biopsy may be utilized if an excisional biopsy is not safe or practical (e.g., retroperitoneal site).
  - FL grade is dependent upon the number of centroblasts within the tumor: grade I: 0–5 centroblasts per high-power field (HPF); grade II: 6–15 centroblasts per HPF; grade III: >15 centroblasts per HPF (patients with grade III FL are approached as high-grade lymphoma).
  - FL has a characteristic immunophenotype that may determined by immunohistochemistry and/or flow cytometry: CD20+, CD10+, CD5-, CD23-, BCL2+, and cyclin D1-; FL is occasionally BCL6+; although FL can be diagnosed on histologic grounds, immunophenotyping should be performed to exclude mantle (CD5+, CD23-) or small lymphocytic lymphoma (CD5+, CD23+).
  - Determination of the proliferation index by the monoclonal antibody Ki-67 has prognostic significance for FL: survival is significantly less for high Ki-67 versus low Ki-67 FL.
  - Presence of t(14;18) can be detected with conventional cytogenetics or via FISH on nodal or marrow specimens.
  - FL expresses CD20, a receptor that is targeted by the chimeric monoclonal antibody, rituximab.

- CBC, LDH, uric acid, and assessment of renal and hepatic function are necessary; serum protein electrophoresis commonly shows monoclonal spike; serum β-2-microglobulin may be useful prognostically.
- Determination of hepatitis B virus (HBV) status with HBV surface antigen (HBSAg) and core antibody (HBCAb)—with quantitative viral load by PCR if either screening tests positive—is required because fatal HBV reactivation has complicated administration of the monoclonal antibody, rituximab; HCV and human immunodeficiency virus (HIV) serostatus should also be obtained prior to treatment.
- Cross-sectional imaging with CT of the neck, chest, abdomen, and pelvis are essential for staging; PET scans are not required in all patients but may be useful on occasion; however, PET may be falsely negative in low-grade FL due to lack of flourodeoxyglucose (FDG) uptake in slowly dividing cells but may identify occult disease in some patients or identify areas of histologic transformation to aggressive NHL.
- Determination of left ventricular function with nuclear gated scan (MUGA) or echocardiography is necessary if anthracycline use is anticipated; periodic assessment of ventricular function should be considered following therapy (or during therapy if cardiac complications occur) and before instituting second-line therapy if additional anthracycline/anthracenedione is considered.
- Bone marrow biopsy and aspirate are essential to exclude marrow involvement (stage IV), which is typically paratrabecular in location; core biopsy should be ≥2 cm.
- Utilization of the FLIPI (Follicular Lymphoma International Prognostic Index) is suggested at determining prognosis but has not been established as a means to determine specific treatment regimens.
  - FLIPI criteria (each 1 point, for maximum of 5 points): age ≥60 years, Ann Arbor stage III/IV, hemoglobin <12 g/dL, serum LDH >normal, involvement of ≥5 nodal areas.
  - Patient with lower scores experience longer survival but patients with higher scores experience shorter survival and increased risk of histologic transformation.

Table 31–1 Ann Arbor Staging Classification

Stage I: involvement of single node region or lymphoid structure (e.g., Waldeyer's ring)
Stage II: involvement of ≥2 node regions on same side of diaphragm
Stage III: involvement of node region(s) or structures on both sides of diaphragm (stage III)
Stage IV: presence of diffuse involvement of ≥1 extralymphatic organs beyond that designated as E (e.g., bone marrow, liver, lung) with or without associated node involvement

Note: the presence or absence of systemic ("B") symptoms should be included with stage designation; A: asymptomatic; B: presence of fever, drenching night sweats, and/or weight loss of >10% of body weight. For stages I–III, apply designation E to refer to involvement of single, extranodal site contiguous to known nodal area; designation S refers to spleen involvement; designation X refers to nodal masses >10 cm in maximal diameter

TREATMENT

- Therapy of FL continues to evolve, and every patient must be assessed individually because many patients may enjoy prolonged survival without treatment; only a general approach will be presented herein.
- Treatment paradigms for FL are stage- and grade-dependent—patients with grade III FL are treated like DLBCL and patients with grade I/II FL are treated according to extent of disease.
  - Stage I/II (limited stage) patients are typically treated with potentially curative radiation therapy, and stage III/IV (advanced stage) may be observed or treated with systemic therapies depending on patient age, presence of comorbidities, symptoms, and organ dysfunction.
  - Patients with nonaggressive, asymptomatic FL may experience spontaneous regression on occasion (15% to 20% of cases), so withholding treatment until B-symptoms, cytopenia(s), bulky disease, or organ impairment occurs is appropriate in many patients.
  - Early treatment with alkylator-based regimens does not improve survival for asymptomatic patients; however, accumulating data suggest benefit of aggressive up-front treatment in patients with advanced-staged FL.
- The GELF (Groupe d'Etude des Lymphomes Folliculaire) criteria are useful in identifying patients who may benefit from early therapy.
  - Involvement of three or more nodal sites, each with diameter ≥3 cm; any nodal/extranodal mass with diameter ≥7 cm; presence of "B" symptoms; splenomegaly; pleural effusion(s) or ascites; cytopenia(s); circulating tumor cells (>5,000 malignant cells/mm^3):
- First-line therapy in symptomatic advanced-stage fit patients typically includes multiagent alkylator-based chemotherapy regimens, which usually includes rituximab, which imparts response rates of 50% to 70% as monotherapy in therapy-naïve patients but with short response duration (<2 years); single-agent rituximab, a chimeric anti-CD20 monoclonal antibody, may be useful for elderly symptomatic patients intolerant of chemotherapy; alternatively, single-agent chlorambucil or cyclophosphamide may be used in elderly/infirm patients.
- Randomized phase III trials have shown improvements in progression-free, event-free, and a trend toward overall survival benefit from up-front chemotherapy plus rituximab regimens in patients with advanced, symptomatic FL; meta-analysis of front-line therapy trials suggest that achievement of CR reduces risk of disease progression.
  - R-CHOP is a widely used regimen for patients with bulky stage II or stage III/IV FL and frequently induces impressive and often complete durable responses.
    - For instance, R-CHOP was associated with a 60% reduction in relative risk for treatment failure, higher overall response rate, and prolonged remission duration compared to CHOP in a German

> study of FL, and R-CHOP improved outcome in elderly FL patients in another study; overall response rates to R-CHOP often exceed 90%.
>> ◦ Use of filgrastim with R-CHOP should be strongly considered, especially in the elderly.
>> ◦ R-CVP (rituximab, cyclophosphamide, vincristine, prednisone) is also an efficacious regimen for FL and is superior to CVP alone, with doubling of time to progression and improved OS.
>> ◦ CHOP followed by radioimmunotherapy (RIT) with ^{131}I-tositumomab imparted a 91% overall response rate and a 69% CR rate in patients with untreated FL; at 5-year follow-up, the 5-year OS was 87%.
> - Interval imaging via PET or CT scan is useful after two cycles and completion of chemotherapy; patients with lack of response or progression should be considered for early salvage treatment; areas of new non-uniform uptake with an SUV uptake >13 are suggestive of transformation.

Table 31–2 Regimens for FL

First-line regimen*†
R-CHOP: cyclophosphamide 750 mg/m^2 IV day 1, doxorubicin 50 mg/m^2 IV day 1, vincristine 2 mg IV day 1, prednisone 100 mg/day by mouth days 1–5, rituximab 375 mg/m^2 IV day 1 every 21 days x 6–8 cycles
R-CVP: cyclophosphamide 800 mg/m^2 IV day 1, vincristine 2 mg IV day 1, prednisone 100 mg by mouth days 1–5, rituximab 375 mg/m^2 IV day 1 every 21 days × 6–8 cycles
R-FND: fludarabine 25 mg/m^2 IV day 1–3, mitoxantrone 10 mg/m^2 IV day 1, dexamethasone 20 mg by mouth days 1–5, rituximab 375 mg/m^2 IV day 1, every 21 days; trimethoprim–sulfamethoxazole 1 tablet by mouth twice daily 3x per week
Rituximab monotherapy: rituximab 375 mg/m^2 IV weekly

Second-line/salvage regimen*†‡
R-FCM: Fludarabine 25 mg/m^2 IV days 1–3, cyclophosphamide 200 mg/m^2 IV days 1–3, mitoxantrone 8 mg/m^2 IV day 1, rituximab 375 mg/m^2 IV day 1 every 21 days x 4 cycles; patients experiencing response can receive rituximab 375 mg/m^2 IV weekly x 4 during months 3 and 9
Radioimmunotherapy: tositumomab or ibritumomab administered in conjunction with nuclear medicine physician

*The role of single-agent rituximab maintenance following first-line R-chemotherapy is still unknown; rituximab should be administered to patients who did not receive it with initial chemotherapy due to prolongation of disease- and event-free survival in this setting.

† Premedicate with acetaminophen 650–1000 mg by mouth and diphenhydramine 50 mg by mouth/IV, 30 minutes prior to rituximab.

*High-dose therapy followed by autologous HSCT should be considered in fit patients who achieve partial or complete response after second-line treatment.

†Extended, or maintenance, rituximab should be considered in second-line setting; several treatment regimens exist based on published trials.

‡Administration of first-line R-chemotherapy regimens can be considered in appropriate patients.

- Relapsed or refractory FL may be treated with chemotherapy plus rituximab regimens, autologous HSCT, or RIT.
  - Multidrug regimens such as FCM-R (fludarabine, cyclophosphamide, mitoxantrone, rituximab) and FND (fludarabine, mitoxantrone, dexamethasone) have shown benefit in some studies in patients fit to receive therapy.
  - Maintenance (four once-weekly infusions of 375 mg/m^2) rituximab following chemotherapy in patients who had received R-CHOP or CHOP prolonged PFS (52 vs. 15 months) and OS at 3 years (85% vs. 77%) compared to observation.
  - Bendamustine, a novel bifunctional alkylating agent, demonstrated a 75% response rate in pretreated, rituximab-refractory FL patients in a recent multicenter study; bendamustine with rituximab produced an overall response rate of 96% (71% of which were CR) in another trial.
  - Autologous HSCT is an option for increasing PFS in patients with relapsed/refractory FL who attain remission with second-line treatment, with 48% of patients in remission at 12-year follow-up.
  - RIT with ^{131}I-tositumomab or ^{90}Y-ibritumomab tiuxetan have demonstrated impressive activity in relapsed FL, with response rates of 80% and CR rates of approximately 25%; due to significant marrow toxicity, patients receiving these agents must have <25% lymphomatous marrow involvement, marrow cellularity >15%, >100,000 platelets/mm^3, neutrophils >1500 cells/mm^3, and no prior HSCT.

COMPLICATIONS OF TREATMENT

- Cyclophosphamide: nausea, vomiting, diarrhea, fatigue, rhinitis, hemorrhagic cystitis, alopecia, skin/nail hyperpigmentation, infusional headache, myelosuppression, hyponatremia/SIADH, gonadal toxicity, secondary malignancies (myelodysplasia, acute myeloid leukemia, bladder cancer).
- Doxorubicin: nausea, vomiting, diarrhea, mucositis, skin/nail hyperpigmentation, photosensitivity, alopecia, extravasation soft-tissue necrosis, myelosuppression, cardiomyopathy (especially with cumulative dose 400–450 mg/m^2).
- Vincristine: neurotoxicity in form of peripheral neuropathy and constipation/ileus (orthostatic hypotension, ataxia, seizures, cortical blindness less common), jaw/parotid pain, limb/back pain, alopecia, rash, vesicant, hyponatremia/SIADH, gonadal toxicity.
- Prednisone: insomnia, irritability/mood changes, appetite stimulation, weight gain, peptic ulceration, infection, myopathy, edema, hypertension, skin breakdown, avascular necrosis, cataracts.
- Fludarabine: nausea/vomiting, fever, rash, pruritis, tumor lysis syndrome, hepatitis, myelosuppression (may be severe and, rarely, permanent), immunosuppression (prolonged risk for cytomegalovirus reactivation, herpesvirus, *Pneumocystis jirovecii*, and fungal infections).

- Chlorambucil: nausea, vomiting, rash, seizures (rare), pneumonitis, myelosuppression (often delayed and prolonged), hyperuricemia, gonadal toxicity.
- Bendamustine: nausea, vomiting, fatigue, diarrhea, fever, headache, stomatitis, constipation, anorexia, rash, myelosuppression, infection.
- Rituximab: infusion reaction (fever, chills, bronchospasm, urticaria, flushing, angioedema, hypotension), tumor lysis syndrome, rash (including Stevens-Johnson syndrome), nausea, cough, rhinitis, sinusitis, lymphopenia, reactivation of HBV or HCV infection with fulminant viremia and hepatitis, progressive multifocal leukoencephalopathy (PML) from reactivation of JC virus (may manifest as confusion/delirium, ataxia, dysarthria, visual changes; diagnosed with PCR for JC virus on cerebrospinal fluid but no effective therapy available with high fatality rate).
- RIT: infusion syndrome (fever, chills, rash, flushing, bronchospasm, hypotension), asthenia, fatigue, infections, myelosuppression, prolonged thrombocytopenia, hypothyroidism (for ^{131}I-tositumomab), secondary myelodysplastic syndromes/acute myeloid leukemia.
- Autologous HSCT: chemotherapy side-effects, prolonged myelosuppression, gondal toxicity, secondary myelodysplasia/acute leukemia in 7% to 19%.

FOLLOW-UP

- Ongoing follow-up following treatment of FL is important because most patients, if not all, eventually relapse despite modern chemoimmunotherapy.
  - Sudden appearance of night sweats, weight loss, and rapidly enlarging lymph nodes is very suggestive of transformation into DLBCL.
- History and physical examination with attention to all nodal areas every 3 months for 2 years, every 6 months for 2 to 3 years, and then at least annually.
- CBC and LDH at 3, 6, 12, and 24 months is reasonable; CT every 6 to 12 months for 2 years following treatment is reasonable, and then as symptoms and signs dictate; routine PET obtained only when clinically indicated.

PROGNOSIS

- The FLIPI is a useful prognosticator even in the rituximab era.
  - Low risk (0–1 factors): 5- and 10-year OS of 91% and 71%, respectively.
  - Intermediate risk (2 factors): 5- and 10-year OS of 78% and 51%, respectively.
  - High risk (3–5 factors): 5- and 10-year OS of 53% and 36%, respectively.
- Patients with localized disease treated with radiation experience 10-year OS approaching 80%.

REFERENCES

Ann Oncol 2009;14:1163.
Blood 2005;105:1417.
Blood 2004;104:1258.
Drugs 2009;69:1727.
J Clin Oncol 2007;25:2544.
J Clin Oncol 2007;25:2554.
J Clin Oncol 2005;23:7565.
J Clin Oncol 1998;16:2332.
Semin Hematol 2008;45:S2.

32 ■ DIFFUSE LARGE B-CELL LYMPHOMA

- Diffuse large B-cell lymphoma (DLBCL) is the most common form of non-Hodgkin's lymphoma (NHL), comprising approximately 35% of all adult NHL cases in the United States.
- The median age at diagnosis is 64 years, with a slight male predominance.
- Untreated, DLCBL is usually rapidly fatal, but is very responsive to multiagent chemotherapy regimens and the anti-CD20 monoclonal antibody, rituximab, which has dramatically changed the outlook for patients with this disease.
- Risk factors: primary immunodeficiency syndromes, HIV infection, autoimmune disease (especially rheumatoid arthritis).

PATHOBIOLOGY

- Despite relatively uniform histology, DLBCL is a heterogeneous disease, with some patients enjoying cure and others experiencing early relapse and death; these differences are due to various genetic and molecular alterations.
- Although most cases of DLBCL arise *de novo*, the oncogenic Epstein-Barr virus (EBV) and HIV are etiologic in some patients.
- DLBCL spreads in noncontiguous nodal fashion (in contradistinction to Hodgkin's lymphoma) and frequently involves extranodal sites and/or organs.
  - Up to one-half of cases involve extranodal sites, most commonly the gastrointestinal tract and bone marrow.
  - Unique subtypes of DLBCL include primary central nervous system lymphoma, the rapidly fatal intravascular DLBCL, and primary effusion lymphoma (PEL), which affects patients with HIV who are infected with human herpesvirus-8 (HHV-8).
- The pathogenesis of DLBCL is complex and is associated with molecular lesions involving tumor suppressor genes and protooncogenes.
- Alterations involving chromosome 3q27 (site of BCL-6 gene) are commonly found in patients with DLBCL and involve translocations between 3q27 and multiple fusion partners such as 14q32 (IgH locus), 2p11 (Igκ locus), and 22q11 (Igλ locus).
  - The BCL6 gene is a repressor of gene transcription, and constitutive activation leads to cell proliferation; expression of BCL6 has been associated with an improved prognosis.

- Increased expression of the antiapoptotic protein, BCL2, due to the presence of the t(14;18) translocation is found in approximately 30% of cases of DLBCL and contributes to the pathogenesis, including increased risk for relapse.
- Overexpression of the tumor suppressor p53 is common.
- Gene profiling with array technology has been utilized to characterize gene expression patterns in various cancers, including DLBCL, which may prove useful in providing prognostification and identification of novel therapeutic targets.
  - Array technology has indentified two subtypes of DLBCL, each associated with different behavior and prognosis: germinal center (GC) phenotype with improved prognosis and activated B-cell (ABC) phenotype with poor prognosis.
  - Immunohistochemical markers have been shown to correlate with gene expression identified on array analysis with regards to DLBCL subtype: GC subtype (CD10+ or BCL6+, MUM1-) and ABC subtype (CD10-, MUM1+ or BCL6-, MUM1-); further research is warranted before treatment decisions are based on these profiles.

CLINICAL PRESENTATION

- Unlike follicular lymphoma, patients with DLBCL are typically symptomatic at presentation, with many noting rapidly growing lymph node(s); patients with extranodal disease may present with sinus pain/aural fullness (Waldeyer's ring), abdominal pain/fecal blood (gastrointestinal tract), or back pain (bone/spine).
- "B" symptoms are common and include weight loss, drenching night sweats, and fever; other systemic symptoms, such as anorexia, fatigue, and weakness, are common.

PHYSICAL FINDINGS

- Localized or widespread lymphadenopathy is the most common finding; splenomegaly and/or hepatomegaly may occur.
- Pallor may signify anemia due to marrow involvement.
- Skin involvement may manifest with erythematous papular/nodular lesions.
- A dull and/or bulging tympanic membrane in a patient with aural fullness or hearing loss should prompt nasopharyngoscopy, which may reveal thickening of Waldeyer's ring tissue due to DLBCL.
- Evidence of pleural effusion (dullness to percussion and decreased breath sounds) may indicate secondary involvement of the pleura, mediastinal lymphatic obstruction from adenopathy, or PEL.
- Cranial neuropathies suggest lymphomatous meningitis, which is more common in patients with spine, marrow, testicular, or sinus/Waldeyer's ring involvement.

DIAGNOSTIC TESTS AND STAGING

- After adequate staging, approximately one-third of patients will have early stage (I/II) and the remainder advanced-stage (III/IV) DLBCL.
- Patients with an isolated or predominant mediastinal mass are categorized as having primary mediastinal (thymic) DLBCL which characteristically affects young females and may be confused with Hodgkin's lymphoma (HL); mediastinal DLBCL has a different gene expression array than typical DLBCL and shares features with HL; management of this type of lymphoma will not be discussed.
- Excisional lymph node biopsy is mandatory, although for intraabdominal or intrathoracic sites, core needle biopsy is acceptable; examination by a hematopathologist is recommended.
  - Histologically, DLBCL consists of a predominance of neoplastic large lymphocytes with vesicular chromatin and prominent nucleoli.
  - The characteristic immunophenotype (via flow cytometry and/or immunohistochemistry) is CD19+, CD20+, CD45+,CD5-, CD23-, and positive for BCL2 and BCL6 in the majority; some cases of DLBCL are CD10+, consistent with transformation from a follicular lymphoma.
  - The variant primary mediastinal DLBCL is typically CD30+.
- Bone marrow biopsy and aspiration are necessary as marrow involvement occurs in 15% to 20% of patients; core of ≥2 cm required.
- Cross-sectional imaging of the neck, chest, abdomen, and pelvis with CT is essential for staging and evaluating response to treatment.
- PET is suggested for accurate staging and assessing response; negative repeat PET after a few cycles of chemotherapy likely portends improved prognosis compared to patients with persistent uptake; most clinicians continue chemotherapy for two cycles beyond PET-negativity or up to a maximum of eight cycles in patients with advanced DLBCL.
- The IPI (International Prognostic Index) is widely utilized to classify patients with DLBCL into four prognostic groups (low, low-intermediate, intermediate, and high risk) based on five parameters identified by multivariable analysis (*N Engl J Med* 1993;329:987); one point is assessed for the presence of each of these for a maximum of 5 points; it is vital to realize that the IPI was devised in the pre-rituximab era and was updated as the revised-IPI by Sehn *et al.* in 2007 as a better predictor of outcome in DLBCL patients treated with R-CHOP (see Prognosis section).
  - Age >60 years, serum LDH above normal, performance status ≥2, involvement of more than one extranodal site, and stage III or IV disease.
- CBC, LDH, uric acid, and assessment of renal and hepatic function are necessary; serum protein electrophoresis commonly shows monoclonal spike; serum β-2-microglobulin may be useful prognostically.
- Determination of HBV status with HBV surface antigen (HBSAg) and core antibody (HBCAb)—with quantitative viral load by PCR if either screening test positive—is required, because fatal HBV reactivation

has complicated administration of the monoclonal antibody, rituximab; HCV and HIV serostatus should also be obtained prior to treatment.

- Determination of left ventricular function with nuclear gated scan (MUGA) or echocardiography is necessary if anthracycline use is anticipated; periodic assessment of ventricular function should be considered following therapy (or during therapy if cardiac complications occur) and before instituting second-line therapy if additional anthracycline/anthracenedione is considered; the cardioprotectant dexrazoxane can be considered in patients undergoing salvage treatment who receive additional anthracycline/anthracenedione (dexrazoxane, IV 30 minutes prechemotherapy at dexrazoxane:doxorubicin ratio of 10:1).

- Lumbar puncture with cytology recommended in patients with HIV infection or marrow, sinus, periorbital, testicular, or spine involvement due to increased risk of meningeal seeding if these sites are involved.

Table 32–1 Ann Arbor Staging Classification

Stage I: involvement of single node region or lymphoid structure (e.g., Waldeyer's ring)
Stage II: involvement of ≥2 node regions on same side of diaphragm
Stage III: involvement of node region(s) or structures on both sides of diaphragm (stage III)
Stage IV: presence of diffuse involvement of ≥1 extralymphatic organs beyond that designated as E (e.g., bone marrow, liver, lung) with or without associated node involvement

Note: the presence or absence of systemic ("B") symptoms should be included with stage designation; A: asymptomatic; B: presence of fever, drenching night sweats, and/or weight loss of >10% of body weight. For stages I–III, apply designation E to refer to involvement of single, extranodal site contiguous to known nodal area; designation S refers to spleen involvement; designation X refers to nodal masses >10 cm in maximal diameter.

TREATMENT

- Treatment of DLBCL is stage-dependent, with early-stage (I/II) patients receiving combination chemoimmunotherapy and involved-field radiation and advanced-stage (bulky stage II/III/IV) patients receiving chemoimmunotherapy.
  - DLBCL is a systemic disease at diagnosis, making chemotherapy the mainstay of treatment; radiation therapy as the sole treatment modality for localized disease results in increased regional as well as systemic relapse, reinforcing the concept of the presence of micrometastases at diagnosis in patients with stage I/II disease.

- Patients with significant disease bulk should receive prophylaxis for tumor lysis syndrome (TLS) with allopurinol 300 mg orally daily; infusion of intravenous dextrose in water with two amples of sodium bicarbonate for urine alkalinization (urine pH >7) is suggested in patients at high risk for TLS; recombinant urate oxidase (rasburicase) rapidly lowers serum uric acid in patients with established TLS and is suggested in patients with renal failure or cardiac arrhythmias (may cause hemolysis in patients with glucose-6-phosphate dehydrogenase deficiency); use of growth factor support with peg-filgrastim 6 mg subcutaneously 24 hours after chemotherapy should be considered, especially in elderly patients and those with bone marrow involvement.

- Treatment of stage I/II disease involves multiagent chemotherapy and involved or extended field radiation.
  - Three cycles of R-CHOP with radiation has been demonstrated to produce excellent outcomes with increased PFS in stage I/II patients; although some European authors have questioned the role of radiation, many U.S. oncologists utilized combined therapy in patients with localized DLBCL.
  - SWOG 8736 demonstrated that three cycles of CHOP followed by radiation produced significantly better OS at 5-years versus CHOP alone (82% vs. 72%), but this difference did not hold with prolonged follow-up.
  - PET should be performed after the three cycles of treatment and those patients with partial response (PR) should be considered for autologous HSCT or completion of therapy with a higher dose of radiation.
- Treatment of stage III/IV disease hinges upon multiagent chemotherapy for six to eight cycles; radiation to areas of disease bulk (>10 cm) can be considered.
  - The standard-of-care regimen for DLBCL is R-CHOP, which induces complete responses in most patients; randomized trials have proven the superiority of eight cycles of R-CHOP over CHOP with regards to disease- and event-free results as well as OS in elderly patients with high- and low-risk DLBCL.
  - Standard R-CHOP is administered at 21-day intervals (R-CHOP-21), but studies comparing a 14-day dosing interval (R-CHOP-14) are ongoing.
  - Patients with bulky (≥10 cm) areas of disease may benefit from six to eight cycles of R-CHOP followed by consolidation locoregional radiation.
  - PET scan should be performed after three to four cycles of chemoimmunotherapy (interim staging) to identify degree of response or those who are refractory to primary treatment—these patients have a poor prognosis and referral to a transplant center should be considered; patients with a CR or PR should receive the remainder of planned treatment; those patients (with local and advanced disease) with PR despite full therapy should be approached as relapsed/refractory disease.
  - PET scan should be performed 8 weeks following completion of systemic therapy.
- Relapsed/refractory disease occurs in 30% to 40% of patients; biopsy should be performed if there is a long remission or if new extranodal disease is present to confirm the diagnosis of DLBCL because up to 25% of patients with late recurrence have low-grade histology.

- Several second-line regimens are available for relapsed disease and patients with PR or CR should receive high-dose induction chemotherapy followed by autologous HSCT, which may result in prolonged disease-free survival or cure.
- Despite several options, no single second-line regimen has emerged as the preferred treatment; individual patient factors

Table 32–2 Regimens for DLBCL

First-line regimen*
R-CHOP: cyclophosphamide 750 mg/m^2 IV day 1, doxorubicin 50 mg/m^2 IV day 1, vincristine 2 mg IV day 1, prednisone 100 mg/day by mouth days 1–5, rituximab 375 mg/m^2 IV day 1 every 21 days x 6–8 cycles

First-line for patients with impaired left ventricle function
R-CNOP: cyclophosphamide 750 mg/m^2 IV day 1, mitoxantrone 10 mg/m^2 IV day 1, vincristine 2 mg IV day 1, prednisone 100 mg by mouth days 1–5, rituximab 375 mg/m^2 IV day 1 every 21 days x 6–8 cycles
R-EPOCH: etoposide 50 mg/m^2/day IV continuous infusion days 1–4, prednisone 100 mg by mouth days 1–5, vincristine 0.4 mg/m^2/day IV continuous infusion days 1–4, cyclophosphamide 750 mg/m^2 IV day 5, doxorubicin 10 mg/m^2/day IV continuous infusion days 1–4, rituximab 375 mg/m^2 IV day 1 prior to infusional agents every 21 days x 6–8 cycles; trimethoprim–sulfamethoxazole DS 1 tablet by mouth twice a day three times per week for *Pneumocystis jirovecii* prophylaxis.

Second-line*†‡
DHAP: dexamethasone 40 mg by mouth or IV days 1–4, cytarabine 2000 mg/m^2 IV over 3 hours every 12 hours for 2 doses day 2, cisplatin 100 mg/m^2 IV continuous infusion over 24 hours day 1 every 21–28 days
ESHAP: etoposide 40 mg/m^2 IV days 1–4, methylprednisolone 500 mg IV days 1–4, cisplatin 25 mg/m^2/day IV continuous infusion days 1–4, cytarabine 2000 mg/m^2 IV day 5 every 21 days
MINE: MESNA 1330 mg/m^2 IV with ifosfamide days 1–3, then 500 mg IV 4 hours following ifosfamide days 1–3, ifosfamide 1330 mg/m^2 IV days 1–3, mitoxantrone 8 mg/m^2 IV day 1, etoposide 65 mg/m^2 IV days 1–3 every 21 days
RICE: rituximab 375 mg/m^2 IV day 1, ifosfamide 5000 mg/m^2 IV continuous infusion for 24 hours day 4, etoposide 100 mg/m^2 IV days 3–5, carboplatin AUC 5 IV day 4, MESNA 5000 mg/m^2 IV continuous infusion with ifosfamide every 21 days; growth factor support with filgrastim 5 µg/kg days 7–14 (pegfilgrastim 6 mg SQ 24 hours after chemotherapy an option)
R-GemOx: rituximab 375 mg/m^2 IV day 1, gemcitabine 1000 mg/m^2 IV day 2, oxaliplatin 50 mg/m^2 IV day 2 every 14 days

*Premedicate with acetaminophen 650–1000 mg by mouth and diphenhydramine 50 mg by mouth/IV 30 minutes prior to rituximab.

*Rituximab 375 mg/m^2 IV can be administered with DHAP, ESHAP, MINE

†Premedicate with acetaminophen 650–1000 mg by mouth and diphenhydramine 50 mg by mouth/IV 30 minutes prior to rituximab

‡Patients achieving PR or CR following second-line therapy who are HSCT candidates should be referred to transplant center for high-dose chemotherapy induction followed by autologous rescue

and physician experience usually determine the regimen; rituximab should be included with these various regimens.

- Patients achieving CR with second-line therapy have a superior OS to those only achieving PR (65% vs. 30%).
- Patients not eligible for HSCT can be treated with any of the second-line regimens, single-agent rituximab, or an oral regimen such as PEPC (prednisone, etoposide, procarbazine, cyclophosphamide) if infusional therapy is not practical.

COMPLICATIONS OF TREATMENT

- Cyclophosphamide: nausea, vomiting, diarrhea, fatigue, rhinitis, hemorrhagic cystitis, alopecia, skin/nail hyperpigmentation, infusional headache, myelosuppression, hyponatremia/SIADH, gonadal toxicity, secondary malignancies (myelodysplasia, acute myeloid leukemia, bladder cancer)
- Doxorubicin: nausea, vomiting, diarrhea, mucositis, skin/nail hyperpigmentation, photosensitivity, alopecia, extravasation soft tissue necrosis, myelosuppression, cardiomyopathy (especially with cumulative dose 400–450 mg/m^2)
- Vincristine: neurotoxicity in form of peripheral neuropathy and constipation/ileus (orthostatic hypotension, ataxia, seizures, cortical blindness less common), jaw/parotid pain, limb/back pain, alopecia, rash, vesicant, hyponatremia/SIADH, gonadal toxicity.
- Prednisone: insomnia, irritability/mood changes, appetite stimulation, weight gain, myopathy, edema, hypertension, skin breakdown, avascular necrosis, cataracts.
- Rituximab: infusion reaction (fever, chills, bronchospasm, urticaria, flushing, angioedema, hypotension), tumor lysis syndrome, rash (including Stevens-Johnson syndrome), nausea, cough, rhinitis, sinusitis, lymphopenia, reactivation of HBV or HCV infection with fulminant viremia and hepatitis, PML from reactivation of JC virus (may manifest as confusion/delirium, ataxia, dysarthria, visual changes; diagnosed with PCR for JC virus on cerebrospinal fluid but no effective therapy available with high fatality rate).
- Second-line/salvage regimens: individual chemotherapy side-effects, prolonged myelosuppression/cytopenias, sepsis, secondary malignancies (especially myelodysplasia and acute myeloid leukemia).
- Autologous HSCT: chemotherapy side-effects, prolonged myelosuppression, gonadal toxicity, secondary myelodysplasia/acute leukemia in 7% to 19%.

FOLLOW-UP CARE

- Following completion of primary treatment, PET scan is indicated to establish remission status.

- History and physical examination with attention to all nodal areas every 3 months for 2 years, every 6 months for 2 to 3 years, and then at least annually.
- CBC and LDH at 3,6,12, and 24 months is reasonable; PET/CT scan when clinically indicated.

PROGNOSIS

- Untreated, survival of patients with DLBCL is less than 1 year.
- Cure rates of approximately 85% to 90% for stage I and 70% to 80% for stage II DLBCL are expected in patients treated with combined-modality therapy.
- Patients with advanced-stage DLBCL are a heterogeneous group with regards to prognosis; in general, 50% to 70% of the 70% to 80% of patients who achieve a CR with first-line chemoimmunotherapy will be cured.
- The revised-IPI (*Blood* 2007;109:1857) is useful for predicting patient prognosis and has been modified to apply to patients receiving R-CHOP.
  - Very good risk (0 factors, 10% of patients): 5-year OS of 94%.
  - Good risk (1–2 factors, 45% of patients): 5-year OS of 79%.
  - Poor risk (3–5 factors): 5-year OS of approximately 55%.
- Generally, patients who relapse after autologous HSCT have a very poor prognosis but some may experience long-term survival with allogeneic HSCT, although at the expense of significant treatment-related morbidity/mortality.

REFERENCES

Ann Oncol 2007;18:1363.
Ann Oncol 1995;6:609.
Blood 2007;109:1857.
Blood 2004;103:3684.
Blood 1998;71:117.
Int J Radiat Oncol Biol Phys 1989;17:767.
J Clin Oncol 2005;23:4117.
J Clin Oncol 1999;17:3776.
J Clin Oncol 1994;12:1169.
N Engl J Med 1993;329:987.

BACKGROUND

- Hodgkin's lymphoma (HL) accounts for approximately 15% of all lymphomas, with approximately 8300 cases and 1400 deaths annually in the United States.
- HL is a prototypic disease of modern curative polychemotherapy—the improvement in overall survival (OS) is superior to all adult cancers, with an overall cure rate of approximately 80%.
  - Due to the very high cure rate of HL, decisions regarding treatment often center on long-term treatment-related toxicity, especially for patients with localized disease treated with radiation; some patients ultimately suffer severe morbidity or mortality years after curative therapy for HL—complications that often include second malignancies.
- HL incidence follows a bimodal age distribution, peaking at ages 15 to 30 and >55 years.
- Risk factors: EBV infection, HIV infection, certain occupations may be at increased risk of HL (farmers, carpenters, meat processors).

PATHOBIOLOGY

- HL is a neoplasm of B-lymphocytes that is unusual in that the majority of cells within a tumor mass are not neoplastic cells, but a reactive pleomorphic infiltration of eosinophils, neutrophils, and plasma cells.
  - Elevated serum levels of interleukins (IL)-6,7,8,9,10 and TNF from immune cells have pathogenic and prognostic implications; elevated IL-6 levels are associated with suboptimal chemotherapy response.
  - Clonal EBV may be detected within Reed-Sternberg cells.
- HL is divided into two major groups: classical HL (95% of cases) and lymphocyte-predominant (LP) HL (5% of cases), which has differing pathobiology, treatment, and prognosis.
- Classical HL is divided into four subtypes: nodular sclerosis, mixed cellularity, lymphocyte-depleted, and lymphocyte-rich, which are characterized by varying numbers of the pathognomic Reed-Sternberg (RS) cell, which exhibits bilobed nuclei with prominent nucleoli ("owl's-eye" cells) and a characteristic immunophenotype: CD15+, CD30+, CD45-, and EMA- (epithelial membrane antigen).
  - Nodular sclerosis (NS) is the most common subtype (60%) and usually affects young females; abundant RS cells are often evident amidst an

inflammatory background surrounded by fibrous bands forming nodules histologically; very responsive to chemotherapy; the RS cell of NS HL has a unique multiobulated nucleus surrounded by a clear region known as the "lacunar cell."

- Mixed cellularity (20%) is characterized by diffuse infiltrate of reactive cells and often affects older males and patients with HIV infection and typically presents in advanced stage (III/IV); most cases have EBV DNA integrated within the genome.
- Lymphocyte-rich is uncommon (15%) and is characterized by an abundant, typically nodular lymphocytic infiltrate; approximately 40% are EBV-associated.
- Lymphocyte-depletion is rare (5%) and is characterized by scant RS cells; most often occurs in elderly males or immunocompromised patients and has a poor prognosis; abdominopelvic adenopathy and/or hepatosplenomegaly are more common than peripheral adenopathy at diagnosis, in contrast to other variants.

- LPHL is characterized by absence of Reid-Sternberg cells but instead by infiltration of lymphocytic and histiocytic (L & H) cells, also known as "popcorn" cells due to the histologic appearance resembling a piece of popcorn.
  - The immunophenotype of L & H cells differs from classical HL: CD20+ and typically CD15- and CD30-; EMA is positive in over one-half of cases.
  - The unique pathobiology of LPHL is exhibited by increased incidence in young males (median age 34 years), localized (stage I/II) disease in three-fourths of cases, and a significant incidence of late recurrence (which usually responds to rituximab), and transformation to DLBCL.
- HL, in contrast to NHL, spreads in contiguous manner, typically spreading in an orderly manner between adjacent nodal basins.

CLINICAL PRESENTATION

- Most patients with HL, especially those with localized disease, present with painless lymphadenopathy, often in the neck or supraclavicular regions.
- Approximately one-third of patients present with "B" symptoms, which include weight loss, fever, and drenching night sweats; uncommonly, HL can manifest as fever of unknown origin (FUO).
  - An unusual fever pattern of HL known as "Pel-Ebstein" fever is characterized by days to weeks of daily fever followed by an afebrile period, followed by fever recurrence.
- Unusual symptoms may occur on occasion: lymph node pain with alcohol ingestion, generalized pruritus, and neurologic symptoms/memory loss due to paraneoplastic antibodies.

PHYSICAL FINDINGS

- The majority of patients with localized HL, especially those with nodular sclerosis variant, present with cervical and/or supraclavicular lymphadenopathy; generalized lymphadenopathy and hepatosplenomegaly are not uncommon and indicate advanced disease.
  - Bulky mediastinal adenopathy may induce superior vena cava compression with facial erythema, conjunctival injection, neck vein distention, and venous collaterals over the upper thorax.
- Pallor indicates anemia due to marrow involvement or, less commonly, autoimmune hemolytic anemia (scleral icterus suggestive of hemolysis).
- Paraneoplastic findings include generalized ichthyosis (scale-like dry skin), erythema nodosum, severe edema (nephrotic syndrome due to minimal change disease), petchiae (autoimmune thrombocytopenia), and ataxia/cerebellar signs (paraneoplastic cerebellar degeneration).

DIAGNOSTIC TESTS AND STAGING

- Excisional lymph node biopsy is essential for diagnosis; core needle biopsy is acceptable for intrathoracic/abdominal nodes; FNA is not acceptable for diagnosis; review of nodal material should be performed by a hematopathologist.
- Bone marrow biopsy and aspiration is important to assess for marrow involvement by HL, which is present in approximately 30% of patients with stage IV disease.
- CBC may reveal anemia, leukocytosis/leucopenia (rare), thrombocytosis, eosinophilia, or lymphopenia.
- Erythrocyte sedimentation rate (ESR) often elevated; shown to be poor prognostic sign.
- Liver function studies necessary prior to chemotherapy; cytokine-mediated elevation of alkaline phosphatase occasionally noted; hypoalbuminemia may signify paraneoplastic nephrotic syndrome.
- Serum calcium may be elevated due to tumor production of vitamin D.
- Staging of HL depends on anatomic location of involved nodes and organs in relation to the diaphragm, as identified on imaging studies and the presence of absence of "B" symptoms.
- CT of the neck, chest, abdomen, and pelvis is usually the initial imaging study and is accurate at identifying areas of involvement by HL, especially lymph nodes, spleen, liver, and bone.
  - Residual masses may persist after chemotherapy and may not indicate active tumor, but residual fibrotic tissue; this is a limitation of CT for assessing treatment response and prognosis.
- PET scanning with F-18 fluorodeoxyglucose (FDG) is emerging as the imaging modality of choice for initial staging, assessing mid-therapy treatment response, and final posttreatment staging.

- PET may be more accurate at assessing bone marrow and hepatosplenic involvement than CT.
  - PET is useful at assessing residual masses following treatment; lack of uptake is compatible with absence of active HL.
  - Normalization of FDG uptake following the first two to three cycles of chemotherapy for advanced disease appears to predict an especially favorable prognosis.
- Echocardiography or nuclear gated (MUGA) scan is essential prior to initiating anthracyclines.
- Pulmonary function tests (PFTs), including DLCO should be obtained prior to use of bleomycin (which can cause pneumonitis or pulmonary fibrosis) or mantle irradiation; patients with preexisting lung disease or who are active smokers should be considered for occasional measurement of vital capacity and DLCO during therapy to monitor for lung toxicity.
- The Ann Arbor staging system has been utilized for over 3 decades; for ease of therapy, HL is generally divided into early stage (nonbulky stage IA/IIA) and advanced (stage III/IV or any stage with "B" symptoms).
  - Stages IA/IIA are considered favorable risk; stages III/IV or any stage with "B" symptoms are considered intermediate risk; and any stage with bulky disease (any mass >10 cm diameter or greater than one-third the transverse diameter of chest at the fifth and sixth vertebral levels) is considered less favorable risk.
- Stages I/II disease is considered unfavorable if any of the following are present: large mediastinal mass, significant splenic involvement, any mass >10 cm, sedimentation rate ≥50 mm/hr, more than three sites of disease involvement, "B" symptoms, or two or more extranodal sites; the presence of any one or more of these is considered unfavorable when determining treatment for localized HL.

Table 33–1 Ann Arbor Staging Classification

Stage I: involvement of single node region or lymphoid structure (e.g., Waldeyer's ring)

Stage II: involvement of ≥2 node regions on same side of diaphragm

Stage III: involvement of node region(s) or structures on both sides of diaphragm

Stage IV: presence of diffuse involvement of ≥1 extralymphatic organs beyond that designated as E (e.g., bone marrow, liver, lung) with or without associated node involvement

Note: the presence or absence of systemic ("B") symptoms should be included with stage designation; A: asymptomatic; B: presence of fever, drenching night sweats, and/or weight loss of >10% of body weight. For stages I–III, apply designation E to refer to involvement of single, extranodal site contiguous to known nodal area; designation S refers to spleen involvement; designation X refers to nodal masses >10 cm in maximal diameter.

Table 33–2 Hasenclever Prognostic Score for Advanced Hodgkin's Disease*†

Serum albumin <4 g/dL
Hemoglobin <10.5 g/dL
Male gender
Stage IV disease
Age ≥45 years
White blood cell count ≥15,000/mm³
Lymphocyte count <600 cells/mm³ or <8% of white blood cell count

*Rate of freedom from disease progression/overall survival (in %) based on number of risk factors
established on multivariate analysis of 5141 patients with advanced Hodgkin's lymphoma treated with
chemotherapy: 0 factors, 84%/89%; 1 factor, 77%/90%; 2 factors, 67%/81%; 3 factors, 60%/78%;
4 factors, 51%/61%; 5 factors, 42%/56%.
†*N Engl J Med* 1998;339:1506.

TREATMENT

- Multiagent chemotherapy is the cornerstone of treatment for HL of all
  stages; generally, patients with IA/IIA may be treated with combined
  chemotherapy and radiation or chemotherapy alone; patients with bulky
  (X) disease typically receive radiation to involved areas following chemotherapy to decrease relapse risk; patients with advanced HL (III/IV, "B"
  symptoms) are treated with chemotherapy alone; involved field radiation
  therapy (IFRT), which involves applying radiation to the lymphoid areas
  involved with disease and not to adjacent lymphoid areas, plays a vital
  role in treatment of early stage HL.
  - The standard of care in the United States is the ABVD regimen, which
    consists of doxorubicin, bleomycin, vinblastine, and dacarbazine (day
    1 and 15 constitute one cycle); advantages of ABVD include ease of
    administration, all intravenous (improved compliance), less cumula-
    tive myelotoxic effects, lower risk of secondary cancers, and relatively
    low infertility risk.
    - ABVD induces CR in approximately 80% of patients with a 5-year
      survival of 70% to 75%.
    - With combined therapy, radiation is usually administered at a dose
      of 30–36 Gy.
  - The Stanford V regimen (mechlorethamine, doxorubicin, vinblastine,
    vincristine, bleomycin, etoposide, prednisone) is not as widely utilized
    but was designed for patients with advanced or bulky stage HL; con-
    sists of a 12-week regimen followed by radiation to bulky sites (the
    radiation must be delivered as described in the original study to avoid
    inferior outcomes).
  - BEACOPP (bleomycin, etoposide, doxorubicin, cyclophosphamide,
    vincristine, procarbazine, prednisone) is a very effective regimen
    for patients with high-risk disease or four or more factors in the
    Hasenclever score but has higher risk of secondary cancers than

ABVD; an ongoing comparative trial of ABVD versus BEACOPP may determine future standard of care.

- Early-stage, favorable stage IA/IIA.
  - Generally, four cycles of ABVD followed by restaging PET and then consolidative IFRT to 30 Gy; alternatively, two cycles of ABVD followed by IFRT can be considered in some patients with favorable stage I/II or low-bulk disease.
  - ABVD alone can be considered in younger patients with favorable-risk HL with a negative PET after two cycles, to avoid the long-term effects of radiation.
  - Stanford V is an option for early-stage disease as well, but the radiation schedule must adhere to published data.
  - Restaging following completion of IFRT is required; patients who remain PET-positive after standard first-line therapy should be managed as relapsed/refractory disease.
- Early-stage, unfavorable stage I/II.
  - Generally four cycles of ABVD followed by PET for a total of six cycles for those who achieve a partial response after four cycles; consolidative IFRT follows chemotherapy; those patients with a partial response after four cycles are administered two additional cycles with repeat staging—consolidation IFRT is administered to PET-negative patients and those with PET-positive disease also receive IFRT, but then end-of-therapy restaging.
- Advanced-stage (III/IV or any stage with "B" symptoms or bulky disease)
  - ABVD is administered for total of six to eight cycles; PET restaging is recommended after four cycles of chemotherapy—those with a CR are administered two subsequent cycles (total of six) and those with PR are administered four subsequent cycles (maximum total of eight).
  - For initial sites of bulky disease within the mediastinum, consolidation IFRT is delivered after six cycles of ABVD followed by two subsequent cycles; IFRT can be administered to other sites of bulky (X) disease to 30–36 Gy following chemotherapy.
    - Sites of bulky disease typically treated with 36 Gy.
  - BEACOPP every 3 weeks is an alternative for advanced-stage HL, especially those with high-risk features (≥4 Hasenclever factors); following eight cycles of chemotherapy, 30 Gy of radiation to initial sites >5 cm in size and 40 Gy to residual PET-positive sites is administered; the reader is directed to other resources regarding BEACOPP, because this is associated with higher toxicity and ABVD remains standard by the majority of most U.S. oncologists.
- Lymphocyte-predominant HL typically behaves indolently and is known for late relapse; due to its rarity; no randomized therapy data are available, but some large groups have published their experiences to guide treatment, with ABVD being the most commonly utilized regimen; because LPHL expresses CD20, some authors suggest use of rituximab alone or with polychemotherapy.

- Stage I/IIA LPHL patients have an excellent response to IFRT alone (30–36 Gy) with 15-year failure-free progression of 84% and 73%, respectively; other studies have demonstrated superior failure-free treatment intervals with combined-modality therapy (ABVD and IFRT) in patients with IB/IIB disease.
- Stage III/IV LPHL should receive chemotherapy with or without IFRT to areas of disease bulk; regimens commonly used at academic centers include ABVD, CHOP, or CVP—with or without rituximab; ABVD remains the most commonly used regimen in this setting due to experience with classic HL.
- Relapsed/refractory HL is not uncommon, occurring in approximately 20% to 30% of patients; patients who relapse following radiation alone for early-stage HL have a 50% to 80% long-term disease-free survival when treated with salvage ABVD.
  - Patients who relapse >12 months after initial therapy may be treated with another combination regimen (e.g., BEACOPP for patients who initially received ABVD).
  - Autologous stem cell transplant is associated with 5-year relapse-free rates of up to 40% in patients who respond to a salvage regimen such as DHAP, ESHAP, or ICE (see NHL section for regimens); however, OS is not improved.
  - Gemcitabine-containing regimens are gaining popularity for both transplant-eligible/ineligible relapsed HL patients.

Table 33–3 Regimens for HL (first-line)

ABVD (standard-of-care): doxorubicin 25 mg/m² IV days 1 and 15, bleomycin 10 U/m² IV days 1 and 15, vinblastine 6 mg/m² IV days 1 and 15, dacarbazine 375 mg/m² IV days 1 and 15, repeat cycle every 28 days

Stanford V: nitrogen mustard 6 mg/m² IV day 1, doxorubicin 25 mg/m² IV days 1 and 15, vinblastine 6 mg/m² IV days 1 and 15, vincristine 1.4 mg/m² IV days 8 and 22, bleomycin 5 U/m² IV days 8 and 22, etoposide 60 mg/m² IV days 15 and 16, prednisone 40 mg by mouth every other day, repeat cycle every 28 days.
Note: patients >50 years reduce vinblastine to 4 mg/m² IV and vincristine to 1 mg/m² IV on weeks 9 and 12. Taper prednisone starting week 10. Prophylactic trimethoprim–sulamethoxazole DS by mouth twice daily and acyclovir 200 mg by mouth thrice daily

BEACOPP: bleomycin 10 mg/m² IV day 8, etoposide 100 mg/m² IV days 1–3, doxorubicin 25 mg/m² IV day 1, cyclophosphamide 650 mg/m² IV day 1, vincristine 1.4 mg/m² IV day 8 (maximum of 2 mg), procarbazine 100 mg/m² by mouth days 1–7, prednisone 40 mg/m² by mouth days 1–14, repeat every 21 days

Escalated BEACOPP: bleomycin 10 mg/m² IV day 8, etoposide 200 mg/m² IV days 1–3, doxorubicin 35 mg/m² IV day 1, cyclophosphamide 1200 mg/m² IV day 1, vincristine 1.4 mg/m² IV day 8 (maximum of 2 mg), procarbazine 100 mg/m² by mouth days 1–7, prednisone 40 mg/m² by mouth days 1–14, repeat every 21 days. Filgrastim 5 µg/kg/day SQ days 8 until neutrophil recovery

COMPLICATIONS OF TREATMENT

- ABVD chemotherapy.
  - Doxorubicin: nausea, vomiting, diarrhea, mucositis, skin/nail hyperpigmentation, photosensitivity, alopecia, extravasation soft-tissue necrosis, myelosuppressin, cardiomyopathy (especially with cumulative dose 400–450 mg/m²).
  - Bleomycin: dermatologic toxicity (hyperpigmentation, rash, vesicles, striae); alopecia; hypersensitivity reactions/anaphylaxis; pulmonary toxicity manifesting as cough, dyspnea, rales, radiographic infiltrates; oxygen toxicity (especially with FIO_2 >40% during surgical procedures) resulting in acute respiratory distress syndrome (ARDS); vascular toxicity (Raynaud's phenomenon, angina pectoris, arterial occlusion/ischemia).
  - Vinblastine: nausea, vomiting, diarrhea, fatigue, stomatitis/mucositis, alopecia, myelosuppression, vesicant, hyponatremia due to SIADH, hypertension (due to autonomic toxicity), neurotoxicity (parasthesia, constipation, orthostatic hypotension, ileus, cranial nerve paresis, ataxia, seizures, cortical blindness), vascular toxicity, pulmonary edema.
  - Dacarbazine: nausea, vomiting (potent emetogen), flulike illness (fever, chills, myalgias, arthalgias), vesicant, myelosuppression, neurotoxicity (parasthesia, headache, delirium, seizures), phlebitis.
- Radiation acute effects (depend on site): fatigue, nausea, vomiting, dermatitis, esophagitis, enteritis, diarrhea, cytopenia.
- Long-term effects are a significant threat to survival in patients cured of HL.
  - Pulmonary toxicity from bleomycin, including interstitial fibrosis.
  - Cardiomyopathy/heart failure from doxorubicin.
  - Non-Hodgkin's lymphoma or acute myeloid leukemia.
  - Secondary solid malignancies, especially >10 years following mantle radiation (13% risk at 20 years): esophageal cancer, lung cancer, breast cancer (especially women receiving radiation prior to age 30; often bilateral), sarcoma, and melanoma.
  - Cardiac toxicity from mantle radiation: valve stenosis/insufficiency, accelerated atherosclerosis, constrictive pericarditis.
  - Cerebrovascular disease/stroke following neck radiation.
  - Endocrine dysfunction: hypothyroidism, hypogonadism/infertility.
  - Lhermitte's phenomenon following thoracic radiation: an electric-shock-like sensation radiating down spine to lower extremities upon neck flexion resulting from spinal cord demyelination.

FOLLOW-UP CARE

- Follow-up of HL continues to evolve and is not supported by grade I evidence, but a rational, evidence-based approach can be applied to most patients, with individualized schedules applied to single patients; a reasonable approach is as follows:

- History, physical examination, CBC, ESR, LDH, liver function tests should be performed every 3 months for 2 years and then every 3 to 6 months until year 5 following treatment.
- CT of the abdomen/pelvis are suggested every 6 to 12 months for 2 to 3 years and then annually until year 5.
- Chest radiograph or CT every 6 to 12 months during first 5 years and then as needed, if symptoms dictate.
- Routine PET scans are not suggested for follow-up surveillance.
- Due to unique long-term effects of HL treatment (especially second cancers and cardiovascular disease), oncologists should follow all patients frequently for the first 5 years following treatment and then at least annually for life.
  - Mammography should begin no more than 10 years following completion of radiation or at age 40 (whichever is earlier); women who received chest irradiation prior to age 30 should be screened with annual MRI and mammography.
  - Annual measurement of TSH should be obtained in patients with a history of chest/neck radiation.
- Ongoing counseling regarding smoking cessation and adaptation of a healthy lifestyle are paramount for all HL survivors.

PROGNOSIS

- HL represents a triumph of modern polychemotherapy, which has imparted an excellent long-term prognosis for many patients with this disease; overall, 80% enjoy long-term survival or cure.
- Interval PET scan after two ocycles of ABVD has powerful prognostic implications: one study demonstrated an 86% relapse rate in PET-positive patients and a 5% relapse rate in PET-negative patients; similarly, interim-negative PET following two cycles of BEACOPP in standard- and high-risk patients demonstrated a 2% relapse rate in PET-negative patients compared to a 27% relapse rate in PET-positive patients.
- Patients with early-stage favorable LPHL has a better prognosis than similar-stage classic HL; patients with stage IA disease have a 100% 5-year OS following treatment with IFRT alone; patients with advanced-stage LPHL have an inferior prognosis to early-stage patients.
- Due to highly effective therapy, many late deaths result from second malignancies such as breast cancer (2.5 to 5 times higher risk if radiation prior to age 30) and lung cancer or cardiovascular disease.

REFERENCES

Ann Oncol 2008;19:iv46.
Acta Haematol 2004;112:141.
Ann Oncol 1996;7:151.
Blood 2004;104:3483.
Blood 2008;111:109.
J Clin Oncol 2009;27:1906.
J Clin Oncol 2006;24:3218.
J Clin Oncol 2004;22:2835.
N Engl J Med 2003;348:2386.
N Engl J Med 2007;357:1916.

INDEX

Note: Page numbers followed by "*f*" and "*t*" denote figures and tables, respectively.

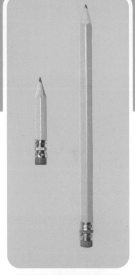

MW00522749

Children develop significantly during early childhood. From infancy to the age of 6, many milestones will occur. One such milestone is learning simple, everyday math. By using this workbook, children can learn to recognize numbers and currency. They will also learn about measurements, number bonds and simple addition and subtraction to get them ready for school.

Holding A Pencil

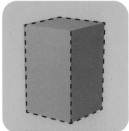

Before getting started, there are a few things your child will need to understand, such as how to hold a pencil. Encourage your child to relax their hand and grip the pencil between their thumb and index finger. Pencil control is an important skill to master. See the images below for the best way to hold the pencil if your child is left-handed or right-handed.

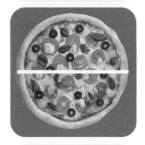

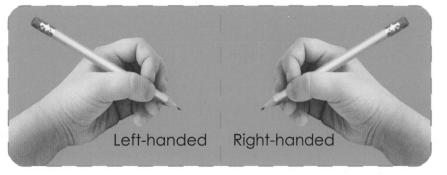

Left-handed   Right-handed

Posture

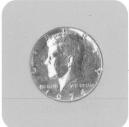

It is best to sit up straight, at a desk or table, with both feet flat on the floor. Position the workbook at a slight angle depending on your child's dominant hand. Angle to the left for right-handers and slightly to the right for left-handers.

Now, let's get started.

Answer key on page 51.

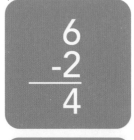

$$\begin{array}{r} 6 \\ -2 \\ \hline 4 \end{array}$$

MEASURE IT

Using a ruler, measure the length of each colored line.
Write your answers in the boxes below.

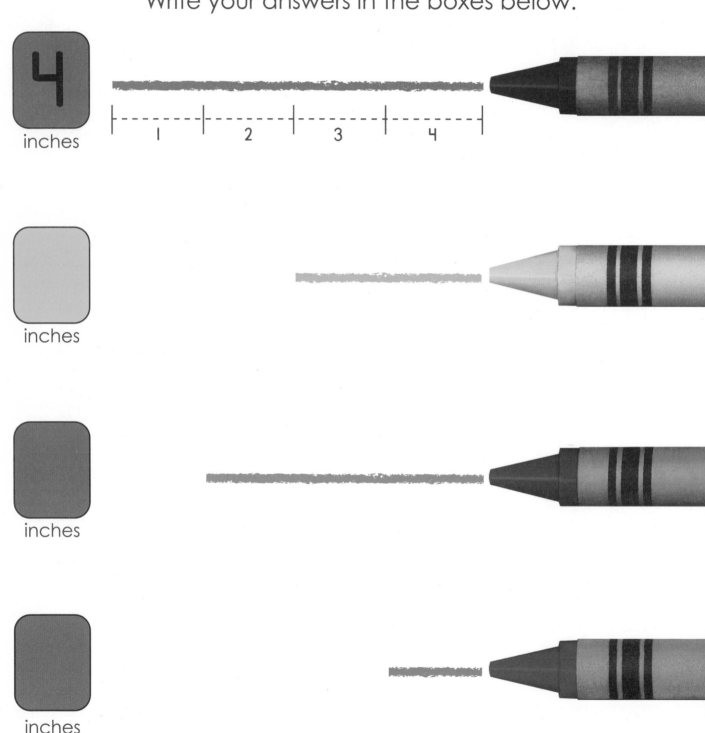

4
inches

inches

inches

inches

Circle the longest line.

Short or Long?

Look at the pairs of objects below.
Circle the shorter object in each box.

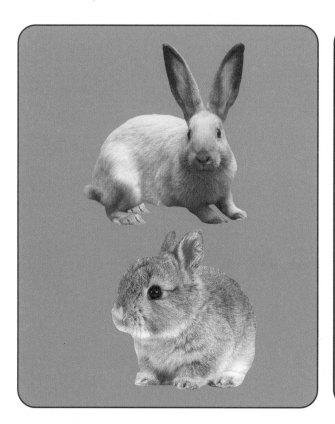

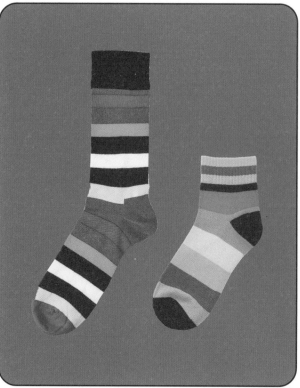

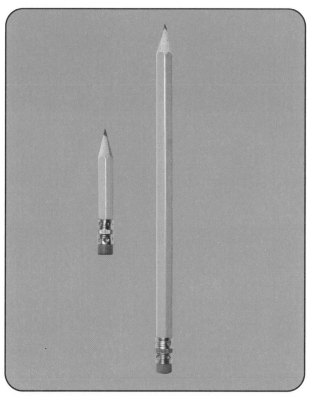

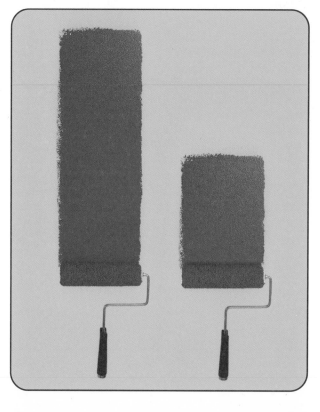

How Do They Stack Up?

Measure each stack and write down its height.

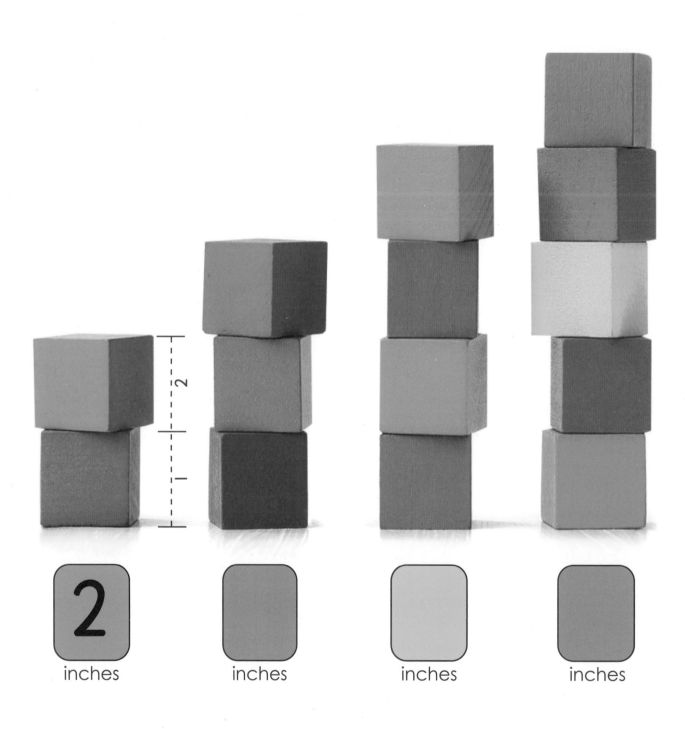

| 2 inches | inches | inches | inches |

Circle the shortest stack.

Practice at Home

Measure the objects below. Then find the same objects at home and measure them. Write your answers in the boxes below.

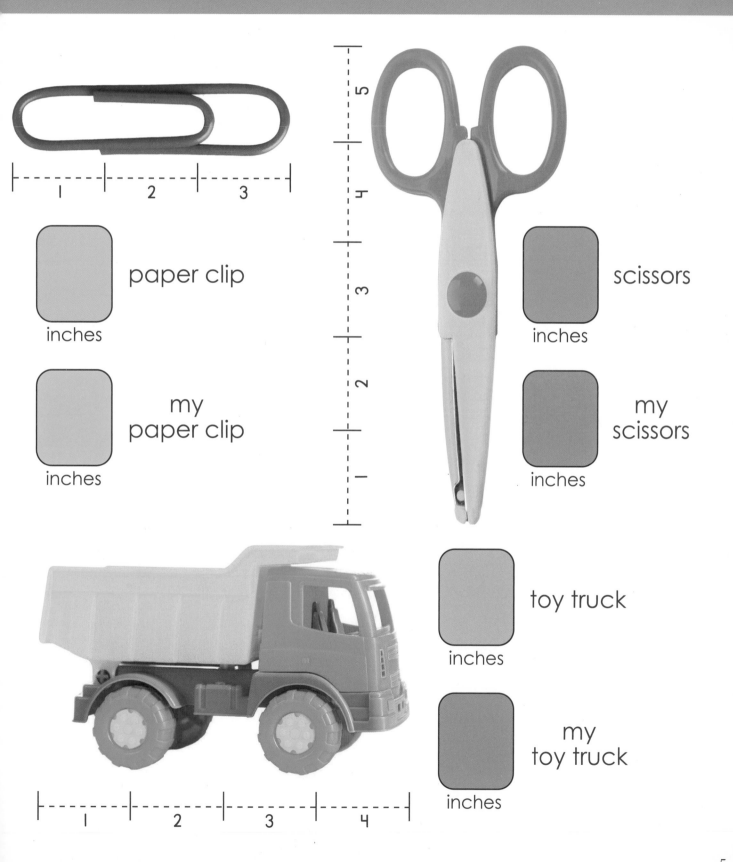

paper clip

inches

my
paper clip

inches

scissors

inches

my
scissors

inches

toy truck

inches

my
toy truck

inches

Practice at Home

Measure the objects below. Then find the same objects at home and measure them.
Write your answers in the boxes below.

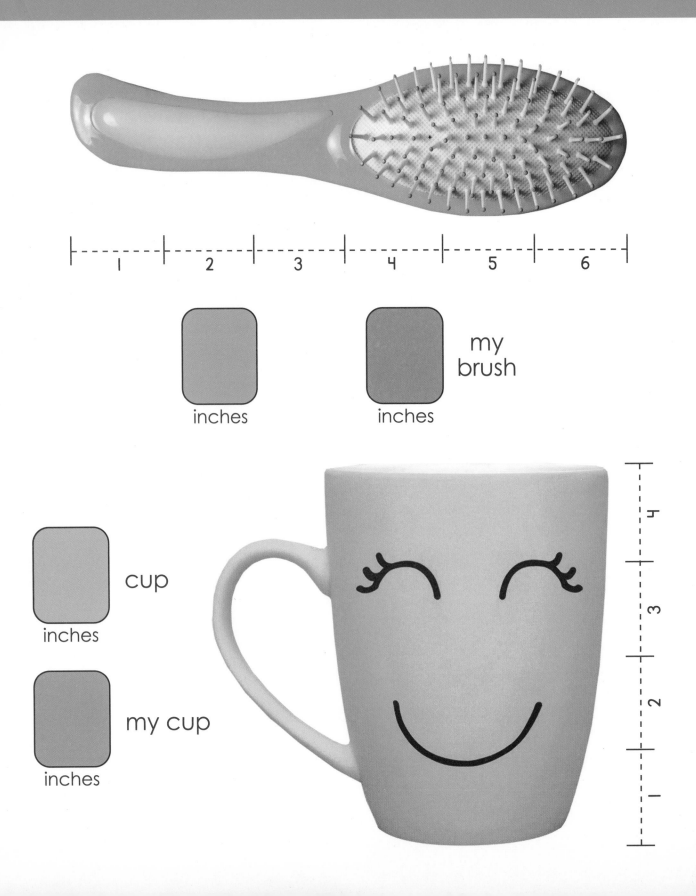

inches

inches

my
brush

cup

inches

my cup

inches

WEIGH IT

Now that you know how to measure with a ruler, let's look at weights. Circle the object you think is lighter in each pair below.

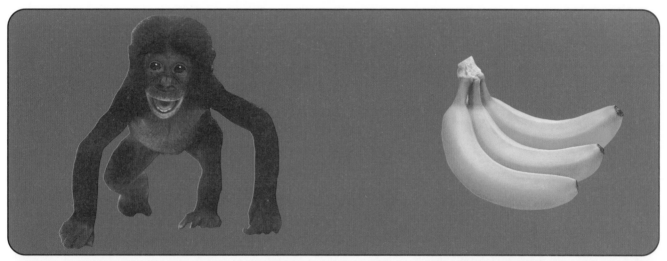

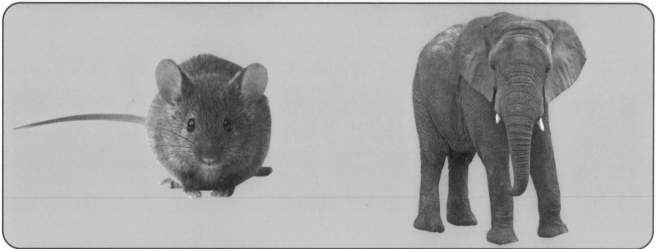

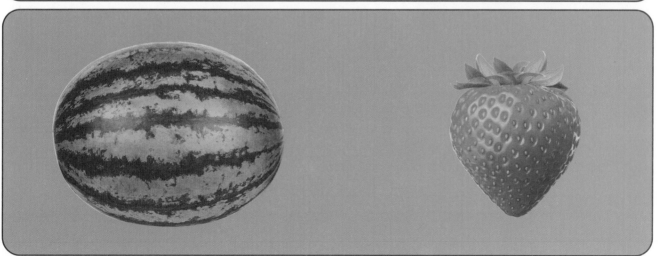

Light or Heavy?

Circle the object that you think is the heaviest.

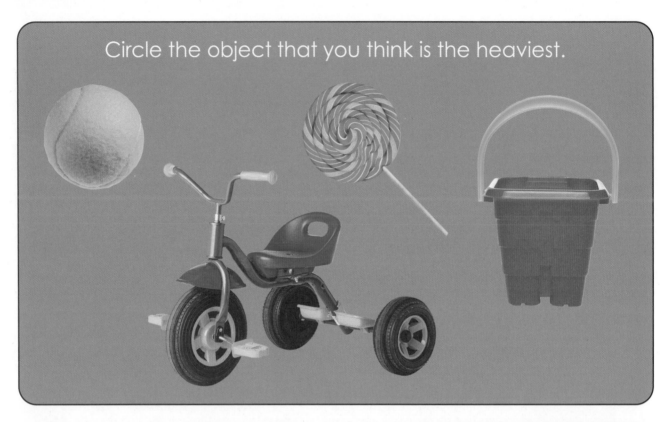

Circle the object that you think is the lightest.

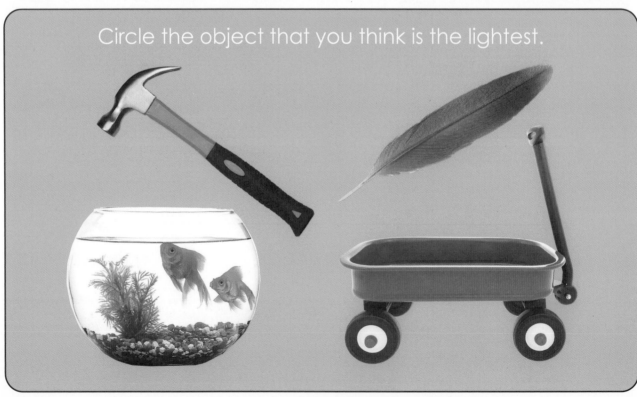

Weighing at Home

With the help of an adult, find the items on the next two pages and weigh them using a kitchen scale.

To start, weigh a full water bottle.
On the next page, circle the objects you think are lighter or heavier than the water bottle.

My water bottle weighs:

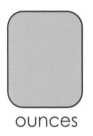

ounces

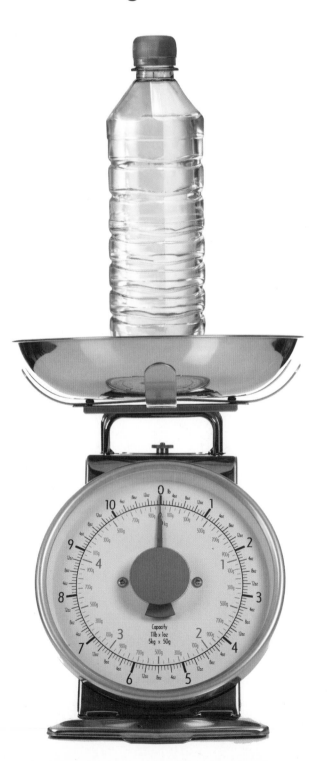

- There are 16 ounces in a pound.

- Ounces are abbreviated as oz.

- If you don't have a scale, hold the objects in your hands to compare weights.

- If you do have a scale, make your estimates first, then check it with scale.

OBJECT	How do you think it compares to your water bottle?	How does it actually compare?
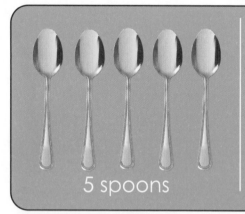 5 spoons	heavier lighter	heavier lighter
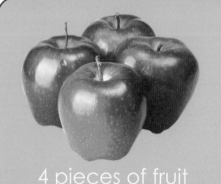 4 pieces of fruit	heavier lighter	heavier lighter
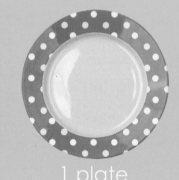 1 plate	heavier lighter	heavier lighter
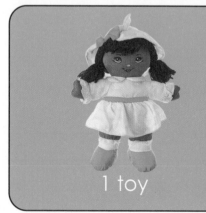 1 toy	heavier lighter	heavier lighter

Equal or Unequal?

When two or more objects have the same quantity,
size or value, they are equal to each other.
Look at the groups below. Are they equal or unequal?

equal parts

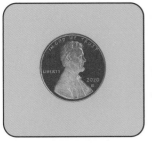 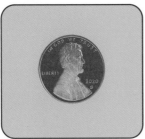

1 penny   1 penny

unequal parts

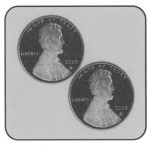 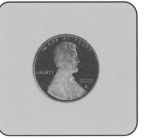

2 penny   1 penny

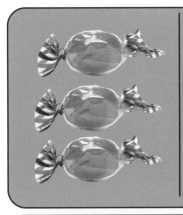 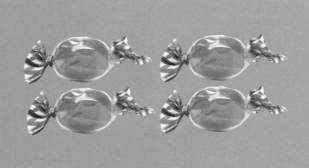

equal

unequal

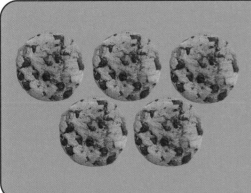 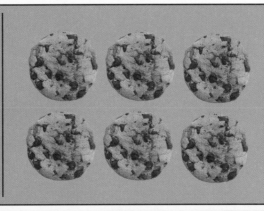

equal

unequal

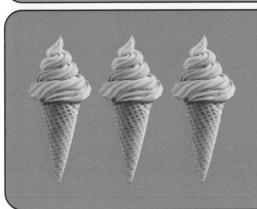 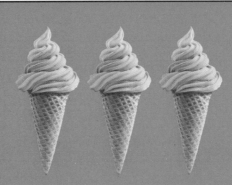

equal

unequal

11

FRACTIONS

A fraction represents a part of a whole.
When something is broken up into a number of equal parts,
the fraction shows how many of those parts you have.

When you have half of something,
it means that something was cut
into two equal parts.
This is a type of fraction.

If you have a whole pizza,
and you cut it into pieces,
each piece is a fraction
of the whole pizza.

This pizza is cut into halves.

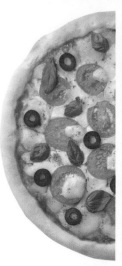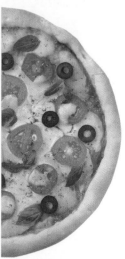

Let's learn how to write a fraction.

1
The top number is one
piece of pizza.

2
The bottom number is how many
pieces the whole pizza is cut into.

Fractions can also be written as words.
Trace the numbers and the words for the fraction below.

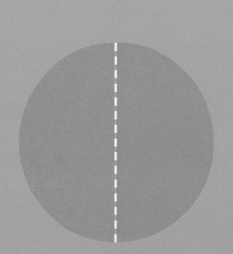

1
—
2
of the circle
is shaded purple.

Half
of the circle
is shaded blue.

Half and Whole

When something is whole, it is complete and uncut. When you cut it into two equal parts, each part is considered a half. Circle the fruits that are a half. Check the fruits that are whole.

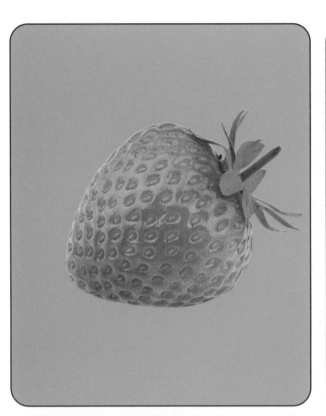

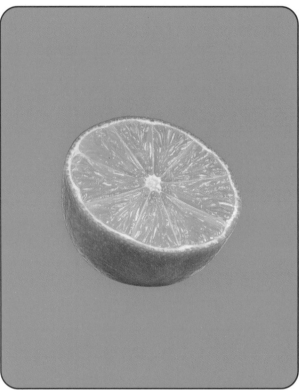

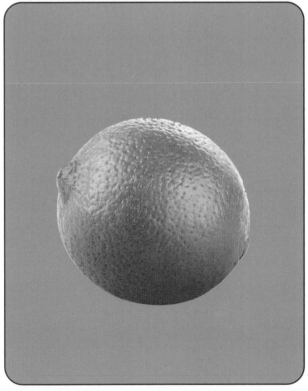

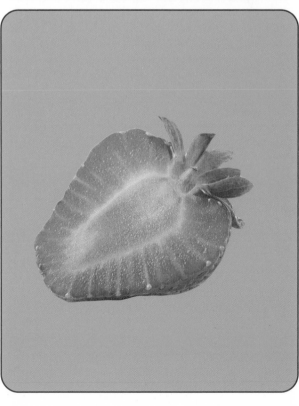

Shading Halves

Each of the shapes below is cut into halves.
Following the first example, use a pen to
shade half of each shape.

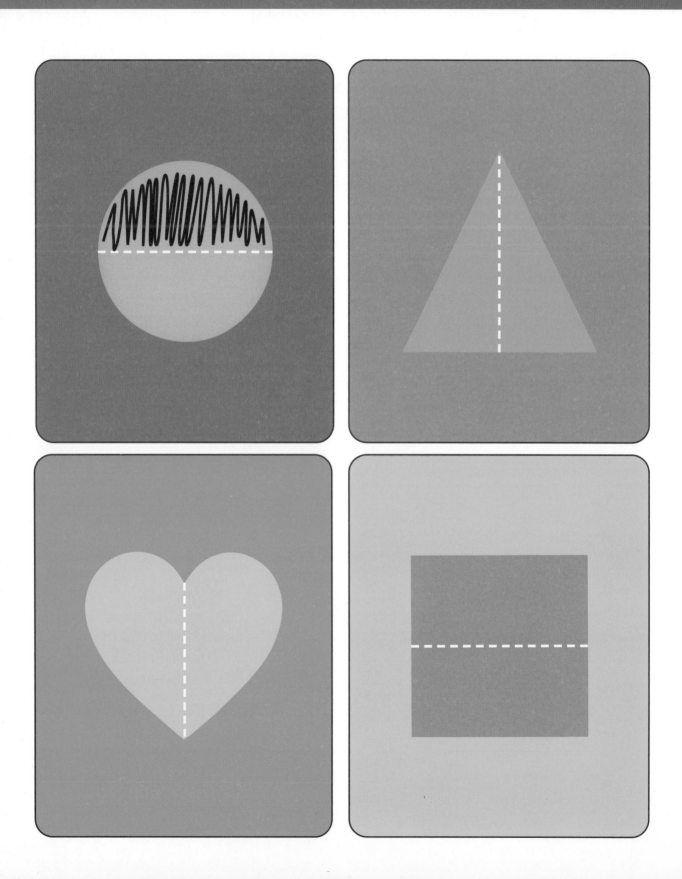

QUARTERS

When you split a whole into more than two equal parts, each part of the whole is another type of fraction.

When you cut something into four equal parts, the parts are called quarters. Four quarters make up a whole.

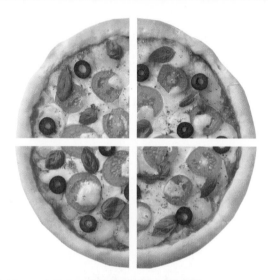

If you have a whole pizza, and you cut it into 4 pieces, each piece is a quarter of the whole pizza.

This pizza is cut into quarters.

Let's learn how to write a quarter as a fraction.

$\dfrac{1}{4}$

The top number is one piece of pizza.

The bottom number is how many pieces the whole pizza is cut into.

Fractions can also be written as words.
Trace the numbers and the words for the fraction below.

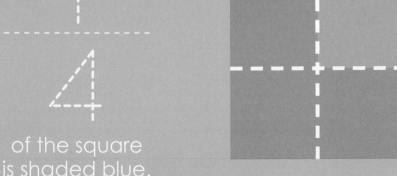

$\dfrac{1}{4}$ of the square is shaded blue.

Quarter of the square is shaded blue.

Shading Quarters

Each of the shapes below is cut into quarters.
Following the first example, use a pen to shade
a quarter of each shape.

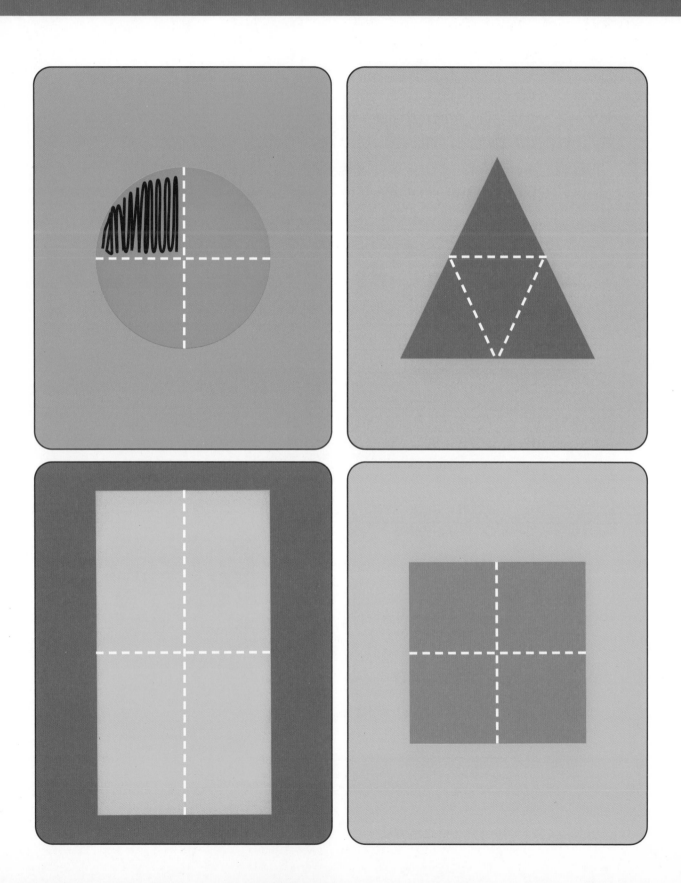

REAL OBJECTS

Look at the objects below. How much is shaded in blue? Write it as a fraction in the boxes below.

$$\frac{1}{2}$$

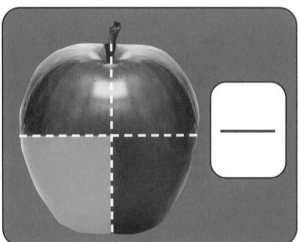

$$\underline{}$$

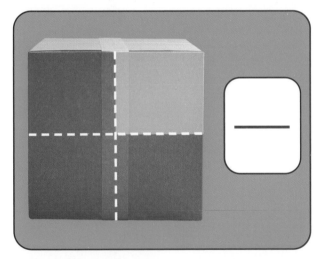

$$\underline{}$$

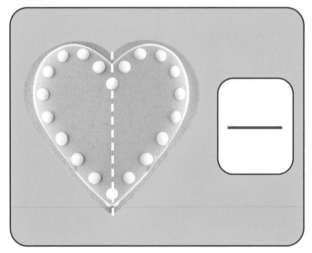

$$\underline{}$$

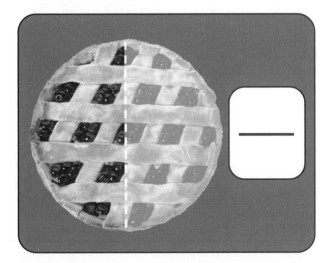

$$\underline{}$$

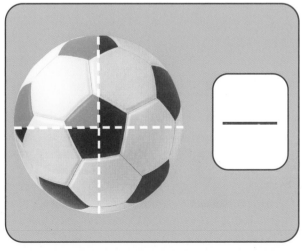

$$\underline{}$$

Match the Fractions

Draw a line from the fractions to the matching shapes.

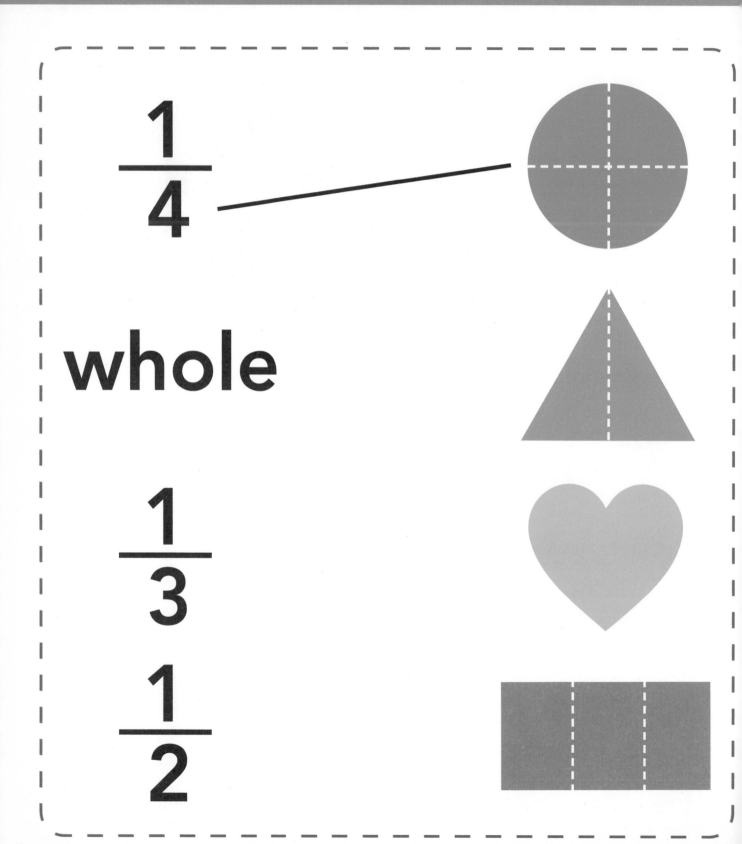

$\frac{1}{4}$

whole

$\frac{1}{3}$

$\frac{1}{2}$

2D SHAPES

A two-dimensional shape is a shape that has length and width but no depth. Trace the names and the shapes below.

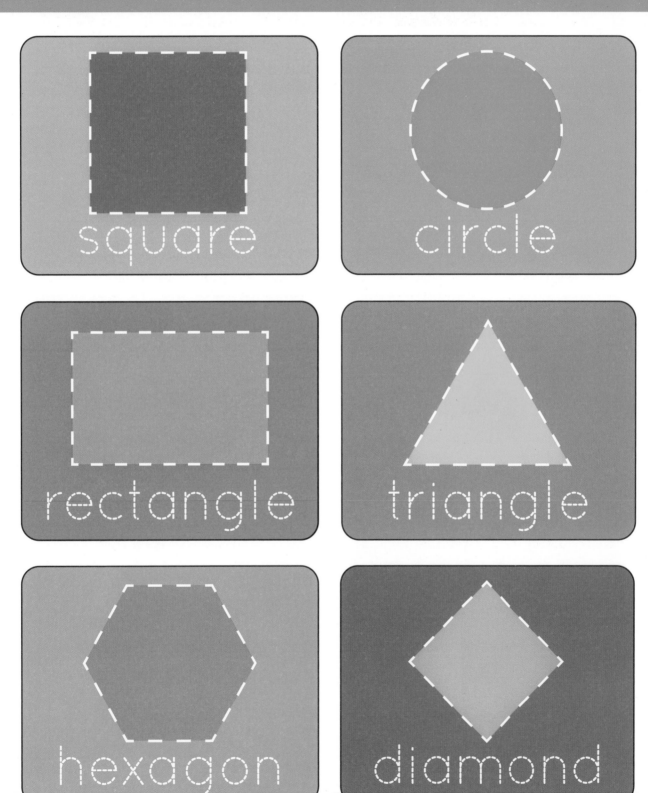

square

circle

rectangle

triangle

hexagon

diamond

3D SHAPES

3D shapes are solid shapes that have three dimensions including length, depth and width.
Trace the names and the shapes below.

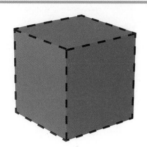

cube
A cube has
six square faces.

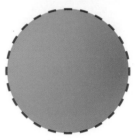

sphere
A sphere is perfectly round.
A ball is a sphere.

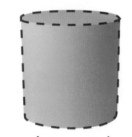

cylinder
A cylinder is like a tube,
with a circle at each end.

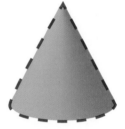

cone
A cone has a circular base
that narrows to a point at
the other end.

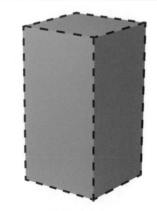

rectangular prism
A rectangular prism has
six faces. Some can be
squares and some
are rectangles.

Match the 3D Shapes

Draw a line from the objects on the left to the matching
3D shapes on the right. Can you see other 3D shapes around you?

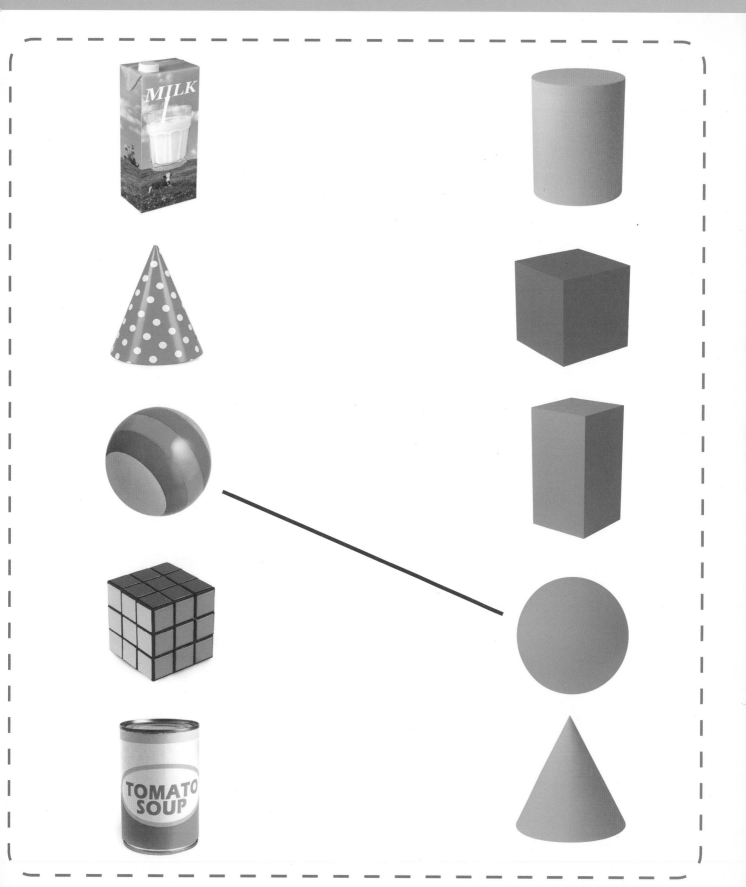

2D OR 3D

Are the shapes below 2D or 3D?
Circle your answers below.

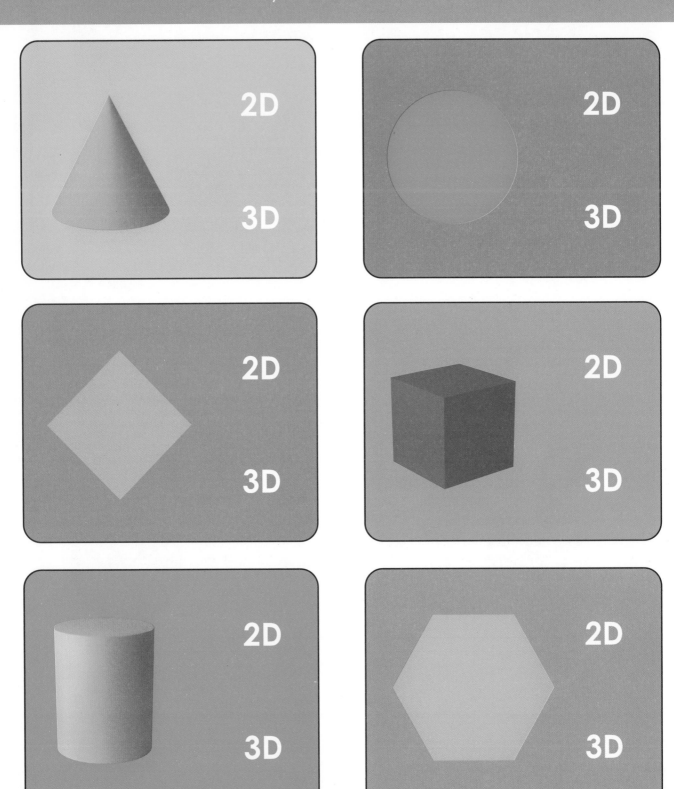

2D

3D

2D

3D

2D

3D

2D

3D

2D

3D

2D

3D

DOUBLES

To double a number, add the same number to itself.
For example, the double of 2 is 2 + 2 = 4.
Trace the numbers below and practice learning doubles.

1 + 1 = 2

2 + 2 = 4

3 + 3 = 6

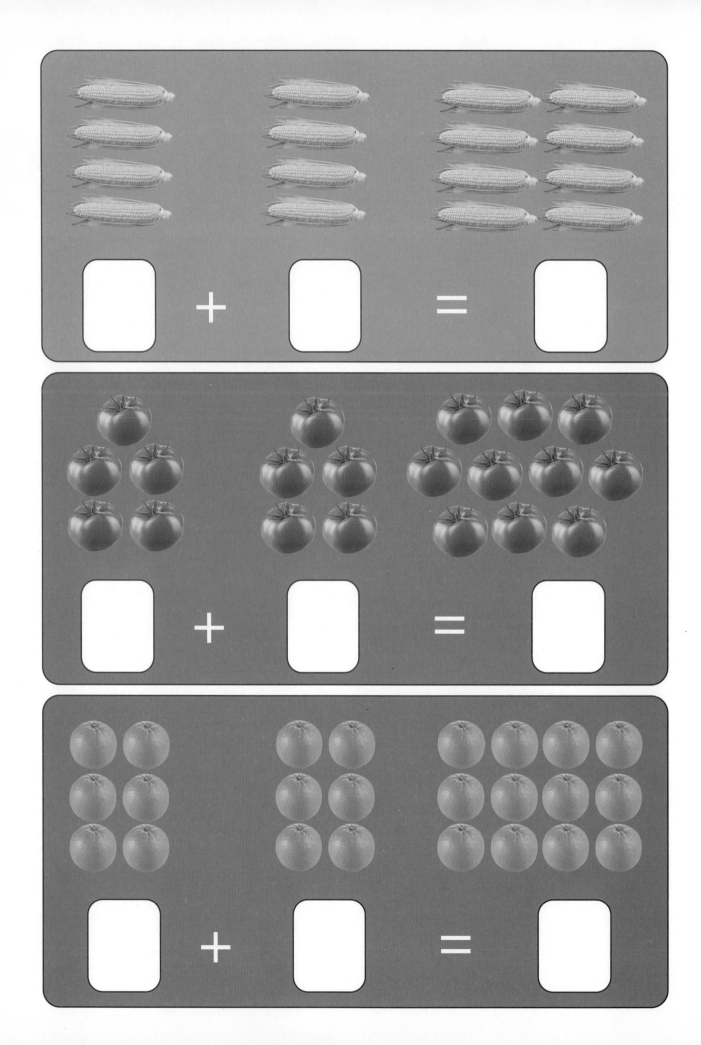

HALVES

To halve a number, the amount you take away is
the same number that's left over.
Trace the numbers below and practice learning halves.

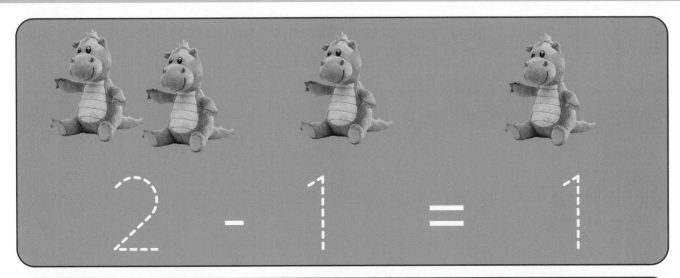

$$2 - 1 = 1$$

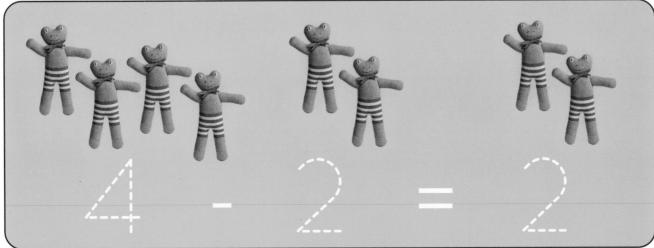

$$4 - 2 = 2$$

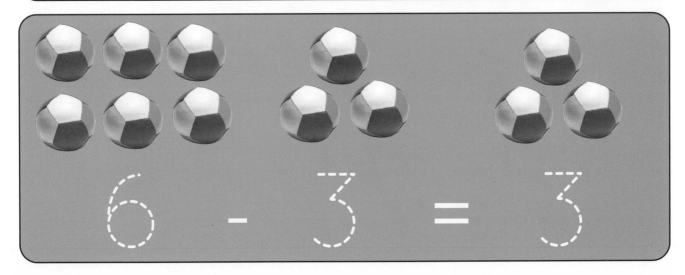

$$6 - 3 = 3$$

Cross out the toys to make **half of 8.**

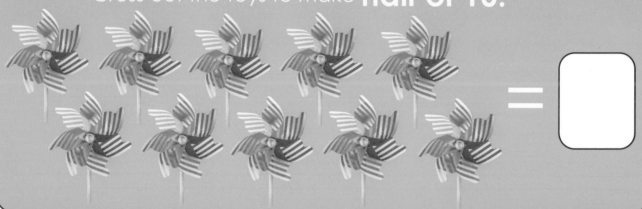

= 4

Cross out the toys to make **half of 10.**

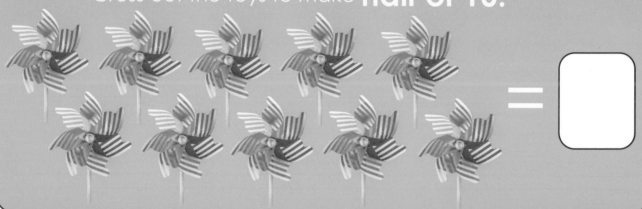

=

Cross out the toys to make **half of 12.**

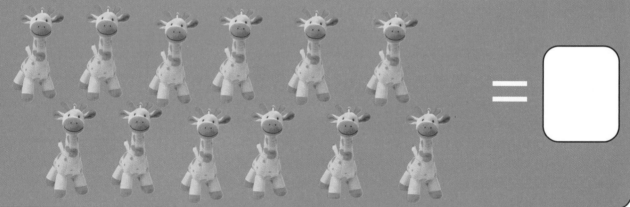

=

Cross out the toys to make **half of 14.**

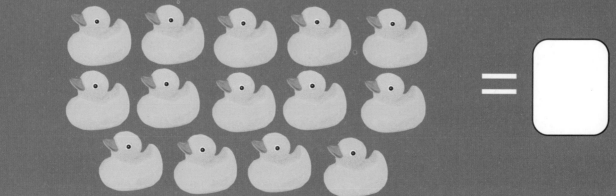

=

COUNTING

Answer the questions below by counting the objects.
Fill in the boxes with your answers.

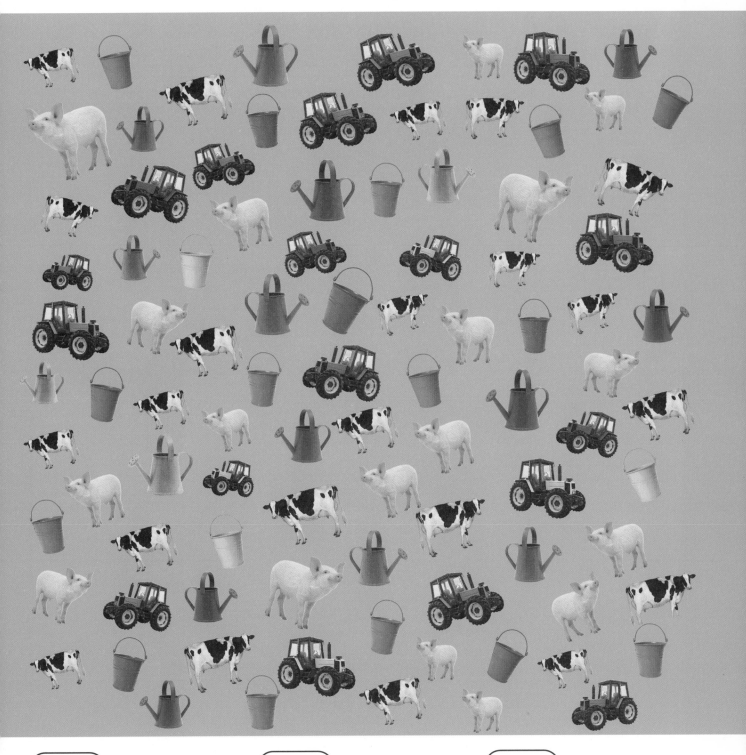

How many
tractors
are there?

How many
cows
are there?

How many
buckets
are there?

COUNTING

Keep counting and fill in the boxes below with your answers.
What other things can you count in the image?

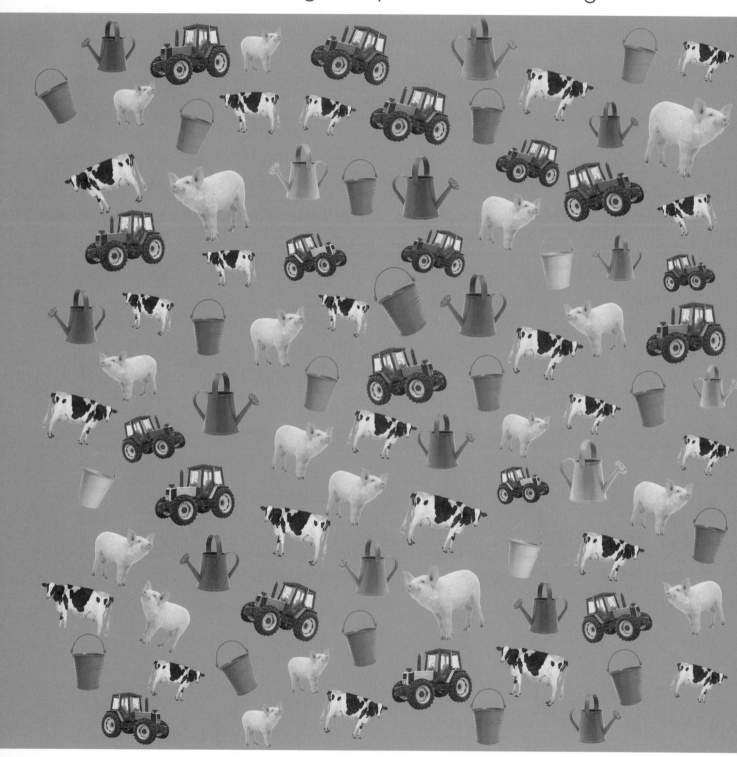

How many
animals
are there?

How many
blue objects
are there?

How many
red objects
are there?

ESTIMATING

Estimating is guessing the value or size based on what you see rather than actual measurement. Estimate the objects below and then count them. Write your answers in the boxes.

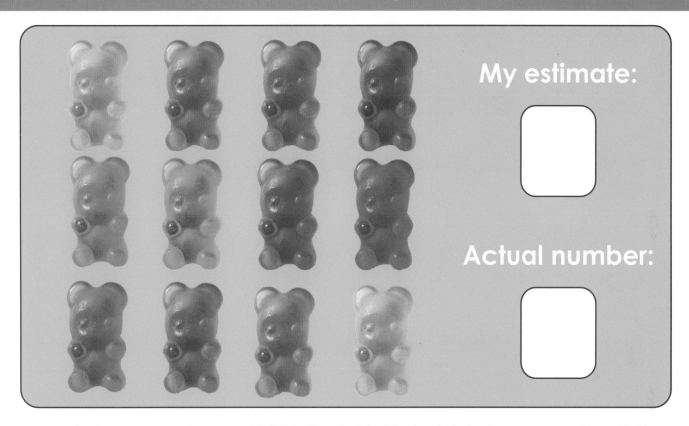

My estimate:

Actual number:

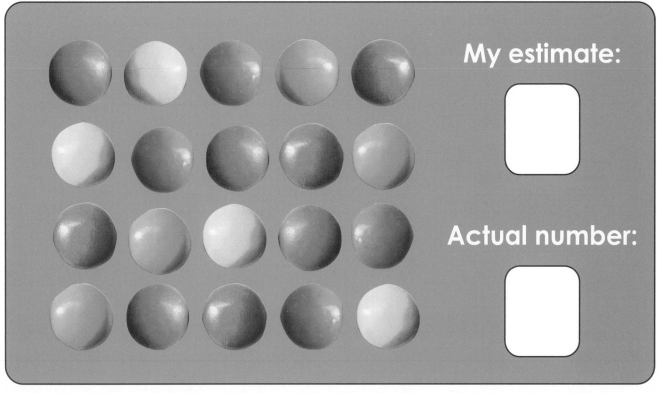

My estimate:

Actual number:

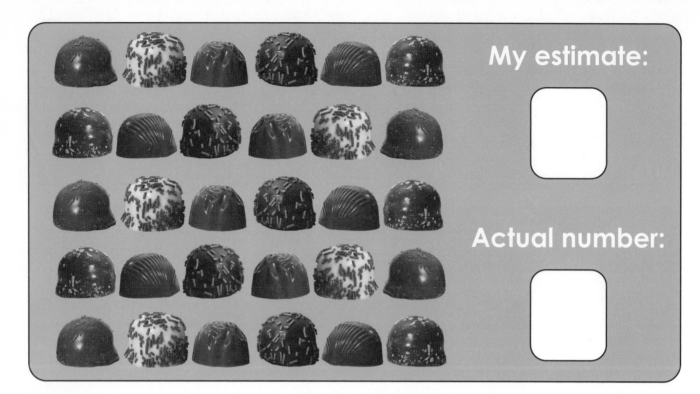

My estimate:

Actual number:

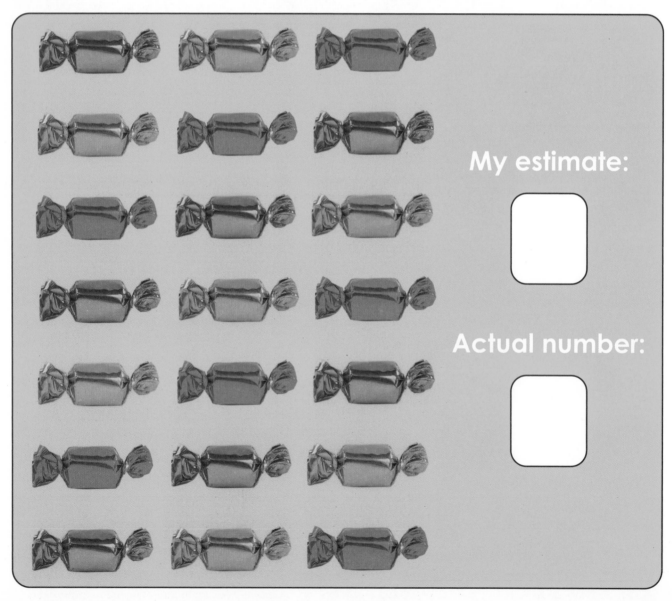

My estimate:

Actual number:

30

NUMBER BONDS

A number bond is a simple addition of two numbers that add up to give the sum. The number bonds below are pairs of numbers that add up to 10.

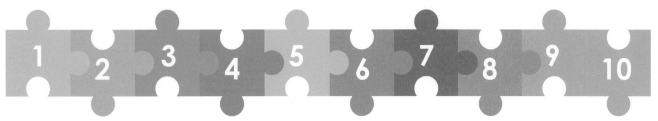

Fill in the number bonds below to get to the number 10.
You can use the number line above to help you.

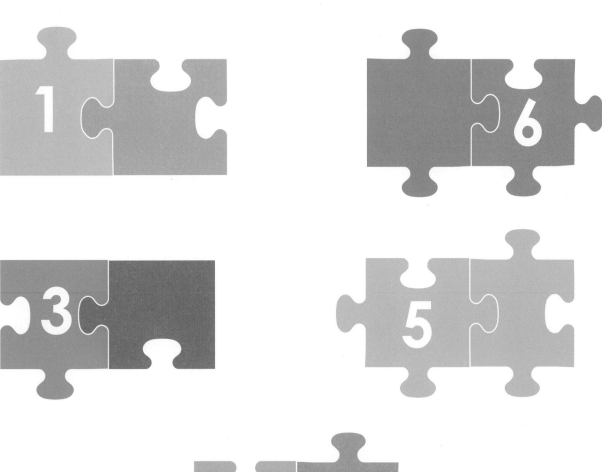

Playing with Number Bonds

Drawing dots on the dominos, finish filling in the
number bonds to 10. An example has been done for you.

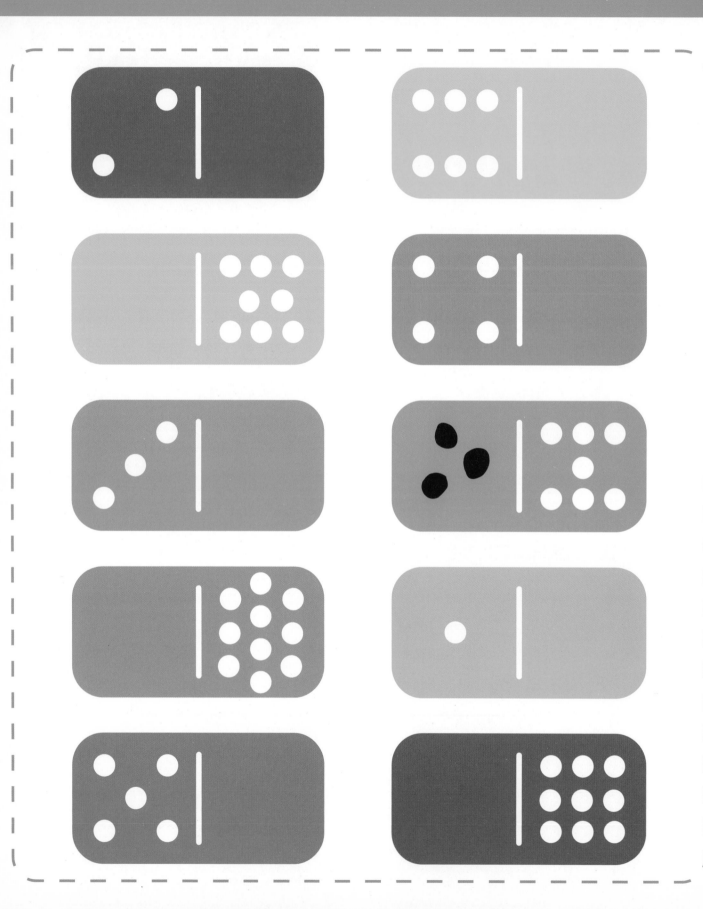

ADDITION

Addition is taking two or more numbers and combining them. That combined number is called the sum. Can you add the buttons below? Use the number line to help you find the sum.

| 1 | 2 | 3 | 4 | 5 | 6 | 7 | 8 | 9 | 10 | 11 | 12 | 13 | 14 | 15 | 16 | 17 | 18 | 19 | 20 |

6 + 4 = 10

7 + 5 = 12

8 + 3 =

☐ + ☐ = ☐

MATH TRICKS

Now, use what you learned about addition to work out larger sums. If a number ends in zero, just add the front two numbers together, then add on a zero.

**If 2 + 1 = 3, then
20 + 10 = 30.**

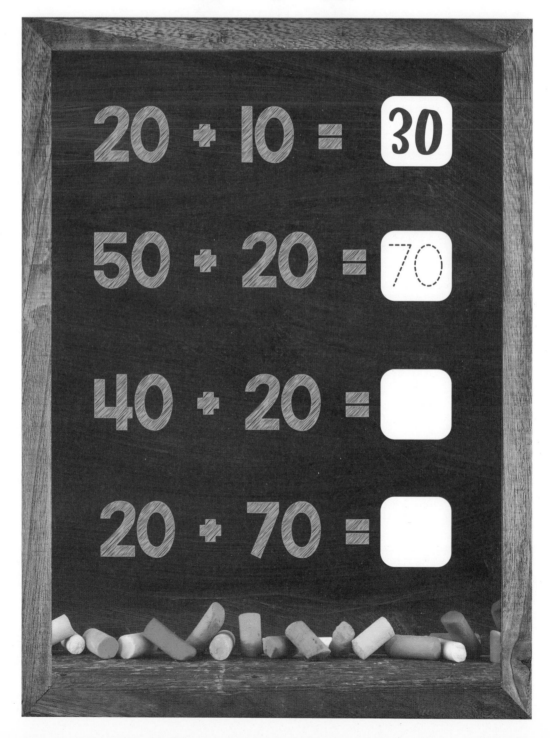

20 + 10 = 30

50 + 20 = 70

40 + 20 =

20 + 70 =

More Addition

Number models can be used when adding to 10.
Trace over the sums below.

0+10=10

5+5=10

1+9=10

6+4=10

2+8=10

7+3=10

3+7=10

8+2=10

4+6=10

9+1=10

Practice your addition to 10 below.

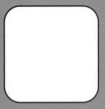 + [ ] = 10

SUBTRACTION

Subtraction is taking one number away from another. That new number is called the difference. Can you subtract the buttons below? Use the number line to help you find the difference.

| 1 | 2 | 3 | 4 | 5 | 6 | 7 | 8 | 9 | 10 | 11 | 12 | 13 | 14 | 15 | 16 | 17 | 18 | 19 | 20 |

8 - 4 = 4

12 - 7 = 5

11 - 3 =

☐ - ☐ = ☐

MATH TRICKS

Now, use what you learned about subtraction to work out the differences of larger sums. If a number ends in zero, just subtract the front two numbers, then add on a zero.

**If 3 - 1 = 2, it means that
30 - 10 = 20.**

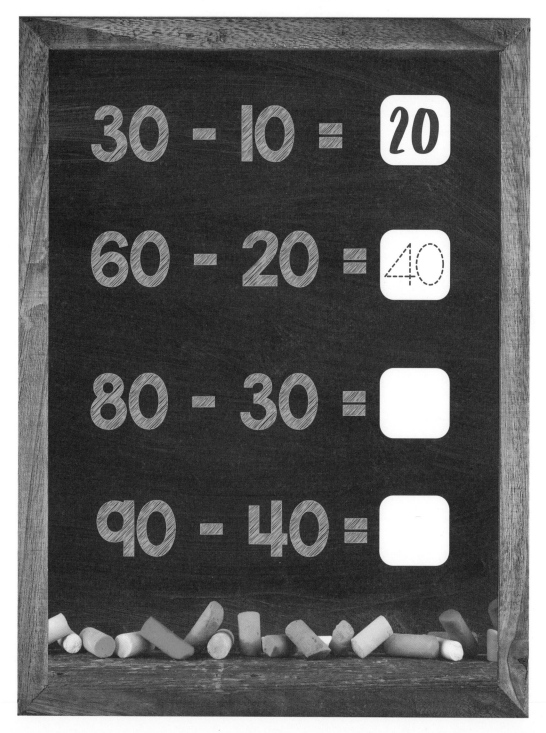

30 - 10 = 20

60 - 20 = 40

80 - 30 = ☐

90 - 40 = ☐

More Subtraction

Number models can be used when subtracting from 10.
Trace over the sums below.

10 - 0 = 10

10 - 5 = 5

10 - 1 = 9

10 - 6 = 4

10 - 2 = 8

10 - 7 = 3

10 - 3 = 7

10 - 8 = 2

10 - 4 = 6

10 - 9 = 1

Practice your subtraction from 10 below.

10 -  =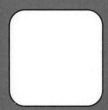

38

MONEY

The currency in the U.S. is called the dollar and we use the symbol "$".
Coins are called cents and we use the symbol "¢".
Trace over the amounts below.

penny

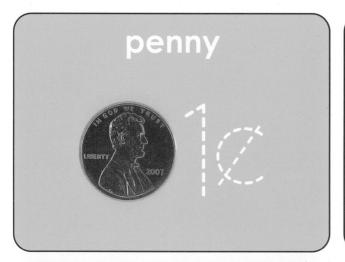

1¢

nickel

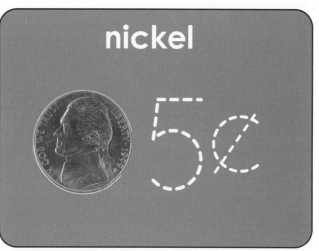

5¢

dime

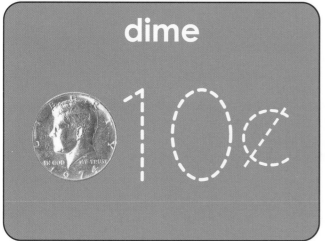

10¢

quarter

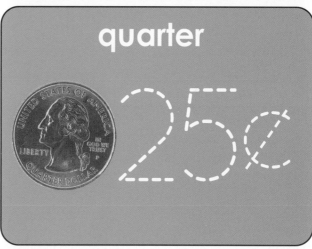

25¢

dollar

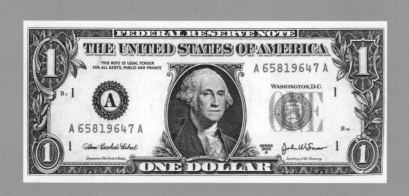

$1

There are 100 cents in a dollar.

Counting Money

Can you count up the value of different coins?
Write your answers in the boxes below.

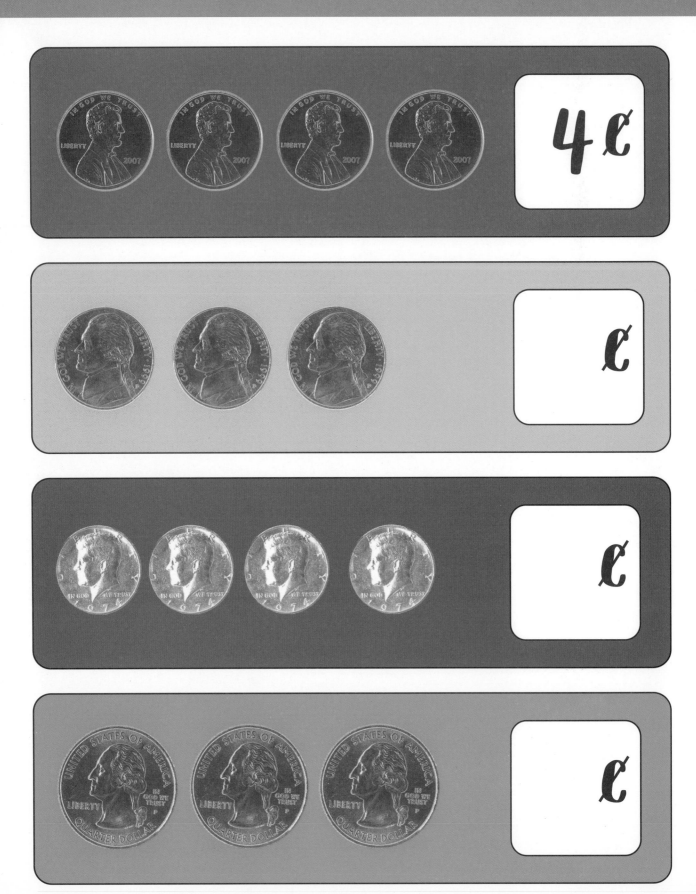

4¢

¢

¢

¢

MORE MONEY

Add up the coin values in each purse. Write the totals in the purses below. Circle the purse that has the most money in it. Draw a check for the one that has the least.

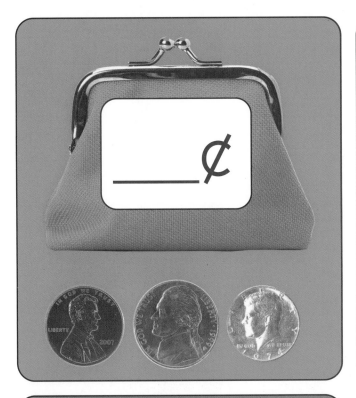

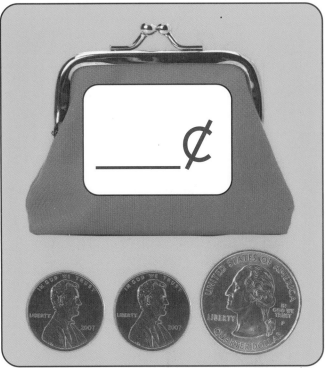

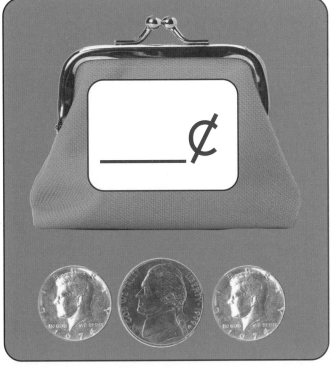

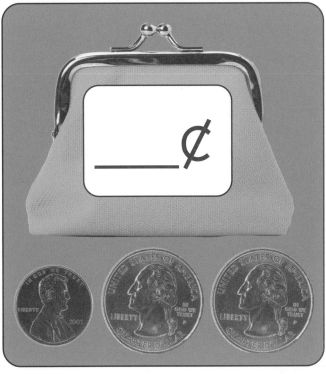

41

Savings Time

Match the coins to the correct piggy bank.
Draw a line between the amount of money
and the piggy bank math that matches.

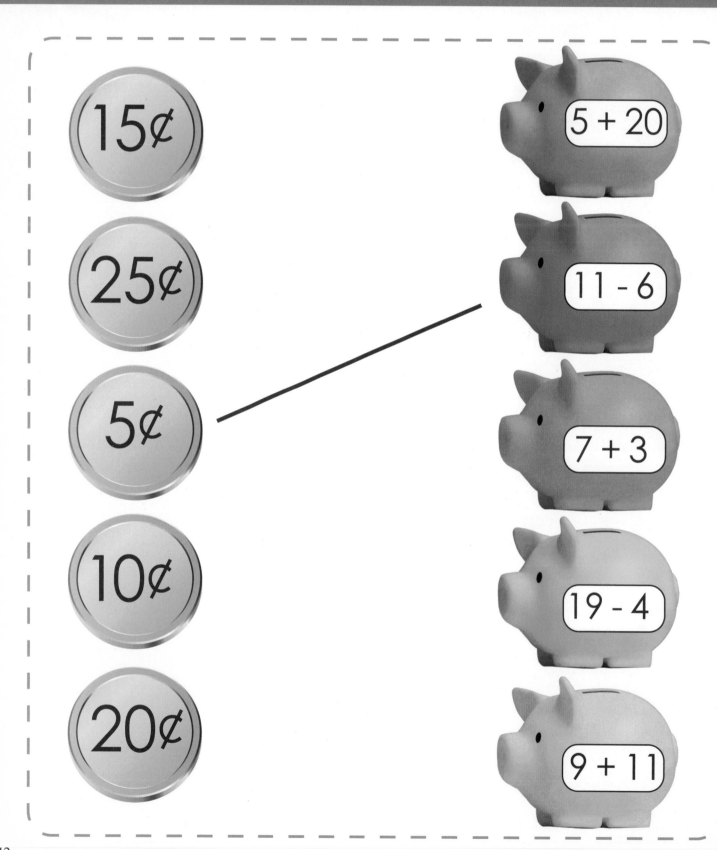

REVERSALS

0 + 10 = 10 is the same as 10 + 0 = 10. These are called reversals and you can write them either way and they are both correct. Trace each number model below.

$$10 + 0 = 10 \qquad 0 + 10 = 10$$

$5 + 5 = 10$	$5 + 5 = 10$
$4 + 6 = 10$	$6 + 4 = 10$
$3 + 7 = 10$	$7 + 3 = 10$
$2 + 8 = 10$	$8 + 2 = 10$
$1 + 9 = 10$	$9 + 1 = 10$
$0 + 10 = 10$	$10 + 0 = 10$

43

SUDOKU

2	3	4	1
1			3
4			2
3	2	1	4

7	6	5	
8		6	7
5	8		6
	7	8	5

FAST MATH +

3 +5	1 +9	2 +4	3 +0	2 +6	1 +8
1 +7	3 +3	2 +3	1 +0	3 +6	2 +8
2 +2	3 +9	8 +4	2 +1	3 +4	13 +2
1 +4	2 +10	3 +7	1 +1	12 +5	3 +2
3 +8	2 +3	1 +5	3 +10	2 +9	3 +6
7 +5	1 +7	6 +7	1 +10	2 +5	1 +3

FAST MATH −

Have an adult set a timer and see how fast you can correctly subtract the numbers below. Erase the answers and try to beat your time.

3 −0	2 −1	7 −1	13 −7	5 −1	8 −2
6 −1	12 −3	8 −6	9 −4	11 −5	8 −3
14 −7	4 −2	6 −4	2 −0	4 −3	13 −2
5 −4	12 −4	15 −7	1 −1	10 −0	3 −1
7 −3	15 −2	11 −7	10 −3	18 −9	7 −4
14 −3	9 −3	6 −2	10 −10	12 −5	6 −3

Practice Page

Have an adult create exercises for you to complete.

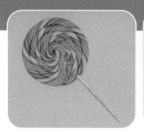 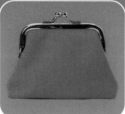 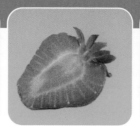 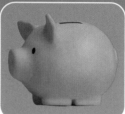

Practice Page

Have an adult create exercises for you to complete.

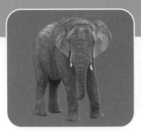 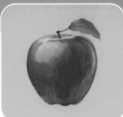 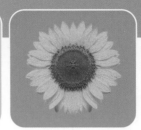 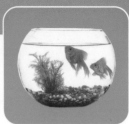

Practice Page

Have an adult create exercises for you to complete.

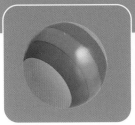 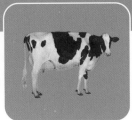 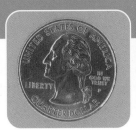 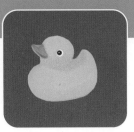

Practice Page

Have an adult create exercises for you to complete.

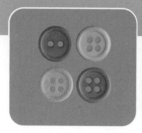 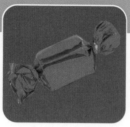 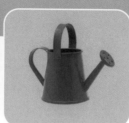 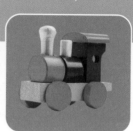

Answer Key

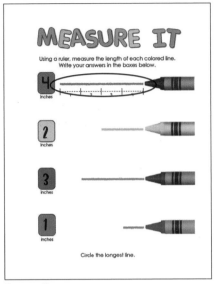

Page 2

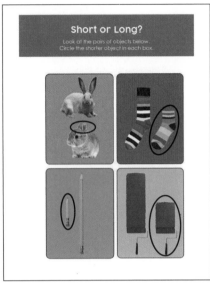

Page 3

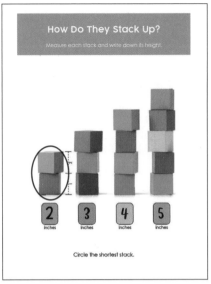

Page 4

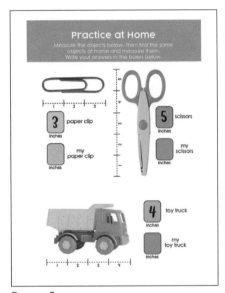

Page 5

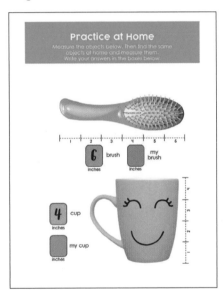

Page 6

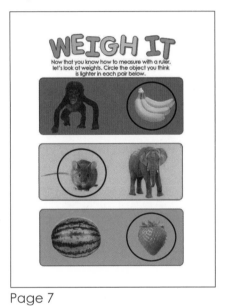

Page 7

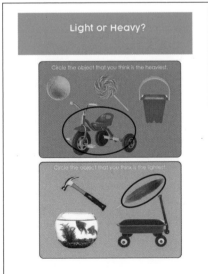

Page 8

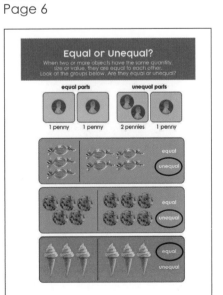

Page 11

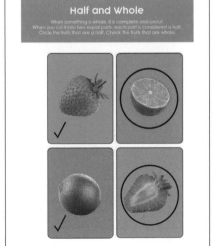

Page 13

51

Answer Key

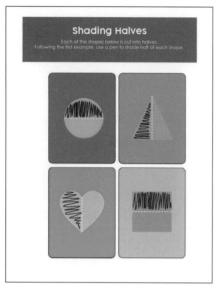

Page 14

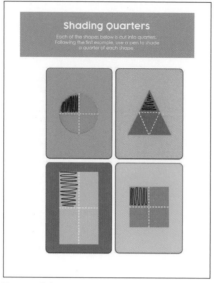

Page 16

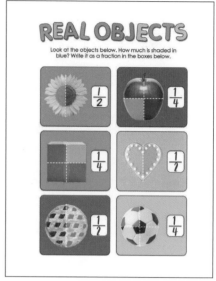

Page 17

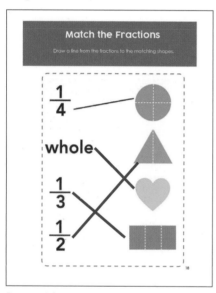

Page 18

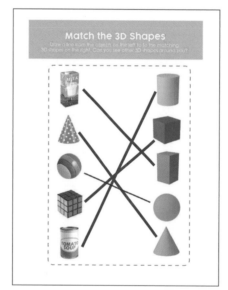

Page 21

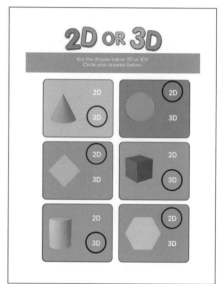

Page 22

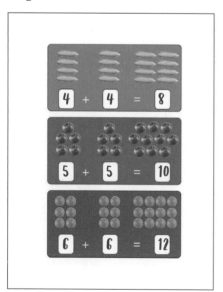

Page 24

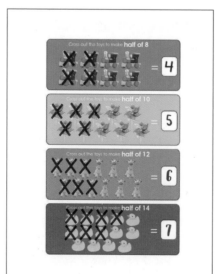

Page 26

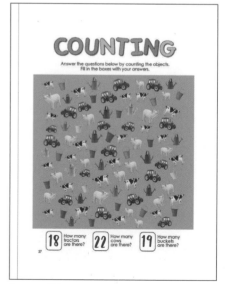

Page 27

Answer Key

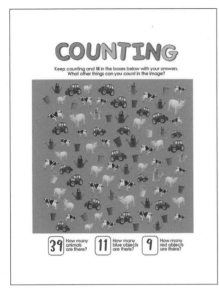

Page 28

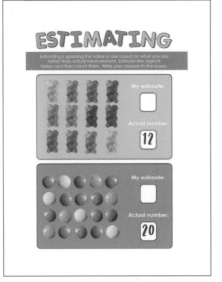

Page 29

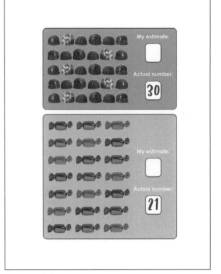

Page 30

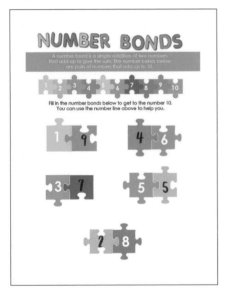

Page 31

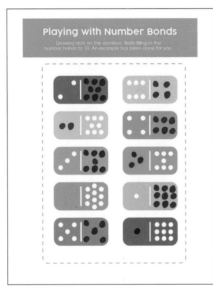

Page 32

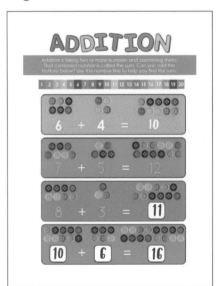

Page 33

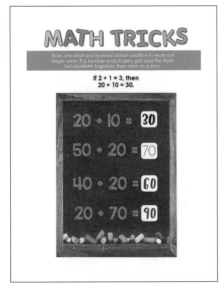

Page 34

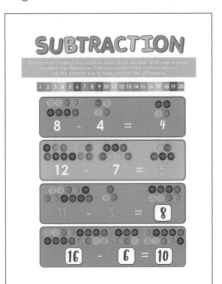

Page 36

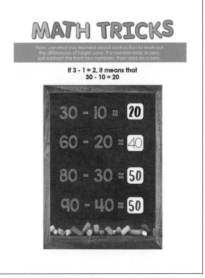

Page 37

Answer Key

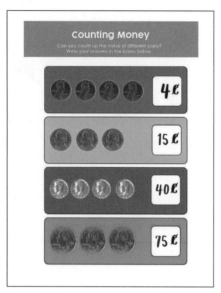

Page 40

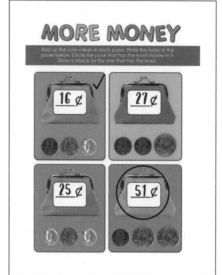

Page 41

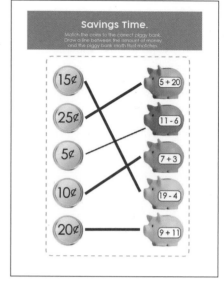

Page 42

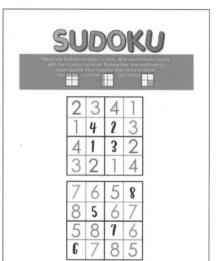

Page 44

FAST MATH +

3 +5 8	1 +9 10	2 +4 6	3 +0 3	2 +6 8	1 +8 9
1 +7 8	3 +3 6	2 +3 5	1 +0 1	3 +6 9	2 +8 10
2 +2 4	3 +9 12	8 +4 12	2 +1 3	3 +4 7	13 +2 15
1 +4 5	2 +10 12	3 +7 10	1 +1 2	12 +5 17	3 +2 5
3 +8 11	2 +3 5	1 +5 6	3 +10 13	2 +9 11	3 +6 9
7 +5 12	1 +7 8	6 +7 13	1 +10 11	2 +5 7	1 +3 4

Page 45

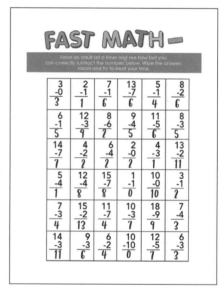

Page 46

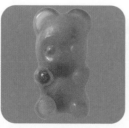
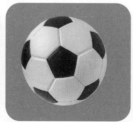
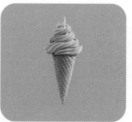
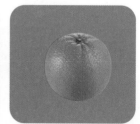

54

+MATH AWARD

This certificate is presented to

_____

for completing and doing a wonderful job of learning Everyday Math.

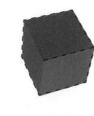

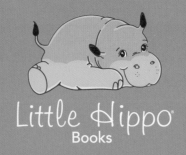

Little Hippo®
Books

Sign up to see what's new at littlehippobooks.com

Follow us on social media to stay up to date on the latest from Little Hippo Books

 @LittleHippoBooks

 @littlehippobooks

Little Hippo Books

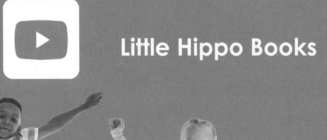

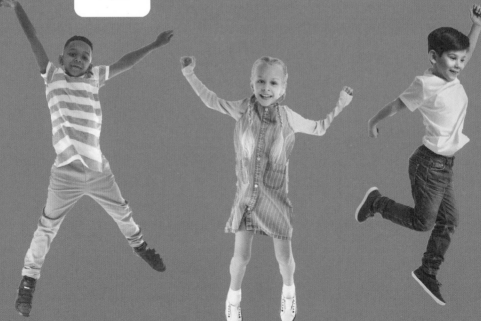